# OVUM IMPLANTATION

## *Its Hormonal, Biochemical, Neurophysiological and Immunological Bases*

M. C. Shelesnyak and G. J. Marcus

*Editors*

Proceedings held at the

**WEIZMANN INSTITUTE OF SCIENCE**
**Rehovath, Israel**

August 1967

Gordon and Breach, Science Publishers

New York London Paris

150 Fifth Avenue, New York, N. Y. 10011
Library of Congress Catalog Card Number: 69-15876

*Editorial office for Great Britain:*

Gordon and Breach, Science Publishers Ltd.
8 Bloomsbury Way
London W.C.1

*Editorial office for France:*

Gordon & Breach
7-9 rue Emile Dubois
Paris 14$^e$

*Distributed in Canada by:*

The Ryerson Press
299 Queen Street West
Toronto 2B, Ontario



Printed in the United States of America

## FOREWORD

Our colleagues who gathered at Rehovoth offer us in this volume the privilege of sharing in the lucid expositions of their formal essays as well as in their uninhibited and wide-ranging discussions. Their approach is at once intensive and yet circumspect. It is this unusual combination which characterizes the Rehovoth sessions.

The moving theme is an effort to completely comprehend special phases of the reproductive process presumably in order ultimately to gain acceptable and effective methods of control. Those who assembled these particular workers were operating from the hard-earned vantage point of a broad and yet penetrating knowledge of reproductive physiology and of those contiguous areas of fundamental physiological study which case new light on their primary field of interest. It is the spark that is struck by such interaction that illuminates these discussions.

Hence, the reader is led to approach the central problem of uterine response not only from the single facet of steroid hormone control but from more searching analyses of the neurohumoral, immunological and morphological factors which may or may not be involved in the primary processes under study. The leader of these sessions has aptly termed this comprehensive approach that of the "biodynamicist."

Spontaneous verbal exchanges of the type recorded

here sometimes include stray threads which superficially appear to mar the basic pattern of the discussions. However, each reader may be able to extract from these accounts some novel approach which affords coherence to previously unconnected considerations.

The Rehovoth group's hard-hitting concentration on nidation strikes at a highly pivotal event in the reproductive process. For through this process the previously free-swimming mammalian "larva" acquires a completely new set of environmental factors which constitute the feto-maternal relationship. The conferees have very appropriately sought the view of colleagues who are not immediately involved in work on this process for stimulation and direction.

It is a privilege to be called upon to forward this instructive volume to colleagues seeking not only new mortar for their own research efforts but also a new orientation and design.

Roy Hertz

# PREFACE

The aim of the Biodynamics Department has been to implement an interdisciplinary approach to exploring mechanisms of actions involved in the biology of reproduction. A special interest of the Biodynamics group has been the study of nidation—ovum implantation—which, in its extreme complexity, involves many basic biological mechanisms.

The Biodynamics Workshop on Ovum Implantation was convened in order to view progress in selected areas of current research which have relevance to ovum implantation, and to integrate results of current investigations on the mechanism of nidation into the general framework of recent advances in biology. It was also the intent to expose and reveal the actual and potential usefulness of nidation as a model system for biological research in areas other than those specifically related to nidation.

## Acknowledgments

It is a pleasure to express our appreciation to all who helped in making this Workshop possible. The Population Council, The Ford Foundation, and the SABA Foundation have all been liberal in their support of the research program of the Biodynamics Department. The Workshop was supported, in part, by grants from the President's Fund of The Weizmann Institute of Science, Organon, Ortho Products, Sandoz, Schering, and Syntex.

All the staff of the Biodynamics Department worked zealously; special credit must be given to Mrs. Betty Shechter, Mrs. Pat Levinson, Mrs. Rina Yitzhaki, and Mr. David Meir. Mr. Benjamin Deutsch of the San Martin Faculty House displayed his usual excellent and abundant hospitality.

Finally, Mrs. Shelesnyak deserves special thanks for her superb help.

M. C. Shelesnyak,[1] Ph.D., Head
Department of Biodynamics
The Weizmann Institute of Science
Rehovoth, Israel

[1] Present address:
Director, Interdisciplinary Communications Program, Smithsonian Institution, 1025 Fifteenth Street, N. W. Washington, D. C. 20560

## PARTICIPANTS

| | |
|---|---|
| Barnea Ayalla | Research Assistant, Dept. of Biodynamics, Weizmann Institute of Science, Rehovoth Israel |
| Billingham, R. E. | Wistar Prof. of Zoology, University of Pennsylvania, Philadelphia, Pennsylvania, U. S. A. |
| Everett, John W. | Prof. of Anatomy, Duke University, Durham, North Carolina, U. S. A. |
| Gorski, Jack | Prof. of Physiology & Biophysics, University of Illinois, Urbana, Ill., U. S. A. |
| Gruber, Fredy | Dept. of Biodynamics, Weizmann Institute of Science, Rehovoth, Israel |
| Joshi, Madhusudan | Dept. of Biodynamics, Weizmann Institute of Science, Rehovoth, Israel |

| | |
|---|---|
| Katsh, Seymour | Prof. & Acting Chairman Dept. of Pharmacology, University of Colorado Medical Center, Denver, Colo., U. S. A. |
| Kisch, Eldad S. | Dept. of Biodynamics, Weizmann Institute of Science. Rehovoth, Israel |
| Kraicer, P. F. | Senior Scientist, Dept. of Biodynamics, Weizmann Institute of Science, Rehovoth, Israel |
| Lamprecht, Sergio A. | Dept. of Biodynamics, Weizmann Institute of Science, Rehovoth, Israel |
| Lindner, H. R. | Head, Dept. of Biodynamics, Weizmann Institute of Science, Rehovoth, Israel |
| Lobel, Bertha L. | Senior Scientist, Dept. of Biodynamics, Weizmann Institute of Science, Rehovoth, Israel |
| Marcus, George J. | Research Associate, Dept. of Biodynamics, at present at Johns Hopkins University, Baltimore, Md., U. S. A. |
| Schayer, Richard W. | Research Scientist, Rockland State Hospital, Orangeburg, N. Y., U. S. A. |

| | |
|---|---|
| Shelesnyak, M. C. | Smithsonian Institution, Washington, D. C., formerly Head, Dept. of Biodynamics, Weizmann Institute of Science, Rehovoth, Israel |
| Tachi, Chikashi | Dept. of Biodynamics, Weizmann Institute of Science, Rehovoth, Israel |
| Tachi, Sumi | Dept. of Biodynamics, Weizmann Institute of Science, Rehovoth, Israel |
| Tausk, Marius | Professor, University of Utrecht, Holland |
| Von Euler, U. S. | Professor, Fysiologiska Institutionen I, Karolinska Institutet, Solnavagen 1, Stockholm 60 Sweden |
| Zmigrod, Avraham | Dept. of Biodynamics, Weizmann Institute of Science, Rehovoth, Israel |

CONTENTS

# THE STUDY OF NIDATION

# THE STUDY OF NIDATION

M. C. Shelesnyak and G. J. Marcus
Department of Biodynamics,
Weizmann Institute of Science, Rehovoth, Israel

Nidation is a fundamental process of animal reproduction peculiar to the higher mammals. We view the process as beginning with coitus and ovulation and ending with the implantation of the fertilized egg. The elucidation of the mechanisms of nidation has been a challenging problem for embryologists, anatomists, physiologists, endocrinologists and biochemists for more than half a century and continues to challenge the imagination.

Among the fruits of earlier investigations of the phenomenon is an awareness that nidation involves a sequence of interdependent, hormonally-governed events which includes transport of semen into the uterus, transport of ova down the Fallopian tubes and concurrently, modification of the uterine milieu to facilitate both reception of the fertilized ovum and active penetration by the ovum into the prepared, that is, transformed, endometrial stroma, or deciduum. This transformation of the stroma, designated as decidualization, is pivotal in the nidatory processes of certain mammals, e.g. the primates and rodents. It trans-

In this presentation, the development of our current concept of the mechanism of nidation (in the rat) will be related in the approximate chronological order of the conduct of the research. It thus reveals the realization of the philosophy of biodynamics, an integration of various disciplinary approaches to an exploration of a particular phase of reproduction, in this instance, nidation. It will also show how the subject becomes more complex and involved, and progressively more fundamental problems arise.

The discovery that the decidual reaction can be induced in the absence of the fertilized egg made possible critical investigation of the separate roles of the ovum and uterus (or the fetal and the maternal organism) in nidation. Sixty years ago, Leo Loeb (1907) observed that injury to the progestational guinea-pig uterus provoked a rapid appearance and growth of endometrial cells which were identical to the decidual cells of pregnancy. This discovery made it possible to investigate the physiological requirements which permit the uterus to respond to stimulation and to decidualize; and also to investigate the identity of the "natural" stimulus. Until about fifteen years ago, the only requirements which had been elucidated were that the uterus be under progesterone dominance and that the endometrium be subjected to the non-specific stimulation associated with any form of trauma.

The proposal of a non-specific stimulus for so specific a phenomenon as decidualization was rejected by us and a metabolic mediator or stimulus was sought. Since injury provoked decidualization, consideration was given to metabolites associated with tissue injury, testing the involvement of the postulated metabolites by the use of specific antagonists (Shelesnyak, 1954; 1957). Histamine early became a candidate for test because of its release consistently in response to tissue injury and because of availability of specific antagonists, the antihistamines. In those studies, the pseudopregnant rat was used almost exclusively to provide the basic experimental requirement of a progesterone-dominated uterus. In the initial exploration, both uterine horns were subjected to trauma by scratching or crushing and antihistamine was introduced into one horn. The control horn exhibited a massive decidual reaction whereas the antihistamine treated horn showed no reaction.

Assuming on the basis of this circumstantial evidence that histamine was an inducer of decidualization, that is, that the antihistamine had prevented the decidual reaction by specific antagonism to the local action of histamine, it should be possible to induce decidualization by supplying exogenous histamine by parenteral route. Induction of decidualization by this method was achieved. This finding, bolstered by the similar ability of systemically administered histamine-releasing compound B.W. 48/80, was valuable support for the hypothesis that histamine participated in the induction of decidualization (Kraicer and Shelesnyak, 1958). However, the required doses of histamine were highly toxic and vitiated the value of the systemic administration of histamine as a useful experimental tool. The search for a less toxic and more reliable method of inducing decidualization without direct manipulation of the uterus led to the discovery that the intraperitoneal injection of the antihistamine pyrathiazine into the progestational rat resulted in the decidual response. The apparent paradox of an antihistamine inducing the response presumed to be mediated by histamine was resolved by the demonstration that the antihistamine pyrathiazine acts initially as an histamine-releaser. Proof, in part, of the histamine-releasing action of pyrathiazine was provided by the observation that chronic treatment with pyrathiazine depleted a rat of histamine, so that the rat became resistant to the injection of erstwhile lethal doses of histamine-releaser compound 48/80, although not to challenge by histamine itself (Marcus, Kraicer and Shelesnyak, 1963). Added support for the necessary role of histamine in nidation was revealed by the fact that in rats depleted of their histamine by chronic treatment with chemical histamine-releasers, decidualization, and consequently implantation, was impaired or abolished (Kraicer, Marcus and Shelesnyak, 1963).

Armed with this method for the induction of decidualization, which obviated surgery and uterine trauma, it was possible to study the earliest biochemical and structural stages of the process without the interference of elements of tissue damage. It was now also possible to delineate more critically than was previously possible the time-limits of uterine sensitivity to decidual induction stimulation in the pseudopregnant rat.

Whereas by means of direct trauma to the uterus, variable success in eliciting a decidual response was possible on any of several days during progestation, by use of the systemic method, a very brief period of high sensitivity was discovered to occur on the morning of day $L_4$ of pseudopregnancy, that is the fourth day of leucocyte vaginal smears (Kraicer and Shelesnyak, 1959; De Feo, 1963). Stimulation within this period resulted in maximal decidual responses, but stimulation without this period was ineffective. When sought, the same period of sensitivity was discovered in the pregnant rat. That is, in fact, the period in which the decidual response is induced by the blastocyst in pregnant rats as indicated by histological studies (Krehbiel, 1937; Psychoyos, 1961).

The finding of the very sharply defined period of uterine sensitivity drew our attention to the immediately preceding period. We sought uterine changes which might be associated with the establishment of uterine susceptibility to decidual induction. Earlier study had shown that a decrease in the uterine mast cell population in the pregnant rat occurred at just this time, suggesting that histamine-release had taken place (Shelesnyak, 1959a). This was later confirmed by measurement of uterine histamine content (Shelesnyak, 1959b). At this time, it was demonstrated by Spaziani and Szego (1958), and, independently, by us (Shelesnyak, 1959c), that the injection of oestrogens causes histamine-release in the uterus of the ovariectomized rat. Consequently, we suspected that a spurt of oestrogen, secreted at the time in question, produced the mast cell depletion and the histamine-release observed in the pregnant rat. Perusal of the literature revealed that follicular activity reportedly occurred in the ovaries of the pregnant rat just prior to the time of maximal uterine sensitivity, that is on days $L_3$ and $L_4$ (Nelson, 1929; Swezy and Evans, 1930).

Postulating that brief exposure of the progestational uterus to ovarian oestrogen on day $L_3$ was the critical influence in establishing uterine susceptibility to decidual induction, we sought to substantiate our hypothesis by applying the classical techniques of extirpation of the ovaries, hormonal replacement therapy and pharmacological intervention. Accordingly, removal of the source of oestrogen, the ovaries, or administration of the oestrogen antagonist, MER-25, prevented decidualization and implantation in the pregnant rat if performed early on day $L_3$, that is before the suspected oestrogen-surge. On the other hand, if treatment was delayed until late on day $L_3$ or thereafter, that is until after the oestrogen-surge was assumed to have occurred, decidualization and implantation did occur. Similar effects on the induction of decidualization in pseudopregnant rats by systemic administration of pyrathiazine were demonstrable. It was also demonstrated that when the ovaries were removed early on day $L_3$, the administration of exogenous oestrogen, as a substitute for the oestrogen-surge, permitted decidualization and ovum-implantation to ensue (Shelesnyak, Kraicer and Zeilmaker, 1963).

Hypophysectomy before the expected surge, in pregnant rats, also prevented implantation, which was then induceable by administration of oestrogen (Zeilmaker, 1963). Hypophysectomy later did not interfere with implantation provided adequate progesterone was supplied (Varavudhi, 1965). We concluded, therefore, that ovarian oestrogen secretion during progestation was under pituitary control. However, subsequent study revealed that injection of various organ extracts or even proteolytic enzymes would induce implantation in the hypophysectomized rat (Varavudhi, 1965). Thus, it appears that some apparently undetermined factors can influence ovarian oestrogen secretion. We remain at a loss to understand or explain this phenomenon.

The concept of the oestrogen-surge received additional support from biochemical, histological and cytochemical studies which elucidated a constellation of changes occurring between days $L_3$ and $L_4$ of progestation. These included increased uterine vascularity, the appearance of oedema, infiltration by eosinophilic granulocytes, increased glandular activity and the sudden occurrence of stromal DNA synthesis indicated by incorporation of labelled thymidine (Lobel, Tic and Shelesnyak, 1965a). There was a parallel, pronounced increase in total uterine mass, in protein and in nucleic acids (Shelesnyak and Tic, 1963a; De Feo, 1963b). In the absence of a stimulus to induce decidualization, all of these activities subside within 24 hours; and, significantly, they are abolished (prevented) by the prior administration of the oestrogen-antagonist, MER-25 (Shelesnyak and Tic, 1963b; Lobel, Tic and Shelesnyak, 1965b). Clearly, a brief period of pituitary-directed oestrogen-secretion occurs on day $L_3$ of progestation. However, conclusive proof awaits direct measurement of ovarian oestrogen output in ovarian venous blood, a feat as yet unattained (in the case of the rat) due to technical limitations.

The conditions resulting from the oestrogen-surge, appear to be a take-off state, for the transformation of the uterus into decidual tissue. Biochemical and histological studies have also given us some insights into the changes characterizing the decidual transformation. After induction, an exponential increase in uterine mass, protein and nucleic acids takes place, beginning at the oestrogen-induced peak on $L_4$, and, as much as $3\frac{1}{2}$ grams of decidual tissue are produced within 72 to 96 hours (Shelesnyak and Tic, 1963a). This corresponds to a tenfold increase in uterine tissue mass. Dramatic changes in enzymic activities, e.g. dihydroorotic dehydrogenase and aspartate transcarbamylase, become apparent in the transformed stroma (Kaye, 1961; 1968) and glycogen, lipids and RNA accumulate in the areas of decidualization (Christie, 1966; Lobel, Levy and Shelesnyak, 1967). During the singular growth of the decidual tissue in the pseudopregnant rat, a remarkable parallel to the formation of the implantation chambers of pregnancy occurs: the decidual reaction is initially localized in discrete nodes in the anti-mesometrial stroma, then spreads radially and mesometrially but remains sharply delineated from the basal endometrium and from the internodes (Lobel, Levy and Shelesnyak, 1967).

At this stage in our investigations, we had formulated a well rounded hypothesis: we proposed that oestrogen secreted by the ovary as a surge during progestation causes release of histamine in the uterus; the released histamine acts on sensitized sites in the endometrium and stimulates the induction of the transformation into decidual tissue, enabling the blastocyst to implant (Shelesnyak, 1959d). Our hypothesis was supported by the evidence for an oestrogen-surge; by the demonstration of histamine-release in the uterus of the spayed rat following oestrogen-injection; and by the finding that histamine-release takes place in the uterus of the pregnant rat just after the oestrogen-surge occurs. Szego and her collaborators had proposed that histamine-release was an obligatory response of the uterus to oestrogen action and that histamine was the mediator of oestrogen action. They also presented evidence that histamine alone, could mimic some of the actions of oestrogens (Szego, 1965).

The validity of these hypotheses was jeopardized when evidence was obtained that an oestrogen surge occurs in the pseudopregnant rat (Shelesnyak and Tic, 1963a; Shelesnyak, Kraicer and Zeilmaker, 1963).

Consequently, it would be expected that the oestrogen would cause histamine-release and hence the induction of decidualization. However, spontaneous decidualization does not occur, normally. When direct chemical analyses showed that the uterus of the pseudopregnant rats contained only minimal quantities of histamine, we rationalized away objections to our hypothesis by concluding that in the pseudopregnant rat uterus, the small amounts of histamine present were not amenable to release and that the induction of decidualization by pyrathiazine or trauma was mediated by extrauterine histamine or "induced histamine", respectively (Marcus, Shelesnyak and Kraicer, 1964).

Subsequent findings, however, forced us to abandon the idea that surge-oestrogen induced histamine release and thus, indirectly, decidualization. We had turned to an analysis of the factors responsible for the differences in histamine levels in the pregnant and pseudopregnant rat uterus. By the use of vasectomized male rats to induce pseudopregnancy instead of electrical stimulation of the cervix, we established two conditions in the uterus: one subject to sperm-free male components and one free of all male components. We were able to show that exposure of the rat uterus to seminal plasma following sterile mating resulted in elevation of the histamine content of the uterus. However, in the rats in coitally-induced pseudopregnancy, in spite of the occurrence of an oestrogen-surge, histamine-release did not occur. The elevated histamine levels persisted (Marcus and Shelesnyak, 1968).

Additional experiments then revealed that an anti-oestrogen, which prevents decidualization and implantation, does not antagonize histamine-release; conversely, an antihistamine which prevents decidualization and implantation, does not antagonize oestrogen action. The oestrogen antagonist, MER-25, which, by antagonizing surge-oestrogen prevents decidual induction and also prevents the spurt of uterine activity resulting from surge-oestrogen (Shelesnyak and Tic, 1963b), does not prevent the histamine-release associated with the oestrogen-surge in the pregnant rat, although it does prevent oestrogen-induced histamine-release in the uterus of the spayed rat (Marcus and Shelesnyak, 1967a). On the other hand, we found that antihistamine, administered intraluminally before the oestrogen-surge, prevents decidualization, but does not prevent or interfere with the action of surge-oestrogen on the uterus; only the synthetic activity characterizing decidualization, but not the other manifestations of the oestrogen-surge, is affected (Tic, Marcus and Shelesnyak, 1967).

We have concluded, therefore, that although both oestrogen and histamine are essential to the decidual transformation, neither alone is sufficient; histamine is not a mediator of oestrogen action, nor is histamine-release caused by oestrogen in the uterus of intact rat. Since histamine-release does not occur during progestation in the absence of the blastocyst, other things being equal, it seems most likely that the fertilized ovum is in some way responsible for the histamine-release.

During the course of studies on the antihistaminic inhibition of decidualization, it was discovered that inhibition of decidualization could be produced by administration of the antihistamine as early as the prooestrus introducing progestation, but, however, not if given only 24 hours before that (Shelesnyak and Kraicer, 1964). We were later able to demonstrate that a significant amount of tritium-labelled antihistamine can be recovered from the rat uterus on day $L_4$ if the antihistamine be instilled on or after the prooestrous which introduces progestation, but none can be recovered if administered even one day prior to prooestrus (Marcus and Shelesnyak, 1967b). We thus showed that the intervention of an oestrus abolishes the inhibitory action of the antihistamine by disposal or removal of the drug. Since the onset of vulnerability to inhibition coincides with a phase of uterine growth induced by oestrogen of prooestrous, we have interpreted these observations as indicating that the "priming" oestrogen secreted at prooestrus has stimulated the turnover and/or formation of uterine components which bind antihistamine and confer upon the uterus vulnerability to inhibition of decidualization. These uterine components formed by priming oestrogen, in fact, establish the potential for decidualization.

A further step in the interpretation of these findings was the formulation of the concept of labile uterine receptors for decidual induction. In accordance with the experimental findings these receptors would be formed in response to "priming" and would require activation by surge-oestrogen before stimulation of decidualization becomes possible; but, these receptors, following the administration of histamine antagonists, bind irreversibly the antihistamine, thereby becoming refractory to stimulation. Finally, assuming histamine to be the mediator of stimulation and that stimulation requires the association of the stimulant with the receptor, then it should be possible to demonstrate an association of histamine (or a metabolite thereof) with the receptor. Such association or binding should occur only when the receptor is susceptible to stimulation, i.e. after activation. In attempting to demonstrate this, our first approach was to investigate the retention of radioactivity following parenteral administration of $^{14}C$-labelled histamine at the time of maximal uterine sensitivity to decidual induction, comparing the time-course of retention in the uterus with that in other organs and tissues. Except for uterus, all tissues exhibited similar exponential decay curves. In the uterus, however, a pronounced plateau lasting until about three hours post-injection was observed. We regarded this behaviour of the uterus as indicative of an unique affinity for either histamine or one of its metabolites. In subsequent experiments, we found that significantly greater amounts of radioactivity were retained by the uterus when the labelled histamine was administered when the uterus was sensitized to stimulation, than at other times (Marcus and Shelesnyak, 1967*c*). Similarly, after administration of labelled histamine on day $L_4$, more radioactivity was retained in the uninhibited horn of a uterus unilaterally treated with antihistamine than in the antihistamine-treated horn. If the antihistamine, however, had been administered before proestrus, so that no inhibition of the ability to respond to stimulation of day $L_4$ was inflicted on the uterus, then both horns retained the greater amounts of radioactivity. Thus, experimental albeit indirect evidence for the existence of histamine-associated receptors for decidual induction formed in response to the action of priming oestrogen of prooestrous has been provided.

The possible identification of such receptors with recognizable, morphologically distinct entities in the uterus requires careful analysis of the dynamics of morphological changes occurring in the uterus following prooestrus, mating, oestrogen-surge and the beginning of the decidual response and implantation. To this end, a critical histological study of the uterus of the pregnant rat was undertaken using autoradiographic technique to aid in the interpretation of observations and in tracing the origins of tissue elements. A salient finding was the observation that infiltration of the uterus by eosinophilic granulocytes, which is a normal feature of oestrus, dependent upon prooestrous oestrogen (Lobel, Levy, Kisch and Shelesnyak, 1967), is greatly augmented, in the event that coitus takes place, by intense infiltration with neutrophilic leucocytes (Lobel, Levy and Shelesnyak, 1967). Following coitus, during oestrus, the neutrophils were found in great numbers in the epithelium and in the lumen, where they were engaged in phagocytosis of spermatozoa. Between day $L_0$ and $L_1$ monocytes gradually replaced the polymorphic leucocytes in the uterus. Cellular degeneration in the luminal and glandular epithelium took place on days $L_0$ and $L_1$. During this period, only epithelium exhibited incorporation of labelled thymidine, parallelling the incorporation observed during the oestrous cycle: the greatest incorporation occurred on day $L_1$. By day $L_2$ the neutrophilic infiltration had largely subsided, epithelial repair had been completed and lymphocytic infiltration had begun. Although oedema did not occur, the picture presented by the uterus was one of acute inflammation and recovery therefrom.

By day $L_4$, widespread incorporation of labelled thymidine in the uterine stroma had occurred, primarily on the antimesometrial side of the lumen. This proliferation of stromal cells was presumably a response to the oestrogen surge. At the same time renewed leucocytic infiltration became apparent and there was generalized endometrial oedema with vascular dilation. Lymphocytes were prominent in the subepithelial and glandular areas, eosinophiles and neutrophiles in the deeper stromal regions. By late on day $L_4$ of pregnancy stromal oedema had become localized to areas near blastocysts and stromal cells in these regions exhibited increased RNase-labile basophilia. Such cells did not incorporate labelled thymidine whereas adjacent stromal cells did. If, however, the tissues were examined many hours after the administration of the label, then labelled decidual cells were found in the niduses indicating that the decidual cells had been formed by division and differentiation of stromal cells, but the decidual cells themselves do not proliferate, at least at this stage. By day $L_5$, lymphocytes, which had incorporated labelled thymidine administered during the previous day, congregated about the periphery of the decidual nodes. By this time, areas of epithelium in contact with the blastocyst have become eroded, trophoblastic cells have penetrated between and under epithelial cells, detaching them and engulfing them by phagocytosis. As the epithelium was disrupted, neutrophils also infiltrated the epithelial areas and aided in phagocytosis of the epithelial debris.

We would invite attention to the rather striking similarities between certain aspects of progestation, that is, early pregnancy and the production of cutaneous delayed hypersensitivity (cf. Waksman, 1960). The production of sensitivity, involving application of an antigen to the skin and the tissue changes in response to the presence of the antigen, is closely mimicked by the deposition of sperm and associated seminal constituents in the uterus and the uterine response to this stimulation as just described. The phase of reexposure, which elicits the delayed response of characteristic of delayed hypersensitivity reactions, is parallelled by the entry of the fertilized ovum into the uterus and the occurrence of a delayed uterine reaction to the presence of the ovum.

If, indeed, there is an immunological aspect to the uterine response to mating and to blastocyst-uterus interactions (*cf.* Tyler, 1961), it is probable that the antigenic material is associated with semen deposited in the uterus after mating and is borne on the fertilized egg which enters the uterus late on day $L_5$. In fact, at this time, sperm fragments may be seen in the blastocyst, lying on it or embedded in it (Tachi and Kraicer, 1967). In the absence of the blastocyst, i. e. in pseudopregnancy, the infiltration of the uterus occurring at $L_4$ is mainly eosinophilic, without the predominance of lymphocytes. It appears, therefore, that the pattern of infiltration observed during pregnancy is the basic hormonally directed infiltration, augmented by the response to antigenic material. The augmented infiltration may account for the increased histamine level in the pregnant uterus, the histamine being imported by the infiltrating leucocytes. Such accumulation of histamine is associated with the sensitization period in the induction of delayed hypersensitivity (Inderbitzen, 1956; 1961). Whatever the precise function of the infiltrating leucocytes be in the decidual response, it may be an essential one; preliminary experiments have shown that drug-induced leucopenia produced prior to entry of the ova into the uterus prevents implantation (A. Horan, M. Goldman, P. Levinson and G. J. Marcus: unpublished findings). Whether the leucopenia and implantation failure are directly related require more extensive investigation.

In summary, we may consider nidation as a sequence of overlapping phases, each characterized by predominating events. The first phase, priming, which includes proestrus and estrus, is characterized by estrogen dominance, which stimulates turnover of uterine components and the formation of new elements, conferring upon the uterus the potential to respond to decidual induction and, as well, vulnerability to inhibition of decidualization. Priming gives way to the second phase, which we prefer to call sensitization. This phase is characterized by coitally augmented infiltration of the uterus by leucocytes and the concomittant accumulation of histamine. The phase is completed by the oestrogen-surge which produces the phase of sensitization and uterine sensitivity is now established. In this stage, the blastocyst enters the uterus, sheds its zona pellucida and induces histamine-release which initiates decidualization. Once decidualization is under way, the blastocyst begins penetration of the uterine epithelium and embeds itself in the nidus. Proliferation of trophoblastic and embryonic tissues has begun with implantation and nidation is complete.

This presentation, in spite of its length, is only a skeleton which will serve this workshop as a basis for more detailed elaborations by members of the group; as a basis for probing into tangential and contiguous fields of enquiry and as a basis for inviting exploration of the subject by our visitors. It should serve to indicate some of our problems and queries. Critical evaluation of our views should reveal the necessity of examining the individual processes as basic natural phenomena which invite the attention of specialists concerned with the particular processes *per se*, rather than in relation to nidation. We hope, then, that from this will come at least an attempt to incorporate specialized knowledge in synthesizing a better understanding of nidation.

## REFERENCES

Christie, G. A. (1966) Implantation of the rat embryo— glycogen and alkaline phosphatases. J. Reprod. Fertil. 12, 279.

De Feo, V. J. (1963a) Determination of the sensitive period for the induction of deciduomata in the rat by different inducing procedures. Endocrinology 73, 488-497.

De Feo, V. J. (1963b) Temporal aspect of uterine sensitivity in the pseudopregnant or pregnant rat. Endocrinology 72, 305-316.

Interbitzen, Th. (1956) Hautallergie und histamin. Dermatologica 112, 435-443.

Inderbitzen, Th. (1961) The mechanisms involved in histamine release and histamine increase in allergic reactions. Int. Arch. Allergy 18, 85-99.

Kaye, A. M. (1961) Pyrimidine biosynthesis in the presence of carcinogenic concentrations of ethyl carbamate (Urethan). Bull. Res. Council Israel 10A, 32-33.

Kaye, A. M. (1968) Urethane carcinogensis and nucleic acid metabolism: In vitro interactions with enzymes. Cancer Res. 28, 1041.

Kraicer, P. F., Marcus, G. J. and Shelesnyak, M. C. (1963) Studies on the mechanism of decidualization. III. Decidualization in the histamine-depleted rat. J. Reprod. Fertil. 5, 417-421.

Kraicer, P. F. and Shelesnyak, M. C. (1958) The induction of deciduomata in the pseudopregnant rat by systemic administration of histamine and histamine releasers. J. Endocrin. 17, 324-328.

Kraicer, P. F. and Shelesnyak, M. C. (1959) Détermination de la période de sensibilité maximale de l'endomètre á la décidualisation au moyen de déciduomes provoqués par un traitement empruntant la voie vasculaire. C. R. Acad. Sci. (Paris) 248, 3213-3215.

Krehbiel, R. H. (1937) Cytological studies of the decidual reaction in the rat during early pregnancy and in the production of deciduomata. Physiol. Zool. 10, 212-234.

Lobel, B. L., Levy, E., Kisch, E. S. and Shelesnyak, M. C. (1967) Studies on the mechanism of nidation. XXVIII. Experimental investigation on the origin of eosinophilic granulocytes in the uterus of the rat. Acta Endocr. (Kbh) 55, 451-471.

Lobel, B. L., Levy, E. and Shelesnyak, M. C. (1967) Studies on the mechanism of nidation. XXXIV. Dynamics of cellular interactions during progestation and implantation in the rat. Acta Endocr. (Kbh.) 56, Suppl. 123.

Lobel, B. L., Tic, L. and Shelesnyak, M. C. (1965a)

Studies on the mechanism of nidation. XVII. Histochemical analysis of decidualization in the rat. Part 1. Acta Endocr. (Kbh.) 50, 452-468.

Lobel, B. L., Tic, L. and Shelesnyak, M. C. (1965b) Studies on the mechanism of nidation. XVII. Histochemical analysis of decidualization in the rat. Part 5. Uterine manifestations of interference with the hormonal requirements of deciduomata. Acta Endocr. (Kbh.) 50, 560-583.

Loeb, L. (1907) Uber die experimentelle Erzeugung von Knoten von Deciduagewebe in dem Uterus des Meerschweinchens nach stattgefundener Copulation. Zbl. Allg. Path. Path. Anat. 18, 563-565.

Marcus, G. J., Kraicer, P. F. and Shelesnyak, M. C. (1963) Studies on the mechanism of decidualization. II. The histamine-releasing action of pyrathiazine. J. Reprod. Fertil. 5, 409-415.

Marcus, G. J. and Shelesnyak, M. C. (1967a) Studies on the mechanism of nidation. XX. Relation of histamine release to estrogen action in the progestational rat. Endocrinology 80, 1028-1031.

Marcus, G. J. and Shelesnyak, M. C. (1967b) Studies on the mechanism of nidation. XXVI. Proestrous estrogen as a hormonal parameter of nidation. Endocrinology 80, 1038-1042.

Marcus, G. J. and Shelesnyak, M. C. (1967c) Studies on the mechanism of nidation. XXV. A receptor theory for decidual induction. Endocrinology 80, 1032-1037.

Marcus, G. J. and Shelesnyak, M. C. (1968) Studies on the mechanism of nidation. XXXIII. Coital elevation of uterine histamine content. Acta Endocr. (Kbh.) 57, 136-141.

Marcus, G. J., Shelesnyak, M. C. and Kraicer, P. F. (1964) Studies on the mechanism of nidation. X. The oestrogen-surge, histamine-release and decidual induction in the rat. Acta Endocr. (Kbh.) 47, 255-264.

Nelson, W. O. (1929) Estrus during pregnancy. Science 70, 453-454.

Psychoyos, A. (1961) Perméabilité capillaire et décidualization utérine. C.R. Acad. Sci. (Paris) 252, 1515-1517.

Shelesnyak, M. C. (1954) The action of selected drugs on deciduoma formation. Endocrinology 55, 85-89.

Shelesnyak, M. C. (1957) Some experimental studies on the mechanism of ova-implantation in the rat. Rec. Progr. Horm. Res. 13, 269-317.

Shelesnyak, M. C. (1959a) Histamine and the nidation of the ovum. Mem. Soc. Endocrinol. 6, 84-88.

Shelesnyak, M. C. (1959b) Fall in uterine histamine associated with ovum-implantation in the pregnant rat. Proc. Soc. Exp. Biol. Med. (N.Y.) 100, 380-381.

Shelesnyak, M. C. (1959c) Histamine-releasing activity of natural estrogens. Proc. Soc. Exp. Biol. Med. (N.Y.) 100, 739-741.

Shelesnyak, M. C. (1959d) Mechanism of implantation and its control. Proc. 6th Int. Congr. Plan. Parenthood Fed., New Delhi, 151-154.

Shelesnyak, M. C. and Kraicer, P. F. (1964) Studies on the mechanism of nidation. XI. Duration of the inhibition of decidual induction by antihistamine. J. Reprod. Fertil. 8, 287-292.

Shelesnyak, M. C., Kraicer, P. F. and Zeilmaker, G. H. (1963) Studies on the mechanism of decidualization. I. The estrogen surge of pseudopregnancy and progravity and its role in the process of decidualization. Acta Endocr. (Kbh.) 42, 225-232.

Shelesnyak, M. C. and Tic, L. (1963a) Studies on the mechanism of decidualization. IV. Synthetic processes in the decidualizing uterus. Acta Endocr. (Kbh.) 42, 465-472.

Shelesnyak, M. C. and Tic, L. (1963b) Studies on the mechanism of decidualization. V. Suppression of synthetic processes in the uterus following inhibition of decidualization by an anti-oestrogen ethanoxytriphetol (MER-25). Acta Endocr. (Kbh.) 43, 462-468.

Spaziani, E. and Szego, C. M. (1958) The influence of estradiol and cortisol on uterine histamine in the ovariectomized rat. Endocrinology 63, 669-678.

Swezy, O. and Evans, H. M. (1930) Ovarian changes during pregnancy. Science 71, 46.

Szego, C. M. (1965) Role of histamine in mediation of hormone action. Fed. Proc. 24, 1343-1352.

Tachi, S. and Kraicer, P. F. (1967) Studies on the mechanism of nidation. XXVII. Sperm-derived inclusions in the rat blastocyst. J. Reprod. Fertil. 14, 401-405.

Tic, L., Marcus, G. J. and Shelesnyak, M. C. (1967) Studies on the mechanism of nidation. XXX. Selective antihistamine inhibition of uterine responses in relation to suppression of decidualization. Life Sci. 6, 1179-1183.

Tyler, A. (1961) Approaches to the control of fertility based on immunological phenomena. J. Reprod. Fertil. 2, 473-506.

Varavudhi, P. (1965) Studies on the mechanism of nidation and the interrelationships between the central nervous system, the adenohypophysis and the ovary. Doctoral Thesis, Weizmann Institute of Science, Rehovot, Israel.

Waksman, B. H. (1960) A comparative histopathalogical study of delayed hypersensitivity reactions in: Cellular Aspects of Immunity, G. E. W. Wolstenholme and M. O'Connor eds. Churchill, London, p. 280.

Zeilmaker, G. H. (1963) Experimental studies on the effects of ovariectomy and hypophysectomy on blastocyst implantation in the rat. _Acta Endocr. (Kbh.)_ _44_, 355-366.

## DISCUSSION

R. W. Schayer: When you concluded the first stage of your presentation, the hypothesis looked nice and pat, and then you gave some of the opposing evidence. I think that all of these discrepancies might possibly be resolved, because histamine metabolism is such a very complex business.

M. C. Shelesnyak: We haven't distinguished between various types of histamine (i. e. mast cell or nascent, for example). This simplification is important for the understanding of our postulates. As to which histamine is involved, is a point to which you, Dr. Schayer, can probably contribute as much as any one in the field. Histamine, as you say, is a very tricky business. Just two examples of the complexity of things are one, that an antihistamine is a histamine-releaser and two, that when you measure tissue histamine levels and find a reduction in histamine while a process takes place, you come to the conclusion that histamine is acting.

R. W. Schayer: Or that if you raise the concentration of histamine you can get the opposite effect by stimulating a defensive mechanism.

U. S. von Euler: Do you envisage this effect of histamine as a general one, on the whole organ or is it in any way localized? You mentioned something about localized action.

M. C. Shelesnyak: We believe that the natural histamine-associated process during pregnancy is, in fact, localized with respect to the uterus. There are, on the other hand, certain generalized reactions of histamine which are of interest to us, for example, the phenomenon of generalized depletion. Depletion of the uterus alone, would be of great interest to us, but we don't know how to accomplish that. The generalized depletion of histamine is reflected in the failure of local histamine action. The uterus, however, is not depleted as quickly or as readily as are other organs. If I err in this belief, Dr. Schayer will correct me.

One of the fascinating things about the whole field is that very little work has been done on the uterus with respect to histamine, other than, of course, the use of the uterus in bioassays. Dr. Schayer and I were discussing the magnificent treatise on histamine edited by Rocha e Silva (Handbuch der experimentellen Pharmakologie, Vol. 18, part 1, Histamine and Antihistamines, Springer Verlag, Berlin, 1966) which makes no reference whatsoever to histamine and the uterus in relation to nidation. There is discussion of histamine assays on the uterus in vitro and apparently the uterus is all right for such measurements, but there is nothing said about the natural histamine-associated processes in the uterus.

I would emphasize, also, that the uterus is a dynamic organ, different at any moment from what it was before and what it will be the moment after. Even after the significant advance in approach made by differentiating between the pregnant and the non-pregnant uterus, very few measurements are of any help to us, because the non-pregnant uterus, for example, does not represent a definite physiological condition and as you have seen from our studies, is variable with respect to histamine content during the natural estrous cycle and in other conditions even those which have been assumed to be fairly stable, such as pseudopregnancy. A pattern of variation exists.

The phenomenon with which we are concerned is a fairly localized phenomenon; we think this is brought out by the presence of the various infiltrating cells, the presence of specifically localized responses along the uterus, the nodal pattern of early decidualization. Precisely why we get nodal induction is a mystery. It may be explicable in the pregnant animal, where there may be some tactile mechanism, unknown to us, which triggers a reaction, but even in the absence of the blastocyst, in the pseudopregnant rat, a parenteral injection of pyrathiazine induces decidualization in localized areas. Although by the fourth day after the induction, when it is customary to examine the uterus, one finds a massive sausage-like response, but if one were to examine the uterus in earlier stages of decidual development, that is the first or second day after induction, one finds that decidualization invariably starts in discrete foci spaced out along the uterus.

U. S. von Euler: Predilection sites, in other words.

M. C. Shelesnyak: Yes, but the basis for this distribution escapes us.

R. E. Billingham: Does the number of these discrete sites correspond roughly to the number of conceptuses that the rat can bear?

M. C. Shelesnyak: Well roughly, but I would emphasize only roughly. We have never undertaken a statistical comparison. Systemic induction produces no more a completely uniform response than is obtained in pregnancy. Sometimes a massive response is obtained and in other instances in which we look on the fourth day of decidual development we find only four or five nodes. But when there is the same variation in pregnancy, one would be hard put to say there is always a certain number. I don't think that preformed sites exist and always existed. I don't think one can say that there is an anatomical basis for having certain parts of the uterus invariably in this transformation.

U. S. von Euler: A biochemical basis, perhaps.

P. F. Kraicer: This will shed, I am afraid, further confusion. Prof. Shelesnyak mentioned that the time of maximum sensitization of the uterus to decidual induction is identical in the pseudopregnant and in the pregnant animal, the time being ten o'clock in the morning of $L_4$, but in studying changes in the ovum which takes place over this critical period, one finds that the ovum is still in a very active process of morphogenesis, and after ten o'clock in the morning on $L_4$, it will be completing the stages of development required to bring it to the nidation stage. At ten o'clock in the morning, it is still covered with the zona pellucida which it will only lose between two and six hours later. It has not yet developed the trophoblastic giant cells which are the things that attach to the uterus, and, as a matter of fact, if there is one characteristic which distinguishes the eggs at this time it is the fact that they are so variable with respect to their stage of development. One finds everything from the late morula to the fully matured blastocyst without a zona pellucida, so that the problem of how ova in all these various stages may affect the endometrium in what must be a rather uniform fashion, is really mysterious.

# THE MICROCIRCULATORY FUNCTION OF HISTAMINE AND ITS ROLE IN GLUCOCORTICOID AND THYROID HORMONE ACTIONS

# THE MICROCIRCULATORY FUNCTION OF HISTAMINE AND ITS ROLE IN GLUCOCORTICOID AND THYROID HORMONE ACTIONS

Richard W. Schayer
Research Center, Rockland State Hospital
Orangeburg, New York

In recent years substantial evidence has been obtained which indicates that histamine functions as an intrinsic microcirculatory dilator (Schayer, 1962; 1963; 1965). If this conclusion is basically correct, histamine would participate in every aspect of body economy and might be of key significance in a number of phenomena of obscure mechanism.

The simple proposition that histamine is continuously formed within cells of the small blood vessels, catalyzed by histidine decarboxylase showing inducible activity, may provide a major clarification of such seemingly unrelated phenomena as the autonomous dilator activities of the microcirculation, the manifold effects of glucocorticoid hormones, and the action of thyroid hormones on growth, development and energy production.

In addition, the microcirculatory actions of histamine may be of considerable importance in a number of aspects of reproduction; among them are nidation (Shelesnyak, 1957), estrogen action (Szego, 1965), and fetal growth and development (Kahlson and Rosengren,

1968). Evidence for involvement of histamine in these latter cases has been capably presented by others and need not be reviewed here; the primary purpose of this paper is to discuss the possible role of histamine in microcirculatory control, glucocorticoid action, and thyroid hormone action.

## I. HISTAMINE AND AUTONOMOUS MICRO-CIRCULATORY CONTROL

The microcirculatory system shows a rather clearly defined autonomous behavior. Normally, most capillaries are closed but each precapillary sphincter relaxes occasionally so all cells get blood periodically. This process of periodic opening and closing of small vessels, designated as vasomotion, adapts to changes in environment. When a tissue becomes active, e.g., during muscular exercise, many additional capillaries open (post-exercise hyperemia). When a tissue has been deprived of blood for a period of time, small vessels become widely dilated when flow is restored (reactive hyperemia; autoregulation). Conversely, when flow in large vessels increases, there is a tendency for small vessels to close (autoregulation). In systemic stress, small vessels, initially closed by action of released catecholamines, gradually reopen; in extreme cases, dilatation may proceed to development of shock. In inflammation there is a similar slowly developing vasodilatation.

As to the mechanism, an extraordinary situation exists. Despite years of intensive study there is no commonly accepted explanation for even a single one of these events, much less any unifying mechanism.

There is no doubt that some of these events are complex and may involve a number of factors. However, if intrinsically synthesized histamine exists at all, it is an obligatory participant in all the above events. The use of this concept provides a unifying and simplifying principle for this confused field.

For this interpretation three experimentally supported postulates are required:

1. Histamine is continuously produced within smooth muscle and endothelial cells of small blood vessels.

2. It acts primarily on intrinsic or intracellular receptors.

3. The mechanism for histamine production can adapt to environmental requirements, i.e., histidine decarboxylase is an inducible enzyme.

According to these postulates histamine is formed within smooth muscle cells, and diffuses out, undergoing loose binding in passing through the cell wall. Then the microcirculatory events described above might occur as follows:

A. Vasomotion

In the sphincter of a closed capillary histamine would accumulate on the outer surface of the cell. Newly synthesized molecules would become loosely bound in the wall and subsequently the concentration of free intracellular histamine would rise. When its dilator effect overcomes constrictor forces, the muscle would relax. Blood entering the capillary would wash away extracellular histamine and cause a gradual reduction, first in loosely bound, then in free histamine. When constrictor forces become predominant, the muscle cell would contract and the cycle would be complete. Through the adaptive characteristics of histidine decarboxylase activity, the basal rate of histamine synthesis could be adjusted to permit vasomotion in various environments.

## B. Reactive Hyperemia

Occlusion of a vessel should lead to accumulation of histamine molecules on the outer cell surface. Newly synthesized histamine molecules would be held in the cell wall, but the intracellular concentration would subsequently rise and affect dilator receptors. Upon restoration of blood flow, dilatation would be maximal. As the accumulated extracellular histamine molecules are washed away, the concentration in the wall and in the cytoplasm would gradually drop to normal.

## C. Postexercise Hyperemia

The rate of intrinsic histamine synthesis would increase as the tissue temperature increased. This is not a slow adaptive effect but occurs immediately owing to the temperature effect on enzymes. Dilatation would also be immediate (Schayer, 1964). Subsequently, through the process of conducted vasodilatation, the arterioles and small arteries could dilate (Hilton, 1962).

## D. Autoregulation

A moderate increase in tissue perfusion pressure would increase flow in open capillaries, expedite washout of extracellular histamine, reduce the intracellular concentration, cause sphincters to close more rapidly than normally, and thus increase resistance to flow.

Conversely, a drop in perfusion pressure, by reducing the rate of histamine removal in open capillaries, would permit sphincters to remain open for a longer than normal period, and thus reduce resistance to flow. It is not implied that other mechanisms may not also be of importance in autoregulation.

## E. Slowly-Developing Dilator Responses

The microvascular vasodilatation which gradually develops in inflammation or in systemic stress states may be due to a progressive increase in intrinsic histamine production; this process may be an exaggerated manifestation of the same adaptive ability which is essential for maintaining vasomotion in the face of constant changes in internal and external environment.

## F. Slowly-Developing Inflammation

The slowly-developing phase of the inflammatory state includes initial opening of precapillary sphincters, gradual spreading of dilatation to larger vessels, and a progressive loss of responsiveness of smooth muscle to catecholamines; in these respects, the picture is similar to that observed in the decompensatory phase of shock (Zweifach, 1961). Inflammation also involves capillary endothelial cell changes. These cells swell and pull apart, forming gaps through which protein molecules can pass. Endothelial cell changes are not usually found in severe systemic stress; presumably released glucocorticoids and catecholamines protect them. Opening of precapillary sphincters, reflex vasodilatation of larger vessels, and endothelial damage are characteristic histamine effects. There is no evident reason why histamine, produced intrinsically at gradually increasing rates, could not be the primary mediator of the inflammatory reaction. We have recently found that inhibitors of protein synthesis, e. g., puromycin, actidione (cycloheximide) and tenuazonic acid, block activation of histamine synthesis in several tissues, following a variety of stimuli. When tested in turpentine inflammation of rat or mouse paw, such compounds not only blocked activation of histamine production, but also strongly suppressed the inflammation. This result is quite remarkable since turpentine initiates a violent response which is only slightly reduced by the usual anti-inflammatory drugs. Additional support for histamine mediation of inflammation comes from the fact that actinomycin D, which blocks activation of many inducible enzymes, fails to prevent activation of histamine synthesis and is also devoid of anti-inflammatory action (Schayer, 1967a).

## II. HISTAMINE AND GLUCOCORTICOID ACTION

From the postulates listed in I, that is, that histamine is formed intrinsically by an adaptive mechanism, it is possible to unify many major glucocorticoid effects. It is believed that glucocorticoid hormone molecules attach to microvascular smooth muscle cells and thus reduce the dilator effect of intrinsically produced histamine. Basically, glucocorticoid effects may be derived from their tendency to close precapillary sphincters for longer than normal periods (Schayer, 1964a; 1967).

## A. The Physiological Function of Glucocorticoids

These hormones are essential for survival only during stress. They have profound effects on metabolism but there is no substantial evidence that they have a metabolic function. In fact adrenalectomized animals show rather normal metabolic patterns provided they are not stressed. In stressed animals sympathetic nervous system activity is increased and blood flow is reduced in certain vascular beds. In accordance with its function in maintaining an adequate nutritive blood flow, the adaptive histamine-producing mechanism is activated. In the intact animal, this process aids homeostasis. However, in the adrenalectomized animal the microcirculatory system is extremely sensitive to histamine, and the typical picture of stress-induced circulatory failure results from the compensatory activation of histamine synthesis.

## B. The Catabolic Effect of Glucocorticoids

Excessive doses of glucocorticoids produce a catabolic effect in virtually every tissue except liver. This state could arise from corticoid antagonism of the dilator action of histamine in vasomotion (I-A). Prolonged closure of precapillary sphincters, by reducing nutritive blood flow to the majority of body cells, could result in the observed loss of tissue constituents and decreased uptake of isotopic precursors. It is not excluded, however, that prolonged corticoid dosing might not increase a tissue constituent. If for a certain substance, degradative processes were inhibited to a greater degree than synthetic processes, the substance would accumulate.

## C. The Anabolic Effect of Glucocorticoids in Liver

Two major factors may be involved in the seemingly anomalous anabolic response of liver to glucocorticoids. First, it is a major function of hepatic cells to activate their metabolic capabilities when exposed to a high nutrient concentration; second, the liver sinusoidal system lacks shunts of large diameter. Therefore, if hepatic microvascular sphincters were closed for a longer than normal period, blood would presumably flow faster through those sinusoids remaining open, and the bordering cells would receive an abnormally large number of nutrient molecules. Triggering of metabolic activation may occur rapidly although full development may require several hours. In accordance with the proposed mechanism of vasomotion, each sphincter cell would eventually relax and the process of local over-perfusion of hepatic cells, a few at a time, would spread throughout the liver. The same mechanism could operate in isolated perfused liver.

## D. The Effect of Glucocorticoids on Water Distribution

Glucocorticoids have a specific effect, not shared by mineralocorticoids, which causes tissue water to enter the vascular system (Russell, 1965). This effect is presumably due to the factors described by Starling's Principle (Landis and Pappenheimer, 1963). When a precapillary sphincter is relaxed, the fluid within the capillary is exposed to arterial pressure and water molecules of blood are forced through the capillary barrier into the tissues. Conversely, when a sphincter is constricted, hydrostatic pressure within the capillary is low; owing to the osmotic effect of plasma proteins, water molecules passing from tissues to blood will tend to be retained. Since it is postulated that glucocorticoids act primarily to reduce the dilator effect of histamine and to close sphincters, transfer of water from tissues to blood should predominate in the glucocorticoid dosed animal.

## E. The Anti-Inflammatory Effect of Glucocorticoids

As indicated in section I - F, slowly-developing inflammation involves changes in endothelial cells as well as in smooth muscle cells. Glucocorticoids block both changes. If histamine mediates the progressive alterations in both endothelium and smooth muscle, a unity in glucocorticoid action is maintained. In later phases of inflammation, the suppression of repair in corticoid-treated animals is probably largely due to curtailment of blood flow to the affected tissue (Ashton and Cook, 1952).

## F. Other Glucocorticoid Effects

Although space does not permit a more complete discussion, the histamine theory is also capable of coping with a number of other observations on glucocorticoids. These include (a) the protective effect of these hormones in endotoxin and septic shock but their ineffectiveness in traumatic shock, (b) their permissive role in stress, (c) their close functional relationship to catecholamines, and (d) the neutralization of certain corticoid effects during stress, i. e., levels of corticoids required for homeostasis in stress, would produce deleterious changes in a non-stressed animal. These, various other points, and an amplification of the above discussion, have been presented elsewhere (Schayer, 1964a; 1967).

## III. HISTAMINE AND THYROID HORMONE ACTION

After the experience with the histamine theory of glucocorticoid action I wondered if the intrinsic histamine concept might help in understanding action of other hormones. In seeking candidates it was necessary to eliminate hormones which produce in vitro effects comparable to the in vivo effects. Thyroid hormone, despite its multitude of in vitro actions, showed in vivo actions in which histamine might have a significant role. Of particular interest was the large body of evidence indicating that thyroid hormone sensitizes the cardiovascular system to catecholamines (Brewster, Isaacs, Osgood and King, 1956; Barker, 1964).

According to leading authorities, the basic mechanism of thyroid hormone action is unknown. As in the case of glucocorticoids, there seems to be a widespread belief that the hormone primarily affects some aspect of metabolism which should be subject to in vitro verification. But if metabolic effects were secondary to circulatory changes, the initial interaction of hormone molecules with receptors on vascular or cardiac tissue might be difficult or impossible to demonstrate in vitro. A number of writers have reviewed the available in vitro data and discussed its inadequacy in explaining the major in vivo effects of thyroid hormones (Tata, 1964; Wolff and Wolff, 1964).

The present discussion is based on the postulate that thyroid hormone is required for the normal function of vascular smooth muscle (and possibly cardiac muscle) so that reactivity of the muscle to its physiological regulators will vary in rough proportion to the number of attached thyroid hormone molecules. The lag between thyroid administration and effect is viewed as the time required for thryoid-induced changes in vascular smooth muscle to occur.

In order to simplify the presentation, the ideas on thyroid hormone action are shown in outline form.

A. Statement: Theory of Thyroid Hormone Action

1. Thyroid hormone may be required for the normal function of vascular smooth muscle. Presumably thyroid hormone molecules attach to receptors on these muscle cells and enhance their responsiveness to substances which regulate contraction and relaxation.

2. The principal physiological regulators of vascular smooth muscle are the constrictors norepinephrine, epinephrine, and the unidentified "tone-force." Opposing the constrictors are the dilators; of these, intrinsically synthesized histamine is of primary importance in control of the small vessels.

3. Cardiac muscle may also be affected directly; however, certain thyroid effects on heart may be secondary to a circulatory change.

B. Possible Sequence of Events Leading to Thyroid-Induced Increase in Basal Metabolic Rate (BMR) During Cold Adaptation

Cold exposure seems to be the only condition, other than those involving growth and development, in which there is a physiological increase in thyroid hormone output (Barker, 1964).

1. Thyroid activity increases; thyroid hormone initiates gradually-developing changes in vascular smooth muscle rendering it hyper-reactive to norepinephrine, "tone force" and histamine.

2. Vasoconstriction due to cold-induced sympathetic nervous system activity (norepinephrine) is intensified.

3. Smooth muscle cells of the smallest vessels (precapillary sphincters) relax because of their enhanced responsiveness to intrinsically-produced histamine; they are much less affected by the sympathetic nervous system than are larger vessels (Zweifach, 1961).

4. Through the process of "conducted vasodilatation" (Hilton, 1962) arterioles relax but the venous system remains partially constricted. Sympathetic vasodilator fibers probably also make some contribution to arteriole relaxation.

5. There is increased heart action and increased pulmonary blood flow. However, blood flow to most other vascular beds may be reduced by sympathetic activity (Folkow, Heymans and Neil, 1965).

6. The overall circulatory pattern consisting of (a) strong heart action, (b) an open arterial system, (c) open precapillary sphincters, and (d) a partially constricted venous system, results in a marked increase in capillary blood flow through skeletal muscle.

7. Because of the abundant supply of nutrients reaching skeletal muscle cells, metabolite-induced activation of certain enzymes occurs; other enzymes may be more active due to greater saturation with substrate molecules or to increased availability of co-factors. A generalized increase in resting metabolism follows. The energy produced is largely used to maintain body temperature.

C. Hyperthyroidism in Homeotherms

1. A moderate "physiological" increase in thyroid hormone levels presumably causes sensitization of vascular smooth muscle and a circulatory pattern favoring enhanced blood flow in capillaries. However, unlike the situation in cold exposure, there is no significant stimulus for sympathetic discharge. Thus hyperperfusion may occur in virtually all tissues. Thereafter, as suggested by others (Pitt-Rivers and Tata, 1959) the response of cells depends on their genetically predetermined capabilities.

2. In the mature animal there is no potential for growth. Therefore, thyroid-induced metabolic activation produces heat.

3. In the immature animal the cells do have potential for growth. Hence the generalized cellular overnutrition may produce both growth and energy.

4. Large "toxic" doses of thyroid hormone probably constitute a stressor and activate the sympathetic nervous system. Blood flow is now diverted to heart, lungs and skeletal muscle, and drastically reduced to most other tissues, no doubt including a number of endocrine glands. Depending on the dose of thyroid hormone, growth might be retarded, stopped, or even reversed. However, the calorigenic effect would presumably remain roughly proportional to the level of thyroid hormone.

D. Increased Thyroid Effects in Amphibians

1. Increased thyroid hormone levels, endogenous or exogenous, sensitize vascular smooth muscle and tissue hyperperfusion occurs.

2. In the immature amphibian, the enzymic potential of the cells is directed toward metamorphosis. The abundant supply of blood borne metabolites triggers enzyme activation, and the subsequent transformations occur in accordance with the genetic information.

3. In the mature amphibian there is no longer a possibility for further development or growth. Since the cells evidently have no enzymic mechanisms

significantly concerned with heat production, thyroid hormone now does virtually nothing (Barker, 1964).

E. Hypothyroidism

1. The responsiveness of vascular smooth muscle to regulators is subnormal; consequently, the circulatory system is inefficient.

2. Weakness, poor growth and development, cold intolerance, and metabolic disturbances could result from impaired nutritive blood flow and inadequate cell nutrition.

F. Evidence Supporting a Vascular Function of Thyroid Hormone

1. Excessive levels of thyroid hormone, endogenous or exogenous, sensitize the vascular system to catecholamines (Brewster, et al., 1956; Barker, 1964).

2. When thyroid output is increased during prolonged exposure of animals to cold, injected norepinephrine is much more potent than epinephrine in increasing heat production (Hsieh and Carlson, 1957).

3. Norepinephrine is almost exclusively a vasoconstrictor; unlike epinephrine, it has very little ability to stimulate metabolism directly.

4. Heat production in hyperthyroid animals is reduced by a variety of drugs which block the vasoconstrictor actions of catecholamines.

5. In hyperthyroid animals adrenergic blockade reduces the BMR to euthyroid levels, not to hypothyroid levels. This, and other evidence, indicates that metabolic effects of thyroid hormone can not be entirely attributed to action of adrenergic amines (Barker, 1964). The present view suggests that vasoconstriction is essential for increased BMR, but that there is an alternative to mediation by catecholamines. A vasoconstrictor "tone-force" exists which is not referable to any known blood-borne substance (Barcroft, 1963) and which is unaffected by any drug acting through reduction of catecholamine action. This tone-force is particularly strong in skeletal muscle, the major site of energy production in hyperthyroidism (Tata, 1964).

6. From the evidence in 2, 3 and 4, above, it seems highly probable that thyroid-induced heat production relates to vasoconstriction.

7. However, vasoconstriction *per se* strongly reduces nutritive blood flow in a resting animal. In order to provide extra energy for prolonged periods, nutritive blood flow must rise above resting levels. In working muscle, for example, sympathetic vasoconstriction is overcome, presumably initiated by increased histamine production (Schayer, 1964) and a pronounced hyperemia ensues. Accordingly, to reconcile thyroid-induced vasoconstriction with the observed activation of metabolism, there must also be a mechanism for opening precapillary sphincters.

8. Thyroid hormone sensitizes animals to the lethal effects of histamine (Spencer and West, 1961).

Since this enhanced sensitivity is blocked by glucocorticoids, it seems probable that the point of sensitization is microvascular smooth muscle.

9. If thyroid hormone does in fact sensitize precapillary sphincters to histamine, and if histamine does in fact cause relaxation of sphincters during exercise, then thyroid hormone excess plus exercise should yield an exceptionally great blood flow in skeletal muscle. This prediction is actually observed; hyperthyroid patients performing a standard exercise show a markedly exaggerated postexercise hyperemia (Barcroft, 1963).

10. Metamorphosis in amphibians presumably requires activation of a vast number of metabolic processes, all within a relatively short period of time. Since elevated nutrient levels are a primary stimulus for enzyme induction and for a general acceleration of cell metabolism, and since the availability of <u>all</u> normal nutrients could be markedly enhanced by the circulatory pattern described in III-B-6, it seems quite reasonable that the transformation of a tadpole into a frog could result from the sequence:

thyroid hormone → increased local blood flow → elevation of nutrient levels in cells → triggering of enzyme activation → metamorphosis.

In contrast to this simple picture, it is difficult to envisage how a primary hormone action directed, for example, toward some change in carbohydrate or protein metabolism, or to an effect on the permeability of certain cells to certain nutrients, could produce a transformation which seems to involve responses of all cells to all nutrients.

11. An antihistamine drug is reported to have prevented thyroxin-induced, and spontaneous metamorphosis in tadpoles (Hahn and Poupa, 1951). In mice desensitized to histamine, the BMR is said to rise much less after thyroxine administration than in control mice (Fabinyi-Szebehely, Gyermek and Szebehely, 1950).

## CONCLUSION

The picture of histamine now emerging is that of an intrinsic microcirculatory dilator which indirectly influences every aspect of body economy. A moderate histamine excess increases nutritive blood flow and permits cells to reach their full potentialities. Conversely, a histamine insufficiency will lead to impaired cell nutrition and to development of abnormalities in cell chemistry and function. It is by the latter process that the side effects of glucocorticoid hormones may arise.

An attempt has been made to interpret thyroid hormone action in terms of a primary circulatory effect, in part involving histamine. This, and other evidence relating histamine to hormone action, suggests that a number of hormones which are present in vertebrates, but not in invertebrates, may participate in distribution of nutrients by modulation of the complex circulatory system of higher animals. The fact that lower forms, even single celled organisms, possess essentially the same metabolic machinery as mammals, does not afford much comfort to those who believe hormones function by direct involvement in some metabolic process.

## ACKNOWLEDGMENT

This work was supported by USPHS Grant AM-10155.

## REFERENCES

Ashton, N. and Cook, C. (1952). In vivo observations on the effects of cortisone upon the blood vessels in rabbits' ear chambers. Brit. J. Exp. Pathol. 33, 445-450.

Barcroft, H. (1963). Circulation in skeletal muscle. In Handbook of Physiology, Sect. 2, Vol. II, pp. 1353-1386. Washington, D.C., American Physiological Society.

Barker, S.B. (1964). Physiological activity of thyroid hormones and analogs. In The Thyroid Gland, Ed. R. Pitt-Rivers and W.R. Trotter. Vol. 1, pp. 199-236, Washington, D.C., Butterworth, Inc.

Brewster, W.R., Jr., Isaacs, J.P., Osgood, P.F. and King, T.L. (1956). The hemodynamic and metabolic interrelationships in the activity of epinephrine, norepinephrine and the thyroid hormones. Circulation, 13, 1-20.

Fabinyi-Szebehely, M., Gyermek, L. and Szebehely, J. (1950). Effect of histamine desensitization upon thyroxine sensitivity. Nature, 165, 155-156.

Folkow, B., Hemans, C. and Neil, E. (1965). Integrated aspects of cardiovascular regulation. In Handbook of Physiology, Sect. 2, Vol. III, pp. 1787-1824. Washington, D.C., American Physiological Society.

Hahn, P. and Poupa, O. (1951). Antihistamines and thyroxine metamorphosis in tadpoles. Nature, 167, 84.

Hilton, S. (1962). Local mechanisms regulating peripheral blood flow. Physiol. Revs. 42, Suppl. No. 5, part II, 265-275.

Hsieh, A.C.L. and Carlson, L.D. (1957). Role of adrenaline and noradrenaline in chemical regulation of heat production. Am. J. Physiol., 190, 243-246.

Kahlson, G. and Rosengren, E. (1968). New approaches to the physiology of histamine. Physiological Reviews. 48, 155-196.

Landis, E.M. and Pappenheimer, J.R. (1963). Exchange of substances through the capillary walls. In Handbook of Physiology, Sec. 2, Vol. II, pp. 961-1034, Washington, D.C., American Physiological Society.

Pitt-Rivers, R. and Tata, J.R. (1959). The Thyroid Hormones, Chapter 5, New York, Pergamon Press.

Russell, J.A. (1965). The adrenals. In Physiology and Biophysics, Ed., T.C. Ruch and H.D. Patton, p. 1133, Philadelphia, Pa., W.B. Saunders, Co.

Schayer, R.W. (1962). Evidence that induced histamine is an intrinsic regulator of the microcirculatory system. Am. J. Physiol., 202, 66-72.

Schayer, R.W. (1963). Induced synthesis of histamine, microcirculatory regulation and the mechanism of action of adrenal glucocorticoid hormones. Progress in Allergy, 7, 187-212.

Schayer, R.W. (1964). Histamine and hyperaemia of muscular exercise. Nature, 201, 195.

Schayer, R.W. (1964a). A unified theory of glucocorticoid action. Perspectives in Biology and Medicine, 8, 71-84.

Schayer, R.W. (1965). Histamine and circulatory homeostasis. Federation Proceedings, 24, No. 6, 1295-1297.

Schayer, R. W. (1967). A unified theory of glucocorticoid action, II. Perspectives in Biology and Medicine, 10, 409-418.

Schayer, R. W. (1967a). Suppression of histidine decarboxylase activation and inflammation by inhibitors of protein synthesis. The Pharmacologist (In press).

Shelesnyak, M.C. (1957). Some experimental studies on the mechanism of ova-implantation in the rat. Recent Progress in Hormone Research, 13, 269-322.

Spencer, P.S.J. and West, G.B. (1961). Sensitivity of the hyperthyroid and hypothyroid mouse to histamine and 5-hydroxytryptamine. Brit. J. Pharmacol. 17, 137-143.

Szego, C.M. (1965). Role of histamine in mediation of hormone action. Federation Proceedings, 24, No. 6, 1343-1352.

Tata, J.R. (1964). Biological action of thyroid hormones at the cellular and molecular levels. In Actions of Hormones on Molecular Processes, pp. 58-131, Ed. G. Litwack and D. Kritchevsky. New York, N.Y., John Wiley and Sons, Inc.

Wolff, E.C. and Wolff, J. (1964). The mechanism of action of the thyroid hormones. In The Thyroid Gland, Ed. R. Pitt-Rivers and W.R. Trotter. Vol. 1, pp. 237-282, Washington, D.C., Butterworth, Inc.

Zweifach, B.W. (1961). Functional Behavior of the Microcirculation. Springfield, Ill., Charles C. Thomas.

## DISCUSSION

M.C. Shelesnyak: I just want to express a few words of admiration, Dick, about the presentation, the theories and the ideas, because, in a sense, the most beautiful things in science and in nature are the simplest ones and when you can really develop a unified singular concept to explain something, it is so much more attractive than when you have an infinite number of small bits and pieces. We hope you are right, as you feel, and so far I haven't heard anything on this program of "Devastating Destruction of Theories," hereafter referred to as "DDT," but we shall see. We have before us the task of relating your ideas and findings to some of ours; I hope we will be able to accomplish this.

G.J. Marcus: Any opinions expressed by myself and probably also by other members of our department, are not necessarily those of the management. Dr. Schayer, would you comment on a curious phenomenon, that is, in regard to the response of cold-adapted rats to tourniquet shock? If rats be adapted to cold, then brought into room temperature, a tourniquet applied to the leg for a suitable period, and then removed, the rats survive, at worst, longer than do non-cold-adapted rats. You have referred to temperature-inhibition and temperature effects on the activation of histamine decarboxylase, but would such effects be involved in this case?

R.W. Schayer: The first thing that comes to mind is that cold-adapted animals become relatively insensitive to norepinephrine. Then the tourniquet isn't nearly as much of a stress as it was. The release of norepinephrine which occurs as a consequence of fluid loss or pain accompanying the tourniquet would be well tolerated and there would be no particular stimulus for activation of histamine release.

G.J. Marcus: What is the mediator of the stimulus that affects the animal after the tourniquet is released?

R.W. Schayer: I think it is believed to be a combination of the catecholamine release plus low blood volume; they lose a lot of fluid into the damaged leg.

G.J. Marcus: Do specific metabolic inhibitors of the histidine decarboxylase interfere with the inflammatory response or with vasodilation?

R.W. Schayer: No. When you say inhibitors you mean things like the in vitro inhibitors of histidine decarboxylases?

G.J. Marcus: Some have been used recently in vivo, I believe [R.J. Levine, Science, 154, 1017, 1966].

R.W. Schayer: Well, they don't show anything, but we don't think they get to the microvascular sites. But if you mean inhibitors of protein synthesis, they certainly do block both inflammation and histidine decarboxylase activation.

M. Tausk: I listened with very great interest to this paper. As Prof. Shelesnyak said, it is always very fascinating to see that somebody has a theory which can explain a diversity of phenomena by a single effect. I agree, but it is my experience that these theories seldom apply in endocrinology. On the contrary, as I propose to illustrate in my own paper tomorrow, I believe that hormones often have a variety of sites of attack and a variety of mechanisms and still, and that is the remarkable thing, these various effects seem to converge towards certain functional targets. But that is philosophy, perhaps and only an introductory remark. May I ask a few very specific questions? You said that it would be a sort of funny coincidence if the antihistaminic preparations should have a pharmacological constricting effect on the precapillary spincters. And you find it less funny that they all have in common antagonizing the effect of histamine on that very sphincter. That is what the antihistamines have in common, they antagonize histamine.

R.W. Schayer: That is what I am saying.

M. Tausk: That's right.

R.W. Schayer: That indicates histamine is acting in the sphincters.

M. Tausk: Well, that is the thing to be proven. But one isn't any less funny than the other. If they have in common antagonism of the effects of histamine on that sphincter, they may just as well have in common a constricting effect on that sphincter. Now, in regard to the effect on the bronchial muscles, we know that we are dealing with very clear-cut effects of histamine on the one hand, and of the corticoids, at least in cases of asthma, on the other hand. Would that antagonism be due to the same mechanism in your hypothesis?

R.W. Schayer: Relative to the first question, my point was that these drugs are called antihistamines because they block all the actions of histamine except that on gastric secretion, or virtually all of them; that is how drug companies find them. Now, there need be no similarity in structure at all or no similarity in side effects, but if one puts any of them on a precapillary sphincter and they all close it, the safest thing to assume is that the precapillary sphincter is being affected by histamine, and antihistamines are showing no new action at all. The constriction is not a direct action but an indirect one due to the blockage of histamine. That's the conservative view.

M. Tausk: It doesn't convince me, but I won't insist on it.

R.W. Schayer: Now about asthma. I am not a physician and don't know too much about asthma, but it's believed by some clinicians that the component upon which the glucocorticoids work is not bronchiolar smooth muscle but the microvascular system: seepage of fluid and that sort of thing.

M. Tausk: What about the effects of histamine?

R.W. Schayer: Well, histamine has two effects, one as a microcirculatory dilator and the other as a bronchiolar constrictor.

M. Tausk: You suggested that the catabolic effect of the glucocorticoids could simply be explained by the greater need of the organism for nutrients. I thought you said something to that effect.

R.W. Schayer: I think glucocorticoids reduce the amount of nutrient molecules the organism gets. They reduce nutritive blood flow; the capillaries are closed longer than they would be normally.

M. Tausk: Then you suggest that because its needs for nutrients are not satisfied it is breaking down proteins. That's what I would have to conclude from what you said.

R.W. Schayer: Well if you're starving, then yes, you'd have to start breaking down proteins, but I don't think I said specifically that they broke down proteins.

M. Tausk: No, but catabolic means breaking down proteins. Well, we know that glucocorticoids have several effects which cannot be separated from each other and others that can be separated.

R.W. Schayer: You'd have to tell me of ones that can be, I don't know of any.

M. Tausk: Well, sodium and water retention.

R.W. Schayer: That's not a glucocorticoid action.

M. Tausk: But cortisone has that effect. I thought you meant to say that all the effects of cortisone could be explained in that way.

R.W. Schayer: No, what I am talking about is hypothetical pure glucocorticoid with no effects on mineral metabolism. I should have made that clear. But I think it is in common usage. It didn't originate with me. When people say a glucocorticoid they are eliminating the mineral aspects.

M. Tausk: Yes, but cortisone is the prototype of the glucocorticoid, but cortisone has a number of effects including water and salt retention. If you introduce one double bond between $C_1$ and $C_2$ you eliminate, as we all know, salt and water retention. So at least two effects can be separated.

R.W. Schayer: I certainly agree on that.

M. Tausk: And there are some indications, although I must admit they are not very strong and very conclusive, but lots of people, as you know, are working in that direction, that there may be some separation between, for instance, pituitary inhibition and anti-inflammatory effects. I say this with great caution and things are not very clear-cut but lots of people are working in that direction. Furthermore, corticoids have an effect that is antagonistic to insulin in practically every respect and that can be shown *in vitro*. It seems to me that it is not, *prima facie*, probable that those effects should be due to the same mechanism, antagonism on the sphincter.

R.W. Schayer: I know there is a lot of *in vitro* evidence for target cells for glucocorticoids but I don't think it is very convincing. I think the main thing that we have gleaned over the years is the woeful lack of any meaningful evidence of in vitro activity of glucocorticoids despite thousands of experiments, no doubt many more unpublished than are published, and the inability of these experiments to cope with any of the major facts. When you stop to think about it, there is a strong possibility for unconscious bias in these experiments; biochemists feel that anything you see in vivo should be demonstrable in vitro because so many things have proven to be. This is a fallacy, it doesn't need to be so. If corticoids act on sphincters, for example, you would not be able to demonstrate this in vitro. So, they may test systems for years and finally after six hundred experiments that don't work or, go in the opposite direction, they get one that does. This is supposed to be evidence, you see, but I don't accept it.

J. Gorski: I'd like to interject something here. There are three very good reports of glucocorticoid effects on cell cultures. These are not tissue slices, but cultures of liver cells. They are minimal deviation tumor cells which have all the characteristics of liver cells and do anything liver cells do. They respond by induction of enzymes, such as tyrosine transaminase. They behave just like normal liver cells. This is in cell culture, with no blood supply. This has now been reported by three different laboratories. [E.B. Thompson, G.M. Tomkins and J.E. Curran. Proc. Nat. Acad. Sci. 56, 296, 1966; V.R. Potter, M. Watanabe, J.E. Becker and H.C. Pitot, Advances in Enzyme Regulation 5, 303, 1967; C.B. Hager, J.R. Reel and F.T. Kenney, unpublished observations, cited in J. Biol. Chem. 242, 4367, 1967].

R.W. Schayer: I don't doubt the results at all. I think they are undoubtedly correct, but I think we must remember that these hormones are surface active and they are going to attach to things, and in tissue culture if you get the right conditions, they may well let in more nutrients.

J. Gorski: Why doesn't progesterone do it? Progesterone is a better agent for this. It binds to the cells to an even greater extent.

R.W. Schayer: I don't know whether people have any incentive to try to find conditions under which progesterone will do it.

J. Gorski: But they do, this is a common control in these experiments. I think this is important because you can't set up a criterion and then ignore a large body of literature.

R.W. Schayer: Excuse me, but most of the attempts to demonstrate induction of enzymes in normal liver, all of them, I think, have failed. You have to go to tumor cells.

J. Gorski: Haynes has also reported stimulation of gluconeogenesis in liver slices by glucocorticoids *in vitro* [R.C. Haynes, Endocrinology 71, 399, 1962].

R.W. Schayer: Well, yes, but I believe his findings varied with conditions. But the point that Prof.

Tausk made, that one cannot separate the anti-inflammatory effects from any of the side effects suggests a single primary point of action; I think this is a reasonable conclusion to draw from that.

J. Gorski: That doesn't mean they don't work differently in different tissues.

M.C. Shelesnyak: Yes, but look. There is one point I think that Schayer has made a number of times, in regard to the in vitro story. He is talking about sphincters and apparently feels that it is part of an organic system, that if you separate it from the organic system the test method is not valid. Am I correct?

R.W. Schayer: Yes, it wouldn't show anything.

J. Gorski: But Haynes is explaining catabolism in the liver.

R.W. Schayer: Anabolism. Prof. Tausk asked about catabolism in other tissues. Well, these in vitro findings have to be reckoned with, but one must always remember how many of them have been unsuccessful or have gone the wrong direction. I am quite aware that this is a big mouthful to swallow, that there is a unity to glucocorticoid effects, but I believe it.

H.R. Lindner: I enjoyed your provocative lecture. It was indeed provocative, and therefore useful, because there is a widely held, almost dogmatic belief among investigators interested in the mechanism of action of hormones that these agents must in some way interact with the genetic control or regulation of protein synthesis at the level of transcription or translation. I, myself, and I believe Prof. Gorski, have adopted this view as our working by hypothesis. Now there are a number of features of hormone action that have troubled us in this respect. One, for instance, is the observation that in response to ACTH injection one gets within minutes, if not seconds, a large increase in blood flow through the adrenal and a steep rise in cortisol production, without any important change in the concentration of cortisol in the blood, and this almost immediate vascular response cannot possibly be explained by an action on the genetic processes of transcription or translation. We don't know today whether this really reflects an increase in nutrient blood flow. A similar early hyperemic effect has been described for estrogen in the uterus. So these things must make us question the validity of some of our current concepts of hormone action.

R.W. Schayer: Every trophic hormone is said to cause almost immediate hyperemia.

H.R. Lindner: Well, it's not so readily demonstrable if you test this with LH on the testis, or even on the ovary. But for ACTH and estrogen, there is no doubt about it. On the other hand, as pointed out by Prof. Tausk and Prof. Gorski, there are observations of an apparent immediate or direct action of cortisol on cells in tissue culture; for instance the inhibitory effect on proliferation of fibroblasts has been shown by Berliner to be mimicked in tissue culture [D. Berliner, personal communication]. I think similar observations with regard to the inhibitory action of cortisol on lymphocytes in vitro have been reported [M.H. Makman, B. Dvorkin and A. White, J. Biol. Chem. 241, 1646, 1966; A. White and M.H. Makman, Adv. Enzyme Regulation 5, 317, 1967]. Also there is at least one report that estradiol enhances the mitotic rate in cultured endometrial tissue [H.R. Maurer, D.E. Rounds and C.W. Reiborn, Nature, 213, 182, 1967].

Earlier, you said that glucocorticoids are not essential for near normal life. Which species did you refer to?

R.W. Schayer: Virtually any. If you take care of an adrenalectomized animal, you can keep him in the complete absence of glucocorticoids, and he can live as long as a normal animal. You may have to supply DOCA in some species, but others don't require any support but saline.

H.R. Lindner: Sheep do not manage to live that way: we have been unable to maintain adrenalectomized or even hypophysectomized sheep under any conditions without giving cortisone, even when environmental temperature was carefully controlled, salt offered, and deoxycorticosterone actetate administered.

R.W. Schayer: Yes. But even if there are only a few species which can do it, it proves glucocorticoids are not essential.

S. Katsh: How normal is "near normal?" They are pretty protected, aren't they?

R.W. Schayer: The point is that life is possible in the absence of glucocorticoids. The only time glucocorticoids are essential is for survival in stress. This is a well-known, but much-forgotten fact, a clue to the nature of their action.

H.R. Lindner: There also seem to be striking differences between species in the action of histamine on smooth muscle, particularly on the uterus.

R.W. Schayer: In the rat uterus, the anomalous behaviour is due to release of catecholamines [S. Tozzi and F.E. Roth, Fed. Proc. 26, 785, 1967].

H.R. Lindner: Well, yes. One thing I'd like to know a little bit more about is the mechanism you propose for the induction of histidine decarboxylase. You talk of this enzyme as an adaptive or induced enzyme. What do you suggest is the immediate inducing agent? You talked about reactive hyperemia, about endotoxin effects and so on, and a variety of other circumstances bringing about increased histamine formation. Which is the common denominator, the immediate inducing agent in these instances?

R.W. Schayer: I don't know what the common inducing agent is.

H.R. Lindner: Also, when you examine a tissue a couple of hours after giving turpentine and measure the enzyme activity, have you really got an induced enzyme or have you got a different cell population? Are any migratory cells present at that stage?

R.W. Schayer: No, it has nothing to do with new cells. You can even activate the enzyme by putting a mouse in a cold room. There is no influx of leucocytes here.

H.R. Lindner: The other thing I'd like more detailed information about is the time relations of the inhibitory effect of actidione on the inflammatory response to turpentine. If I understood you correctly, it was evident after half an hour or one to two hours.

R.W. Schayer: No, the experiments were done such that the actidione was given at zero and two hours and the turpentine was given at 0.5 hours, and the whole experiment I think was terminated at 4.5 hours. We keep these experiments fairly short because other effects come into being if you carry them too long. You do get a little redness in the paw and a slight increase in weight, but it's remarkably different from the untreated animal, which is hugely inflamed.

H.R. Lindner: How do you explain the relative ineffectiveness of cortisol in suppressing this inflammatory response? Why is it so markedly less effective than actidione?

R.W. Schayer: Well, I think that cortisol is a moderate antagonist of histamine. It doesn't block activation, it just reduces the effect. I think that's what it's there for.

H.R. Lindner: When you have increased metabolic activity, say increased muscular work, do you believe the hyperemia is the primary event? May it not occur in response to the accumulation of some metabolite, lactic acid or increased $CO_2$ tension, which in turn gives rise to capillary dilatation, by histamine-release or some other mechanism. In other words, does hyperemia induce increased metabolic activity or vice-versa?

R.W. Schayer: This dilator-metabolite relation has been worked over for so many years, but with no results. For example, there are people who have a genetic defect in the enzyme which produces lactic acid, and they get exactly the same muscular hyperemia as normals [S.M. Hilton, Physiol. Rev. 42, Suppl. 5, part 2, 265, 1962]. Well, I think metabolic activity causes hyperemia, but if hyperemia should come first, as I believe it does with thyroid hormone, metabolic action may be secondary to a forced hyperemia, to an overperfusion which is abnormal. Neither one need be the first; either could be.

C. Tachi: Since velocity is a function of the substrate concentration and I would think that the plasma level of histidine is below the enzyme saturation level and well within the range where a change in concentration of histidine should cause a change in the rate of histamine production, can a change in the plasma level, for example, by the injection of histidine cause an increase in the rate of histamine formation similar to that observed during post-exercise hyperemia?

R.W. Schayer: This has been done in microcirulatory preparations; increasing the concentration of histidine produced hyperemia and histidine is the only amino acid which would give a hyperemia, but I don't think just feeding a lot of histidine would produce a hyperemia.

C. Tachi: While the regulation of the microcirculation certainly plays an important role in the control of cellular metabolic activity, still, the nutrients in tissue fluids must pass through the cell membrane and the membrane may exert a regulatory action by selection of the species of nutrient molecules and by controlling the rate of influx and efflux of molecules. I would think that the activity of cell membranes is complementary to the microcirculatory control. Landon and Forte [E.J. Landon and L. Forte, <u>Fed. Proc.</u> <u>23</u>, 437, 1964] observed a marked decrease in the sodium-potassium ATP-ase activity, the so-called transport or membrane ATP-ase, after adrenalectomy in rats. Chignell and Titus obtained similar results [C.F. Chignell and E. Titus, <u>J. Biol. Chem.</u> <u>241</u>, 5083, 1966] and found that administration of corticosterone in doses mimicking adrenal output restored the normal level of the kidney sodium-potassium ATP-ase within a couple of days. The point is that glucocorticoids can produce changes in certain cellular transport systems and in the absence of the adrenal these may be impaired.

R.W. Schayer: The point I want to make here is that in very carefully controlled studies where the adrenalectomized animal is maintained with great care, nobody to my knowledge has ever shown any marked deviation from normal in any metabolic factor. Where it does occur, it can often be traced to circulatory insufficiency.

H.R. Lindner: Well, there is a marked change in the response to insulin, for example.

R.W. Schayer: Well, they have no adrenalin.

H.R. Lindner: True, but cortisol will reverse this effect.

C. Tachi: How about glomerular filtration?

R.W. Schayer: Normal, if you carefully control the animal. Water balance is normal in an adrenalectomized animal if you give it saline. You see, in the old days there were many metabolic defects found in an adrenalectomized animal which ultimately were found to be traceable to poor conditions. Often, they weren't fed properly. If you keep them very carefully and feed them the same amount as your controlled animals, you can't show much effect of adrenalectomy. This is another reason why I don't believe the hormone has a metabolic function. You can't show that its absence causes any definite metabolic change.

P.F. Kraicer: I am very much impressed by the remarkable influence which generalized theories have had on the course of endocrinology. The most striking example, of course, is the so-called General Adaptation Syndrome theory of Selye which, in being tested, and ultimately rejected, has contributed so much to our knowledge of corticosteroid endocrinology. For this reason, I think Dr. Schayer's presentation was more than stimulating for he provides us with a theory of general relevance to all physiological phenomena of growth and adaptation. And progestation is a period of growth and adaptation of the genital tract. The regulation of the microcirculation and its mediation of endocrine effects in relation to the genital tract vitally concerns us.

In our laboratory we have been engaged in the study of the endocrinology of carbohydrate metabolism, quite unrelated to other work in biodynamics. We have been investigating the physiological response to a rather interesting compound, a 7-carbon sugar, called mannoheptulose, which is obtainable from avocado. [E. Simon and P.F. Kraicer, Israel J. Med. Sci., 2, 785, 1966]. I believe that by using mannoheptulose we have at least gotten a solid clue as to the nature of the response of the liver to glucocorticosteroids. I'd like to discuss a little of the work which Professor Ernst Simon and myself have been doing recently because of the relevance to Dr. Schayer's theory.

Briefly, one can say the following. When we give an injection of mannoheptulose to an animal, what we essentially do is turn off the tap that drains the insulin out of the pancreas and into the blood. This is quite independent of whether the animal is under a tonic stimulation, say a heavy meal, to secrete insulin, or is fasted. As long as the animal has mannoheptulose in its blood, insulin secretion is cut off. As soon as the animal eliminates the mannoheptulose, it will return to a normal metabolic state. What we find is, that when we give a dose of this drug to the animal, it becomes diabetic and it indeed becomes hyperglycemic. We asked when we were just beginning this research: if mannoheptulose turns off the insulin supply temporarily from the pancreas, why on earth does the animal develop hyperglycemia, where does the excess glucose come from, particularly in the fasted animal? The answer was, it comes from gluconeogenesis, out of the liver.

Now, if we remove the adrenal from an animal and we give it our mannoheptulose, we get no gluconeogenetic response. This animal is characterized by two things: before we give it mannoheptulose, it has a blood sugar lower than normal. This we assume is due to the fact that it is hypersensitive to its own insulin and so tonic quantities of insulin produce hypoglycemia. Given the mannoheptulose, the tonic insulin secretion is reduced or abolished, the blood sugar climbs a triffle, almost to the level of the normal fasted animal, and stays there. Glucocorticoids restore the normal hyperglycemic response in a matter of 30 minutes. We have not tried shorter times. Even more striking, if one gradually increases the dose of corticoid hormones, one reaches a level, at about a quarter of a milligram of cortisol, when one gets a response to mannoheptulose which is exactly the same as in a normal animal. Further administration of corticoid hormones causes no further gluconeogenetic response.

What we think we have here then, is that the insulin level in the portal blood reaching the liver controls the level of gluconeogenesis. And in order that the liver be able to respond to the insulin, to be inhibited, it must have an adequate background of corticosteroid, the corticosteroid must be present. In this sense, the corticosteroid action on the liver is permissive, maintaining the liver in "good" state or "bad" state. [D.J. Ingle, Acta Endocr. (Kbh) 17, 172, 1954]. But we then would quibble with the whole argument of anabolic or catabolic action of corticosteroids on the liver. In this response of gluconeogenesis at least we would suggest that the regulatory hormone is insulin, that insulin inhibits the transformation of protein into carbohydrate, presumably deamination of amino acids, and that the corticosteroids perform no direct regulatory action. So, although we don't know exactly what the glucocorticoids affect in the liver, it is apparently not the metabolism *per se.* Enough steroid must be present to ensure normal liver function and response to insulin. Excess steroid has no effect in our system.

R.W. Schayer: Well, I could go along with most of that. But to me the permissive action of a corticoid means that it stabilizes the capillary beds. Mannoheptulose is a foreign substance. Could it be viewed as toxic?

H.R. Lindner: No, as a glucose analogue I would think.

P.F. Kraicer: Yes, I seriously doubt that it acts on the liver as a toxin. As far as we have been able to ascertain, the only action of the material is at the pancreas. Gluconeogenesis is a hepatic response to insulin-lack.

R.W. Schayer: In general, you give substance X and you get a certain response. Substance X may be a stressor. Almost anything is a stressor, if you give enough of it. Now, if you give substance X to an adrenalectomized animal, it doesn't show the same metabolic response at all. This, according to my belief, is because any stressor will cause too many sphincters to open and you won't get the same circulatory patterns. If you have a slight circulatory deficiency, you'll get different metabolic effects. Then if you give enough glucocorticoids to stablize the vascular beds, you'll get the normal response to substance X in your adrenalectomized animals. Thereafter, giving more glucocorticoids will not necessarily change things very much.

U.S. von Euler: If I understood correctly, you said that the antihistamines do produce an effect on the small vessels which could be ascribed to the antihistamine action. But in certain other cases, I think you mentioned that the antihistamines do not antagonize the effects which presumably, according to your theory, are due to the release of histamine.

R.W. Schayer: When you give them systemically, you can't really get a big enough dose to show vasoconstriction. Actually when you give them systemically, they are said to potentiate the effects of catecholamines.

U.S. von Euler: And I understand that your explanation was that they don't enter the places intracellularly where they could act in sufficient concentration. Do they enter all? Have you tried with labelled antihistamines?

R.W. Schayer: No, it's a very difficult experiment, I haven't done that.

U.S. von Euler: It might be of interest to do that histochemically with some labelled substance.

R.W. Schayer: One would need equipment and things that I don't have.

U.S. von Euler: The second question, do you have any evidence that histamine could be stored in some kind of microsome or granule of any kind, except of course in the mast cells, which I exclude? It might be of some interest if that were the case, since possibly the release rates from organelle stores could possibly have a much higher $Q_{10}$. I'd just mention that, for instance, catecholamines in their organelles show a $Q_{10}$ in this region of about 3 to 4.

R.W. Schayer: Usually when people try to homogenize tissues and what-not and get things out, histamine is in the soluble fraction. It doesn't really mean it couldn't attached loosely somewhere.

U.S. von Euler: In the rabbit the responses to histamine are notoriously weak. Do you have any comment to that?

R.W. Schayer: You mean blood pressure and that sort of thing? Well, the only comment I would have there is that histamine can be a vasoconstrictor at the level of large arteries and veins. I just don't think that that is too relevant in normal physiology, because if it were formed in very tiny amounts it would presumably affect only those cells which were not mainly under nervous control and therefore would be mainly centered in the precapillary sphincters. As one gets to vessels of greater diameter, you see, this influence would be relatively small and not too well noted.

U.S. von Euler: One very brief point. Again, as I mentioned to you during the coffee break, against all rules, once when we were doing assay work on the anesthesized cat blood pressure, we noticed that the glucocorticoids had quite a marked immediate increasing effect on the response to catecholamines. I just wanted to mention that.

R.W. Schayer: I think that is very important. Others have found this in different systems. If a hormone which shows no discernible metabolic effects for an hour maybe, but has virtually immediate effects on the circulatory system, you have to be very careful that the metabolic effect is not secondary. The circulatory effect can scarcely be secondary to a metabolic effect which shows up an hour later.

B.L. Lobel: We have observed phenomena in the progestational uterus which we find difficult to reconcile with your theory of microcirculatory control. Just prior to implantation in the rat there is vasodilatation in the uterus and the endometrial stroma in the vicinity of the as yet free blastocyst becomes edematous. Also, mast cells located about arterioles in the mesometrial triangle undergo degranulation at about this time. Now recently, in a study of the ultrastructure of mammalian arterioles and precapillary sphincters, J.A.G. Rhodin [J. Ultrastructure Res. 18, 181, 1967] observed nerve endings in contact with the smooth muscle cells constituting the sphincters. Would you comment on the relation between your theory of microcirculatory control, Rhodin's observations and the mast cells degranulating, hyperemia and edema in the preimplantation uterus?

R.W. Schayer: Firstly, as I have presented it, I can't see that the theory has anything to do with the immediate hyperemia, unless estrogen has somehow changed the responsiveness of the precapillary sphincters to the histamine being formed in them all the time. But other people have shown that estrogens do release histamine very quickly, is that not correct?

G.J. Marcus: Yes, but not in the progestational uterus.

R.W. Schayer: I'm not sure that we know where it occurs. Mast cells are not the only repository of histamine. I think that any microvascular sphincter contains some loosely-bound histamine, and that some stimulus might release it.

M.C. Shelesnyak: Is it correct that you are really not talking about mast cell histamine?

R.W. Schayer: My own theory has nothing to do with mast cell histamine, that's right. I believe that mast cell histamine complements this intrinsic histamine that I am talking about to provide a rapid action whereas intrinsic histamine is usually mobilized slowly.

H.R. Lindner: Do you believe that the two respond to the same stimuli?

R.W. Schayer: In some cases it certainly seems they do, but more work would have to be done to prove it. I have no real experience with estrogen, so I don't know. My whole feeling is that there are so many possibilities here that have not been explored.

B.L. Lobel: What would be the relation between the innervation of the precapillary sphincters and the slow synthesis of histamine as you described it?

R.W. Schayer: Well, the innervation of precapillaries is quite a novelty to me. I mean, most tissues apparently do not show it. This is the general belief. I think one function of this histamine is to prevent prolonged vasoconstriction and curtailment of nutritive blood flow. I'm sorry I can't give you anything more definite.

H.R. Lindner: Prof. Shelesnyak, you told us this morning about the degranulation and disappearance of mast cells and the decrease in histamine content of the uterus on day $L_4$ in the pregnant rat. You also mentioned that you no longer believe estrogen is the cause of the histamine release and I think Dr. Marcus would agree with that. Now, you know that, in mated rats overiactomized on $L_2$ and maintained with progesterone, you can induce implantation at will several days later, say five or eleven days later. Do you think that the same changes in mast cell population and uterine histamine content happen to occur at the time you choose for injecting oestrogen to induce delayed implantation? If not, does this mean that the degranulation of mast cells and fall in histamine content be irrelevant to the induction of implantation?

M.C. Shelesnyak: This has never been measured, but the chances are pretty good that the exogenous estrogen does release histamine in delayed implantation, because you are dealing with a spayed rat. You see, the evidence so far is that estrogen will induce a release of histamine in the uterus provided the uterus is of a spayed animal. In order to induce delay, you spay the rat and you may even do this without giving progesterone during the period of delay so you in fact have a spayed animal in which estrogen should release uterine histamine.

G.J. Marcus: I would like to point out that mast cell degranulation may, in fact, have no immediate relevance to implantation. As Dr. Schayer stated, mast cells are not the only repositories of histamine. In our studies, the uteri which were assayed were invariably trimmed free of mesometrium so that the tissue we analyzed contained few mast cells; therefore, the changes in uterine histamine content which we have discussed do not represent changes in mast cell histamine.

Now, with regard to the exploration of estrogen action on the uterus by invoking effects on the microcirculatory system. As this was originally proposed, I believe by Szego, nothing was actually said then about an effect on intrinsic histamine, but I think we should reexamine the original observations on which the theory was based, theories of estrogen action involving histamine mediation in microcirulatory systems [E. Spaziani and C.M. Szego, Endocrinology 63, 669, 1958; ibid, 64, 713, 1959; C.M. Szego, Fed. Proc. 24, 1343, 1965].

As Astwood pointed out sometime ago [E. B. Astwood, J. Endocr. 1, 49, 1939] if one observes a response of the uterus on proestrus, the estrogen would likely have been secreted by the ovary sometime earlier, that is on the last day of the previous cycle, the diestrus. And Dr. Barnea has experimental evidence that that is the case [A. Barnea, T. Gershonowitz and M.C. Shelesnyak, J. Endocr. 41, 281, 1968]. We are convinced that estrogen is secreted on what we call day $L_2$, that is diestrus, and the next day you see the response of the uterus and the vagina to estrogen action. However, at this time the histamine content of the uterus is maximal. This is, of course, in intact animals. If you deal with a spayed rat an administration of estrogen causes a very pronounced drop in the histamine content of the uterus within hours. But this is in the spayed rat, not the intact rat. Now, we have obtained evidence that estrogen does not act in this way in the intact rat, particularly, in the progestational rat. You have the evidence here of histamine estimations during the estrous cycle with a maximum after estrogen action. During progestation, if you will recall some of the curves presented earlier, there is a decrease in the histamine level between day $L_3$ and day $L_4$ and since this covers the period that estrogen has been acting on the uterus, and we previously assumed that the decrease was due to histamine-release, induced by the estrogen. However, if the animal is treated with MER-25 under conditions of dose and time, such that the conventional parameters of the uterine response to estrogen, that is, increase in mass, protein, RNA and DNA are inhibited, no effect on the release is observed. Of course, this presented a possibility that the MER-25 was in itself causing histamine release, but it does not cause histamine release in the spayed rat. In fact, it inhibits the releasing actions of estrogen in the spayed rat [G.J. Marcus and M.C. Shelesnyak, Endocrinology, 80, 1028, 1967]. This is one of the major reasons that we now believe that estrogen does not cause histamine-release in the normal rat uterus.

Now, with regard to whether histamine may be considered to be a mediator of estrogen action, we have looked into this by demonstrating selective inhibition of the uterine responses to the estrogen of the estrogen surge, during progestation. Normally, if one measures the usual parameters of weight, nucleic acid and protein content, increases are noted on days $L_4$ and $L_5$. These increases are abolished if the animal is given the antiestrogen MER-25 on day $L_3$. If, however, the animal is given an intraluminal injection of antihistamine, the increases are not prevented even though implantation or decidualization, are abolished. We find no evidence that the antihistamine interferes with the uterine responses to estrogen [L. Tic, G.J. Marcus and M.C. Shelesnyak, Life Sci., 6, 1179, 1967]. Therefore, we reject the concept of histamine mediation of estrogen action, and if histamine doesn't mediate it and histamine is not released by estrogen, we cannot see that microcirculatory changes can be invoked as the means of explaining estrogen action on the uterus.

M. Tausk: Does cortisone prevent nidation?

G.J. Marcus: No, not at reasonable dose levels.

J. Gorski: It doesn't affect estrogen action.

M. Tausk: That's not the point. Dr. Shelesnyak said that we need both estrogen and histamine, although the action of one isn't mediated by the other. The other thing he said was that nidation had some similarity with an inflammatory reaction. So I thought then cortisone might inhibit it.

M.C. Shelesnyak: But it doesn't.

P.F. Kraicer: I'd like to ask Prof. Tausk, at what dose level would you expect cortisone to inhibit if it were inhibitory in the manner in which you spoke, in the rats?

M. Tausk: I am sorry, I haven't the slightest idea what doses we would need for that. I think it might be applied locally, topically.

P.F. Kraicer: A dose similar to a dose which would give what effect?

M. Tausk: I think an anti-inflammatory effect. If you can inhibit the inflammation which is caused by a cotton pellet, and if a deciduoma resembles even remotedly the reaction caused by a cotton pellet, the cotton pellet being replaced by the blastocyst, I thought it would stand to reason that cortisone might inhibit that reaction, and so I just wondered whether it would.

M.C. Shelesnyak: In general, to the best of my knowledge, anti-inflammatory substances do not in our hands inhibit implantations.

M. Tausk: But anti-inflammatory substances are not all alike and that is another point which came out during Dr. Schayer's presentation.

M.C. Shelesnyak: I think my answer is based on my understanding of your question as a sort of model dose of cortisone. I am sure that a toxic dose or really massive dose would interfere with implantation but that type of response, that inhibition with implantation can be achieved by a very large number of toxic substances. I mean, if you do anything to upset an animal, it may interfere with implantation, but that's not your question.

J. Gorski: But if this were given periodically through a continuous period, it doesn't block it?

G.J. Marcus: Again no, not at reasonable doses. Only when you get up to daily doses of 5 to 10 mg of cortisone do you begin to interfere with implantation [J.M. Meunier and A.J. Thevenot-Duluc, Bull. Soc. Roy. Belge Gyn. Obstet. 30, 539, 1960].

M.C. Shelesnyak: You see, the problem here is, when you try to evaluate the activity of a substance on nidation, you have to be very careful that you concern yourself with a specific time, in order to relate the possible action to any inhibition. For example, as I said this morning, histamine-releasers will interfere with implantation. But they have to be given over a period of time so that they deplete the animal of histamine. You have to very careful. The type of remark that one might make in Annual Reviews of Physiology, that histamine releasers interfere with implantation, period, is misleading. You have to point out that the depletion of histamine by histamine releasers will result in this. Again, the anti-estrogens or the antihistamines are effective only at certain times, so one has to be very cautious and very precise in this particular area, at least to satisfy us. It's probably true in other areas of investigation, as well.

J. Gorski: The fact is that corticoids block the water uptake response to estrogen but don't block other estrogen responses. Therefore, we have never felt that it was concerned with the initial action of estrogen as such. I always thought, however, that this was pretty important for the total physiological response, particularly the deciduoma formation. I'm a little surprised that cortisone didn't inhibit implantation.

R.W. Schayer: Shelly, excuse me, but histamine-release is a funny subject. Compound 48/80 releases histamine, but, in some tissues at least, (I have never tested uterus) it activates histidine decarboxylase. A paradoxical thing, but true. Continued use of 48/80 can also produce a refractoriness in the microcirculation. Now all this has to be considered. No histamine-releaser is a simple-acting thing.

M.C. Shelesnyak: Even distilled water will release histamine in the rat.

R. W. Schayer: Yes, but, can one say with some assurance that if you instill histamine into the uterus you would get this deciduoma. You said this.

M.C. Shelesnyak: Yes, there is no doubt that if you instill histamine in the uterus, you get a decidual reaction, but there is no doubt that you can instill an infinite variety of substances which may either release histamine or cause enough irritation and produce de novo synthesis of histamine. This whole business of getting the progestational endometrium to decidualize by introduction into the lumen of various substances is one which is fraught with more conflict in the literature and more irrelevant publications than any I know of because it is really meaningless. Take a simple needle and you can't argue that we are not getting a release of histamine. Someone is fascinated by the fact that an injection of air is effective. Well, you distend the uterus, and you know perfectly well you can start things which may involve histamine-release. So it's a circle that you can't get out of by the use of methods which involve the introduction of substances into the lumen.

R.W. Schayer: This is my point, that if you're convinced that any non-specific irritant will do this, and I'm convinced that any non-specific irritant inflammatory action is invariably accompanied by activation of histamine synthesis or release, then as far as I am concerned histamine is the mediator.

M.C. Shelesnyak: Alright, he's on our side. Put his name down.

A. Barnea: You seem to relate the whole inflammatory response to the action of histamine on the microcirculation. It would seem that it would take a certain amount of time for enzyme induction to get under way after application of the inflammatory stimulus. I believe it is well-know that there is an immediate response in inflammation which is probably not dependent on an increase in enzymic activity.

R.W. Schayer: English workers [W.G. Spector and D.A. Willoughby, Bacterio Rev., 27, 117, 1963] have shown that there are two phases in the microcirculatory effect. The first is immediate, lasts about an hour and can be blocked totally with antihistamine. But the slow phase cannot be blocked by antihistamines. That's why they have been reluctant to believe my ideas that histamine has anything to do with it.

A. Barnea: I wondered if this increase in histamine is intracellular, so that upon synthesis the histamine is released from the place where it is synthesized so that it can react with the receptors within the cell. At the same time, it could act on enzymes which inactivate histamine. For example, it is well known if there is a release intracellularly of catecholamines, not by nerve stimuli, but by drugs, these catecholamines may be inactivated intracellularly by monamineoxidase, for example, and these catecholamines won't be active when they are released later on. If you have such a high concentration of histamine released intracellularly, why isn't it inactivated within the cell before reaching the receptor. It seems strange to me that you have such a high concentration of histamine which is not inactivated within the cells by diaminoxidase or any other system.

R.W. Schayer: The distribution of the enzymes which destroy histamine, diaminoxidase and histamine methylating enzymes is entirely different from that of histamine decarboxylase. Methylating enzyme, for example, in the mouse is almost entirely in the liver. Many tissues have very little ability to destroy histamine but they can form it. There is no evidence that anything comparable to catecholamine inactivation takes place with histamine.

# BINDING, UPTAKE AND RELEASE OF ADRENERGIC NEUROTRANSMITTER

# ADRENERGIC NEUROTRANSMITTER

U. S. von Euler
Professor of Physiology, Karolinska Institutet
Stockholm, Sweden

Soon after the identification of the adrenergic neurotransmitter with noradrenaline (NA), it was found that organs and tissues normally contained a characteristic amount of this amine, mostly together with a small quantity of adrenaline (A). This suggested to us that the transmitter was bound in some specific way in the adrenergic nerve fibres. Goodall (1951) showed in our laboratory that degeneration of the sympathetic fibres to the heart caused the NA to disappear but that it returned upon regeneration of the nerves. A comparison of the NA content in the splenic nerve trunk and in the organ suggested that the NA must be accumulated in the nerve endings. The specific binding site was found to be represented by subcellular nerve granules (Euler and Hillarp, 1956) which could be conveniently prepared from bovine splenic nerves by squeezing or homogenization and subsequent differential or gradient centrifugation.

## FREE AND BOUND NA

Using the squeezing or homogenization technique it appeared that only a fraction of the total NA in nerves or organs was granule bound while the remainder appeared as a soluble fraction in the supernatant on high speed centrifugation. Since it was hard to imagine that some 50 per cent of the total NA in nerves should occur in a free form we have looked into this problem further. It was then found that continued treatment of the granule-containing suspension, obtained from a homogenate after removing coarse particles, made an increasing portion of the bound NA appear as soluble. Assuming a similar time course for this gradual alteration of the granules from time zero, the original proportion of granule bound NA would be about 90 per cent of the total. This figure is of course rather approximate but indicates that the greatest part of the NA is granule bound. Whether any free NA in the true sense of the word occurs in the nerve ending is uncertain, it could well be that a small portion is bound to some structure from which it is easily releasable in order to make it ready to act as neurotransmitter upon activation of the adrenergic nerve fibre. Various binding possibilities have been discussed by Green (1962). Data with regard to proportions of bound and soluble NA in organ and tissue homogenates may therefore have to be reconsidered.

Very little is known so far concerning the structural details of the nerve ending or what appears to be its functional unit, the varicosity of Hillarp (Fig. 1). Electron microscopic pictures show granules dispersed within the varicosity but do hardly reveal their interrelationships with each other or with the internal

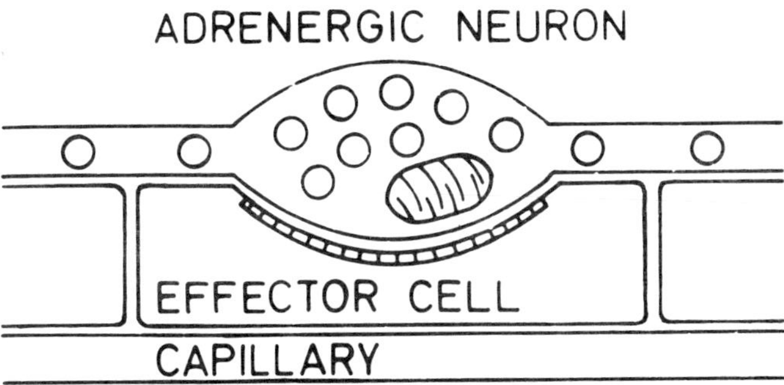


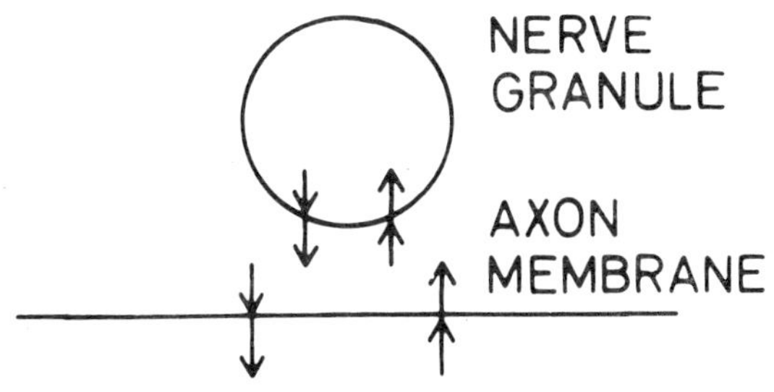


Fig. 1. Upper part: Schematic representation of the terminal part of an adrenergic axon with a varicosity containing transmitter granules and mitochondria. Contact area with effector cell. Lower part: Separate uptake and release processes at axon membrane and nerve granule.

structure of the special axon part involved. Electron microscopy of isolated granules show, however, tube-like extensions which may indicate connection structures with other granules or with the intraaxonal membrane system (Fig. 2). Sometimes granules even appear in chains in preparations of this kind. Obviously the chances to observe such interconnections of a tubular nature are much reduced in tissue sections, for geometrical reasons.

## PHYSIOLOGICAL SIGNIFICANCE OF GRANULE BINDING

The binding of the neurotransmitter to granules in the nerve varicosities appears to constitute an efficient and relatively simple form of storage, particularly if one were to accept the figures given by Euler (1954) or by Dahlström and Häggendal (1966) according to which the terminal parts should contain NA in concentrations of the order of $10^{-2}$ M. At any rate it is clear that by binding in a physiologically inactive form in submicroscopic structures relatively large amounts of transmitter can be stored at strategic points and also—by binding in a large number of separate units--potentially form a very versatile system. One is reminded of the red blood cells which by their great number and large area can rapidly give off or take up their specific loads.

A comparison of some properties of the chromaffin cell granules and the nerve granules reveals differences of an interesting nature. Hillarp and Nilson (1954) showed that adrenal medullary granules release their amine content quite slowly whereas we found

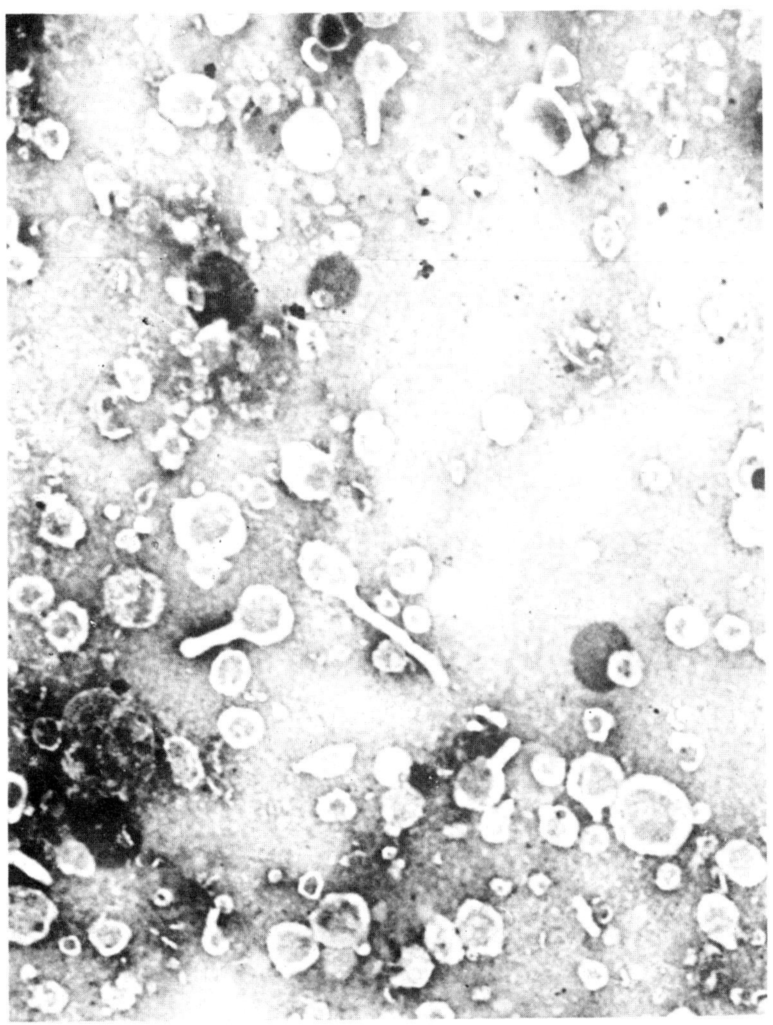

Fig. 2. Isolated nerve granules obtained by squeezing bovine splenic nerves and removal of larger particles. Negative staining with phosphotungstic acid. (x 42000).

(Euler and Lishajko, 1963) that nerve granules when incubated at 37° give off their NA at a remarkable speed, some 10 times faster than the adrenal granules. This we regard as a sign of physiological differentiation by which the two types of granules are singularly well adapted to their specific functions. We might expect from adrenergic nerve granules that they should be able, in principle, to supply the stored transmitter at a fast rate and replace the amount bound to receptors, inactivated by enzymes, or lost by diffusion. This would be necessary since, during certain conditions, such as standing or muscular work, the release of adrenergic transmitter in vasoconstrictor nerves is continuous and considerable.

If we turn to the adrenal medullary granules, on the other hand, one could readily imagine what would happen if the medullary cell granules should be able to give off half of their content in less than 5 minutes. As it is, any explosive liberation of catecholamines from the suprarenals is prevented by the slow release rate. Even in the adrenal medullary cells we may postulate the existence of a small quantity outside the granules serving as an immediately available store. This assumption is also in harmony with the characteristic burst of a small dose of catecholamines from the adrenal medulla when an individual is frightened.

The significance of the slower release rate of NA in granules from male accessory genital organs is at present not clear.

## Uptake and Release in Granules

A prerequisite for the function of the granules is that they have facilities for uptake as well as release of the compounds serving as neurotransmitters. In mammals these consist practically exclusively of NA in the peripheral system.

Isolated nerve granules lend themselves readily to studies on uptake and release of NA and other amines. When prepared by homogenization of suitable nerve trunks, such as the splenic nerves, a suspension of granules is obtained which is relatively homogenous and suitable for practical purposes. Such granules, obtained in a suspension with isotonic potassium phosphate at pH 7 - 7.5, give reproducible results as regards uptake and release. The release of NA at low temperature is very slow, the half time being of the order of 24 hours at ice water temperature. The release rate increases rapidly, however, with temperature, reaching a half time of 3-4 minutes at 37°. This would obviously mean that at low tissue temperature the granules have a built-in mechanism which brakes the release. During hypothermia, either artificial or e.g. in hibernating animals, the release rate of NA from nerve granules is thus kept at bay. Further studies in this field appear desirable. Hyperthermia on the other hand should increase the release rate.

During our studies on the release rate of NA from isolated nerve granules it was observed that it varied with the concentration of soluble NA in the suspension. In order to obtain the basic release rate it therefore became necessary to keep the suspension free from soluble NA which apparently was recaptured and thus gave an apparently lower release rate. In fact we have observed (Euler and Lishajko, 1963) that in the presence of $10^{-4}$ M NA there was no net loss from the granules during incubation, owing to reuptake as shown with radioactive NA (Euler, Stjarne and

Lishajko, 1963). A suitable method for removing free NA in the suspension of granules was found by adding ferricyanide, $5 \times 10^{-3}$M, which effectively inactivated the NA as it appeared during the apparently undisturbed release process. During these conditions reuptake was wholly prevented as checked by adding radioactive NA. A study of the correlation between NA concentration in the medium and the apparent release rate, as indicated by the percentage remaining NA in the granules, showed that from a NA concentration of about $10^{-7}$M on, the apparent release rate diminished and was reduced to almost zero at $10^{-4}$M. The proportion of NA incorporated in the granules by reuptake could be estimated with the aid of radioactive NA.

This relationship suggested that the concentration of free—or functionally free—NA could determine the release rate of NA from the granules, which one might assume to be the process by which the store for immediate use is refilled and maintained saturated. An interaction of this kind would obviously represent a kind of feedback mechanism, presumably serving to control the supply of available transmitter and at the same time save the stores from wasteful leakage. This would also mean that the equilibrium concentration of NA *in vivo* has to be about $10^{-4}$M which does not seem to be precluded by any known facts.

So far, the data of ourselves and others (Potter and Axelrod, 1963) appear to indicate that the release process depends in the first place on temperature, pH of the reaction medium, and the NA concentration in the medium. The release process follows an exponential course and the release rate can therefore be expressed by a 'release constant' from the conventional logarithmic decay equation. During basic release conditions, when no reuptake takes place, the release constant has a value of about 0.02 at 20° and about 0.18 at 37°, corresponding to a release of 2 and 18 per cent per minute respectively of the NA present in the granules at a given moment.

## AMINE UPTAKE IN GRANULES

Three methods have been particularly useful in the study of amine uptake in the tissue stores. The introduction, by Axelrod in 1960 (see Axelrod, 1965), of uptake studies with tracer amounts of NA with high specific activity has been of great importance for the elucidation of the general principles for the uptake. Briefly, the uptake of exogenous NA is dependent in the first place on a rather specific mechanism of uptake through the axon membrane, sometimes called the membrane pump. Once inside the axon membrane, the amines rapidly exchange with the extragranular and perhaps less rapidly with the intragranular amines. When the granular stores have been labelled, the release can be followed and the turnover estimated. Similar results have been reached in experiments on isolated organs and tissue slices.

A second method is more direct in nature and is based on actual refilling after depletion. Usually such repletion has been attempted after depletion of the stores with reserpine, and even if the degree of refilling in this case may be regarded as poor, it has nevertheless been possible to restore the effects of nerve stimulation temporarily (Burn and Rand, 1958).

More conspicuous results have been reached by

refilling the stores after depletion with decaborane (Euler and Lishajko, 1965) or prenylamine (Mackenna, 1965) whereby at least some stores have resumed their normal content for varying lengths of time. Even in these cases it has been established the exogenous NA has rapidly entered the granular compartment of the stores. The remarkable ability of the adrenergic axons to take up the exogenous amine after depletion is illustrated by the fact that an isolated, decaborane-depleted rat heart can be nearly wholly refilled by perfusion for 10 minutes with a solution containing 1 μg NA in 100 ml, of which some 40 per cent is removed by the heart during the perfusion (Bhattacharya, 1967).

A third method pertains to the uptake of amines in isolated granules. It should be noted, however, that the methods mentioned are not strictly speaking comparable since the first two techniques refer to the overall uptake in tissue, involving both the axon membrane and the granules. Although this reservation may not be particularly relevant in this context it will be of great importance as regards the action of drugs on amine uptake. At any rate the expression 'uptake' should be qualified, stating whether it refers to uptake by the axon membrane, the granules or both. Extragranular or extraneuronal uptake may also come into consideration.

## REUPTAKE IN GRANULES

As mentioned above, the release of NA during incubation of isolated nerve granules is accompanied by an uptake of the amine, the rate of which depends on the NA concentration. The reuptake can be strongly enhanced by addition of ATP in the presence of $Mg^{2+}$ (Fig. 3). ADP is almost as active as ATP while AMP has little effect. Some effect is observed also with uridine and other nucleotides but considerably less than with ATP. The ATP-facilitated uptake can be prevented by agents which uncouple oxidative phosphorylation such as dinitrophenol or dinitrophenylhydrazine. The strong action of exogenous ATP on uptake makes it appear probable that the endogranular ATP is of importance for the normally occurring reuptake. In some preparations incubation with ATP in the presence of $10^{-6}$M NA can lead not only to reuptake but also to actual net uptake over and above the original content of NA in the granules.

Very little is known about the actual way of binding of the NA molecules during the uptake process. Even if ATP is involved in this process it is still uncertain to what extent ATP binds amines. At any rate the amine release is considerably faster than the ATP release (Euler, Lishaijko and Stjarne, 1963); and the occurrence of ATP and amine in a molar ratio of about 1 : 4 with an equal number of charges may be fortuitous.

One may ask: How specific is the binding of amines to granules? A comparison between NA, A, and isoprenaline has shown that all three of these catecholamines are taken up by granules to the same extent. Clearly the granules are not discerning between the different $\beta$-hydroxylated catecholamines once they have entered the axon. Under biological conditions isoprenaline hardly reaches the stores, however, since the axon membrane acts like a barrier and also to some extent inhibits the uptake of A. By this mechanism NA

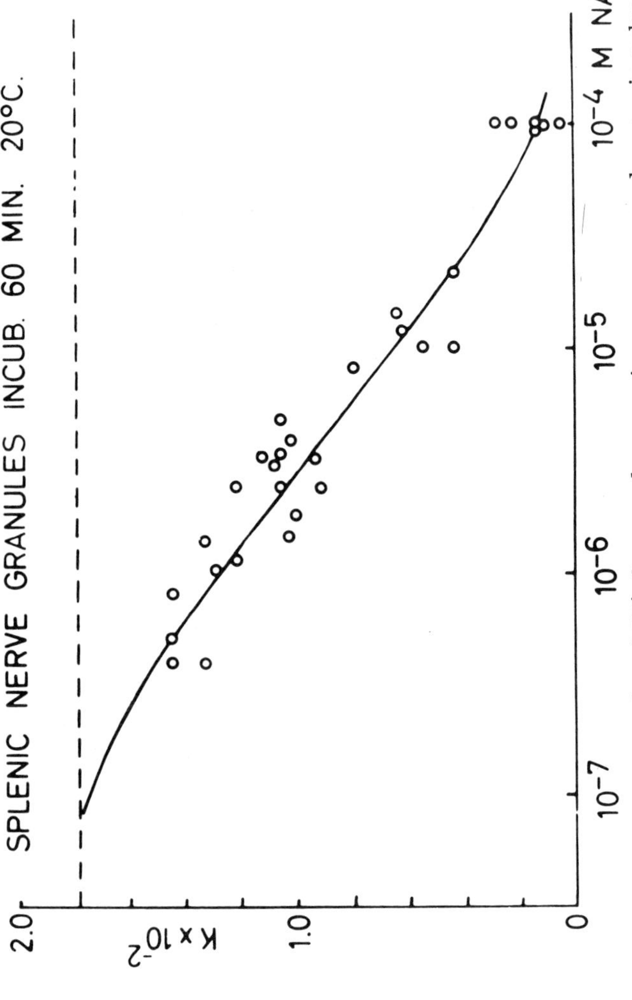


Fig. 3. Release rate of NA from adrenergic nerve granules on incubation in phosphate buffer 60 minutes at 20°, represented by release constant (ordinate). Abscissa: Concentration of NA in incubation medium.

is at an advantage as neurotransmitter and the chance for other amines to compete is thus further reduced.

The rather academic question as to how much of the NA in a given store in an adrenergic axon is produced by synthesis and how much taken up from the circulation has been discussed on some occasions, and figures of 20 percent uptake have been given for the rat heart. This of course does not mean that in the absence of circulating NA the stores in the heart should decrease by 20 per cent, but illustrates that there is a certain exchange of NA molecules within the organism, made possible by the continuous release and uptake.

Although uptake of adrenaline and substitution of a large portion of the NA can be achieved by intravenous injection of a considerable dose of adrenaline (some 10 times the total amount of NA present in the nerves) the uptake of A in axons and granules under physiological conditions is very modest and there is no indication that it is of physiological significance.

## UTERUS

In connection with the profound changes in size and functional activity in the uterus it is hardly surprising that this should be reflected also in the catecholamine distribution (Rudzik and Miller, 1962). As in most other sexual organs the adrenergic fibres supplying the uterus originate from sympathetic ganglia in the vicinity of the organ. Thus cervical ganglionectomy reduces the NA content of the uterus by 80% (Barnea and Shelesnyak, 1965). This is similar to the vas deferens which receives short adrenergic neurons from ganglia just outside the organ (Sjöstrand, 1965). There are no indications, however, that the uterus should be supplied with a rich nerve net of adrenergic fibres like the vas deferens. The NA content of the uterus is quite moderate and apparently the adrenergic fibres are mostly confined to the blood vessels while the smooth muscle receives some adrenergic innervation at least in the rabbit (Owman and Sjöberg, 1966). Surgical or chemical adrenergic denervation does not prevent the estrus cycle or ovum implantation (Barnea and Shelesnyak, 1965). Changes in the NA content were noted, however, during the cycle, and at estrus the NA content was reduced.

The nonpregnant rat uterus contains about 0.23 μg A per g. With increasing weight of the organ during pregnancy and the postparturient period the A content falls to about 0.13 and 0.05 μg/g respectively (Wurtman and Axelrod, 1966). These figures are slightly higher than in most other organs, although it should be recalled that chromaffin cells containing A are generally found in this region. It is possible, however, that A is bound in some other way, particularly in view of the relatively large changes in A content during different functional stages. Thus Barnea and Shelesnyak (1965) reported that A is not bound to neuronal elements and that after adrenergic denervation its content is raised by 100 per cent. Owman and Sjöberg (1966) found no A or dopamine in the uterus of the rabbit, however. During estrus or estradiol treatment the content of A increased, while that of NA fell (Cha, Lee, Rudzik and Miller, 1965). Thus, while a correlation between the uterine NA and the estrus cycle and estrogen level is observed, no such correlation seemed to exist for adrenaline, which is bound and distributed in an uniform way all over the organ. The A content, in contrast to the NA, is not reduced by reserpine, further indicating that the A is not bound in nerves. Although several data are compatible with the assumption that the A is present in chromaffin cells, the observation that the A occurs in the 'soluble' fraction after homogenization of the organ (Wurtman, Axelrod and Potter, 1964) speaks against this assumption.

According to Wurtman and Axelrod (1966) the rat uterus takes up some 4 times as much $H^3$-A during estrus as during diestrus No such changes were observed for $H^3$- NA. It has also been reported that the level of naturally occurring A doubles between diestrus and estrus. In pregnancy the A content of the rat uterus increased 7-fold partly due to increased perfusion and increased A-binding efficiency of the organ. The A content per g of organ falls, however, particularly soon after parturition. The cause of this depletion is not clear.

The finding of uterine A in the soluble fraction after homogenization of the uterus and sedimentation of the granular fraction together with the facts that cocaine has only little action on its uptake, or tyramine on its release, suggests that uterine A is bound in some unusual way.

## ACTION OF DRUGS ON NA RELEASE AND UPTAKE

If the physiological uptake and release sites in the adrenergic nerve endings can be localized to the axon membrane as well as the granules, it appears likely that a variety of chemicals and drugs should interfere with these functions. A large number of drugs have also been described which facilitate or inhibit the processes at the membranes, even if almost nothing is known about the real mechanism of these actions.

I shall here briefly touch only a few examples of drug action, referring to reserpine, adrenergic blockers and indirectly acting amines.

## 1. Reserpine

A dose of reserpine 0.25 mg per kg, given intravenously in the spinal cat, has virtually no cardiovascular effect, although it causes a considerable depletion of the NA stores in the organs within a couple of hours. This has been interpreted as the result of inactivation of the released transmitter by intraaxonal monoamine oxidase (MAO). Why the transmitter released by tyramine and other indirectly acting amines is not inactivated in the same way has not so far been explained, but the findings of Kopin and Gordon (1962) have emphasized these facts. At any rate inhibition of MAO causes a profound change in the reaction pattern in that reserpine, e.g. after nialamide, becomes strongly pressor and cardioaccelerator (Fig. 4). Reserpine retards the direct release of transmitter from granules but blocks reuptake and uptake and can in this way enhance release by a kind of valve effect.

Prenylamine, which releases NA directly from granules acts differently: a dose of this amine which is inactive by itself on the adrenalectomized spinal cat, causes a considerable rise in blood pressure and increased heart rate during a NA infusion but is not influenced by MAO inhibitors.

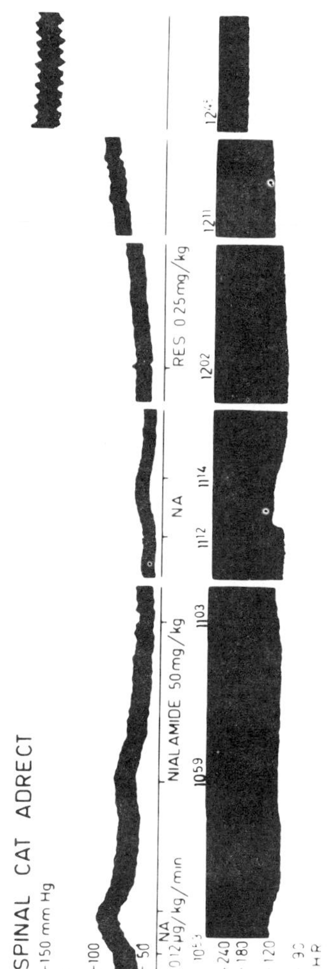


Fig. 4. Spinal cat, adrenalectomized. Upper curve blood pressure, lower curve heart rate. Reserpine 0.25 mg/kg given i.v. 1 hr after nialamide i.v. 50 mg/kg.

## 2. Indirectly Acting Amines

Since the concept of the mode of action of tyramine was first proposed by Fleckenstein and by Burn and Rand in the 50's it has become generally accepted. Only very recently it has been possible to differentiate between two possible mechanisms, however. According to the idea proposed by Schümann and Philippu (1961) tyramine should substitute the adrenergic transmitter in the granules. The other possibility, inhibition of reuptake, suggested by Muscholl (1960) and by Stjärne (1966) has also won acceptance. In experiments on isolated nerve granules it has been possible to show that actually both mechanisms may operate, depending on the tyramine concentration. Thus in a concentration range of $10^{-7}$ - $10^{-4}$M there is a moderate direct release by substitution, while inhibition of uptake becomes more marked from about $10^{-5}$M and is almost total at $3 \times 10^{-4}$M (Fig. 5) (Euler and Lishajko, 1967).

The direct releasing effect on the NA in granules is particularly strong for phenylethylamine and also well marked for amphetamine. Ephedrine on the other hand has only weak effects in these respects and only in a concentration of $3 \times 10^{-4}$ is the inhibition of reuptake well developed. This amine has, like mephentermine, a retarding action on the release. By studying the direct release in the absence of reuptake and the reuptake in the presence of NA it is now possible to characterize the different sympathomimetic amines as regards their indirect action. It is of some interest to note that in a concentration of $10^{-4}$ M, ephedrine, in the presence of NA $10^{-6}$M, appears to have no effect

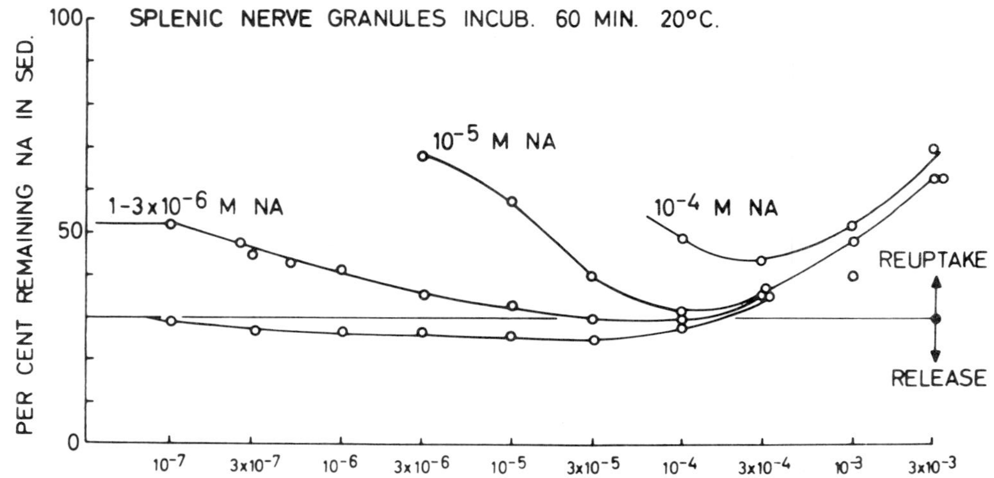


Fig. 5. Effect of tyramine on release and reuptake of NA in nerve granules. Lower level: basic release. Ordinate: per cent remaining NA in granules after incubation 60 minutes at 20 °C. Different levels indicate from below: Absence of NA, 1-3 $\times 10^{-6}$ M NA, $10^{-5}$ M NA, $10^{-4}$ M NA. Abscissa: Concentration of tyramine. Note absolute increase in release rate by tyramine in absence of NA and inhibition of reuptake at 1-3 $\times 10^{-6}$ M NA.

on the release rate. A closer analysis shows that the retardation of release balances the inhibition of re-uptake.

3. Adrenergic Blocking Agents

Axelrod, Hertting and Potter (1962) observed that certain adrenergic blocking agents inhibited the NA uptake in organs after injection of dl-$^{3}$H-NA. In experiments on isolated nerve granules we have shown (Euler and Lishajko, 1966) that a large number of $\alpha$- and $\beta$-blocking compounds retard the NA release and inhibit the uptake of NA in the presence of ATP. This seems to be a general rule with few exceptions, notably MJ 1998 and Inpea, both $\beta$-blockers. It would still be premature to make any statements as to the significance of these findings but it is tempting to speculate that some similar process which disturbs release and antagonizes the uptake of the transmitter in nerve granules also has a similar action on the hypothetic receptors. If this were so, it might also be possible to gain some insight in the chemical organization of the receptor mechanism.

## A CONCEPT OF THE PRINCIPLES FOR ADRENERGIC NEUROTRANSMISSION

On the basis of available data it seems possible to draw a tentative scheme of the transmission from adrenergic nerve terminals. As a result of the nerve impulse the axon membrane becomes depolarized and it seems likely that this disturbance is accompanied by a release of transmitter from the membrane itself and its intraaxonal connections either by an increase in the permeability of the membrane or by liberation of the transmitter from a loosely bound pool, perhaps by ionic shifts.

Assuming that the granule-bound transmitter is in dynamic equilibrium with an extragranular small pool, which serves as the immediate supply of transmitter on nerve stimulation (transport NA), a fall in concentration of the latter would cause a rapid release of transmitter from the granules until a new equilibrium is reached. From the discussion on free and bound NA in the axons it may be inferred that the available pool is small and therefore well suitable to serve as a regulator of the granular store (servo mechanism).

It is well known that the stores maintain their content of NA even during continuous nerve stimulation. This requires a rapid resynthesis which apparently is triggered by the release of transmitter from the granules to the small extragranular pool. The regulatory factor determining resynthesis may be assumed to be the concentration of NA in the granules which would mean that resynthesis or at least the last step, $\beta$-hydroxylation, which takes place in the granules, is regulated by a negative feedback system, presumably product inhibition.

When the NA content of the granules is decreasing as a result of transfer of material to the depleted transport pool, the conditions for increased uptake of dopamine and subsequent transformation to NA are improved. In NA saturated granules dopamine uptake is small and resynthesis inhibited. Dopamine also prevents reuptake of NA into the granules and in this way facilitates the transmitter effect.

ACKNOWLEDGMENTS

Part of the research reported in this document has been supported by the Swedish Medical Research Council, project no. B 67-14 ×-97-03 and by the Air Force Office of Scientific Research under Grant AF EOAR 67-18 through the European Office of Aerospace Research (OAR), United States Air Force, which is gratefully acknowledged.

## REFERENCES

Much of the relevant literature will be found in the monographs of Iversen (1967) and Holtz and Palm (1966).

Axelrod, J. (1965). The metabolism, storage, and release of catecholamines. Rec. Progr. Hormone Res. 21, 597-619.

Axelrod, J., Hertting, G., and Potter, L. (1962). Effect of drugs on the uptake and release of $^{3}$H-norepinephrine in the rat heart. Nature 194, 297.

Barnea, A., and Shelesnyak, M.C. (1965). Studies on the mechanisms of nidation. XV. The effect of cervical ganglionectomy. J. Endocr. 32, 199-204.

Bhattacharya, I.C. (1967). To be published.

Burn, J.H., and Rand, M.J. (1958). The action of sympathomimetic amines in animals treated with reserpine. J. Physiol. (London) 144, 314-336.

Cha, K.-S., Lee, W.-C., Rudzik, A., and Miller, J.W. (1965). A comparison of the catecholamine concentrations of uteri from several species and the alterations which occur during pregnancy. J. Pharmacol. exp. Ther. 148, 9-13.

Dahlström, A., and Häggendal, J. (1966). Studies on the transport and life-span of amine storage granules in a peripheral adrenergic neuron system. Acta physiol. scand. 67, 278-288.

Euler, U.S. v., (1954). Adrenaline and noradrenaline. Distribution and action. Pharmacol. Rev. 6. 15-22.

Euler, U.S. v., and Hillarp, N.-A. (1956). Evidence for the presence of noradrenaline in submicroscopic structures of adrenergic axons. Nature (London) 177, 44-45.

Euler, U.S. v., and Lishajko, F. (1963). Catecholamine release and uptake in isolated adrenergic nerve granules. Acta physiol. scand. 57, 468-480.

Euler, U.S. v., and Lishajko, F. (1965). Uptake of catecholamines in the rabbit heart after depletion with decaborane. Life Sci. 4. 969-972.

Euler, U.S. v., and Lishajko, F. (1966). Inhibitory action of adrenergic blocking agents on catecholamine release and uptake in isolated nerve granules. Acta physiol. scand. 68. 257-262.

Euler, U.S. v., and Lishajko, F. (1967) mechanism of drug-induced catecholamine release from adrenergic nerve granules. Circulation Res. 21, Suppl 3, 63-69.

Euler, U.S. v., Stjärne, L., and Lishajko, F. (1963). Uptake of radioactively labeled dl-catecholamines in isolated adrenergic nerve granules with and without reserpine. Life Sci. 2, 878-885.

Fleckenstein, A., and Stöckle, D. (1955) Die Hemmung der Neuro-Sympathomimetica durch Coclin. Arch exp. Path. Pharmak. 62, 159-169.

Goodall, McC (1951). Studies of adrenaline and noradrenaline in mammalian heart and suprarenals. Acta physiol. scand. 24. Suppl. 85

Green, J.P. (1962). Binding of some biogenic amines in tissues. Advances in Pharmacology, 1 349-422. Academic Press, New York.

Hillarp, N.-A., and Nilson, B. (1954). The structure of the adrenaline and noradrenaline containing granules in the adrenal medullary cells with reference to the storage and release of the sympathomimetic amines. Acta physiol. scand. 31, Suppl. 113, 79-107.

Holtz, P., and Palm, D. (1966). Brenzkatechinamine und andere sympathicomimetische Amine. Biosynthese und Inaktivierung. Freisetzung und Wirkung. In Ergebnisse der Physiologie biologischen Chemie und experimentellen Pharmakologie. 58, Springer-Verlag, Berlin-Heidelberg-New York.

Iversen, L.L. (1967). The uptake and storage of noradrenaline in sympathetic nerves. The University Press, Cambridge.

Kopin, I.J., and Gordon, E.K. (1962). Metabolism of norepinephrine -$H^3$ released by tyramine and reserpine. J. Pharmacol. exp. Ther. 138, 351-359.

Mackenna, B.R. (1965). Uptake of catecholamines by the hearts of rabbits treated with Segontin. Acta physiol. scand. 63, 413-422.

Muscholl, E. (1960). Die Hemmung der Noradrenalin-Aufnahme des Herzens durch Reserpin und die Wirkung von Tyramin. Arch. exp. Path. Pharmak. 240. 234-241.

Owman, C., and Sjöberg, N.-O. (1966). Adrenergic nerves in the female genital tract of the rabbit. With remarks on cholinesterase-containing structures. Z. Zellforsch. 74, 182-197.

Potter, L.T., and Axelrod, J. (1963). Properties of norepinephrine storage particles of the rat heart. J. Pharmacol. exp. Ther. 142. 299-305.

Rudzik, A.D., and Miller, J.W. (1962). The effect of altering the catecholamine content of the uterus on the rate of contractions and the sensitivity of the myometrium to relaxin. J. Pharmacol. exp. Ther. 138, 88-95.

Schümann, H.J., and Philippu, A. (1961). Untersuchungen zum Mechanismus der Freisetzung von Brenzcatechinaminen durch Tyramin. Arch. exp. Path. Pharmak. 241, 273-280.

Sjöstrand, N. (1965). The adrenergic innervation of the vas deferens and the accessory male genital glands. Acta physiol. scand. 65, Suppl. 257.

Stjärne, L. (1966). Storage particles in noradrenergic tissues. Pharmacol. Rev. 18. 425-432.

Wurtman, R.J., and Axelrod, J. (1966). In Endocrines and the central nervous system. Williams & Wilkins Co., Baltimore, p. 354-365.

Wurtman, R.J., Axelrod, J., and Potter, L.T. (1964). The disposition of catecholamines in the rat uterus and the effect of drugs and hormones. J. Pharmacol. exp. Ther. 144, 150-155.

## DISCUSSION

M.C. Shelesnyak: I would like to go back for a moment and point out that in the opening presentation, I attempted to give some background and indicated that my presentation and, in a sense, the whole conference, would to a certain extent parallel the historical development of our investigations. You may have wondered, nevertheless, as to why we have been concerned with catecholamines at this stage. As a matter of fact, our interest in catecholamines was derived from our concern with histamine and an awareness of antagonism between histamine and adrenalin and the observation that adrenalin interfered with nidation. A serious program of investigation was undertaken, however, only when Dr. Barnea began her work here. The work proved to be of great interest, but the interest of the findings, unfortunately, was not entirely matched by the relevance.

A. Barnea: I would like to give a little more of the background regarding our work with uterine catecholamines. Our original approach was to try and see whether uterine catecholamines, or more specifically, the sympathetic nerves of the uterus are associated with reproductive processes in the uterus. The first thing we did was to denervate the uterus by means of cervical ganglionectomy, which produces fairly extensive degeneration of sympathetic nerves in the uterus, and look for interference with the estrous cycle and nidation. No effect was apparent; the estrous cycle proceeded normally and so did nidation. When we checked the uterine catecholamine content we found that the noradrenalin level was reduced by about 80 per cent, but the adrenalin level was not reduced as expected; on the contrary, it rose by about 100 per cent. As is well known from Professor von Euler's studies, in many organs, adrenalin is not concentrated in adrenergic nerves, but in other structures, perhaps chromaffin cells, which are not affected by denervation. This adrenalin may be involved in the reproductive processes.

One thing which suggested that catecholamines may participate in reproductive processes was an interesting observation arising from work on the metabolism of estrogens. During the past 10 years or so, it was found that estradiol may be hydroxylated in the 2 position and, in the presence of S-adenosyl methionine, the resulting 2-hydroxy estrogen will be methylated in the 2- or 3-position, or in both, to give the corresponding methyl ethers. The enzyme which catalyses the O-methylation of estrogens appears to be identical with that which methylates the catecholamines. Breuer [H. Breuer, Proc. IInd Int. Congr. Endocr.; Excerpta Med. Int. Congr. Ser. No. 83, 1106, 1964] and Lucis [O.J. Lucis, Steroids 5, 163, 1965] demonstrated that catecholamines competitively inhibit the O-methylation of estrogen *in vitro*. Breuer has proposed that some regulatory mechanism may affect this inactivation of estrogens and that the catecholamines may be involved. Therefore, we thought that it might be interesting to see whether endogenous catecholamines influence the action of estrogen on the uterus; perhaps, and I say perhaps because we don't have any direct evidence for this, by interaction with some pathway in the metabolism of estrogens.

As I mentioned, we could not deplete the endogenous stores of adrenalin by denervation, so we tried reserpine, which, as you have just heard, is a very potent releaser of catecholamines. We gave a single injection of reserpine to immature of spayed mature rats, followed, at various intervals by a single injection of estradiol-17$\beta$ or estradiol benzoate. The animals were killed five hours after the estrogen administration and the fresh weight of the uterus was determined. We found that the reserpine, if administered long enough before the estrogen, completely blocked the estradiol benzoate-induced increase in uterine weight both in immature and in spayed mature rats (Fig. 1). To our surprise, however, when the experiments were repeated using free estadiol, we were unable to obtain complete inhibition of the uterine weight increase response; we never got more than 50 or 60 per cent inhibition of the increase.

The uterine response to a single injection of estradiol benzoate was inhibited completely only when the hormone was administered within a certain period after the reserpine; between 0-4 hours in immature rats and 16-24 hours in spayed, mature rats. The partial blockade of free estradiol, however, was noted only when the hormone was administered at the beginning of these specific periods. The uterine response to free estradiol, administered 4 (immature) or 24 (mature, spayed) hours after the reserpine, was not inhibited.

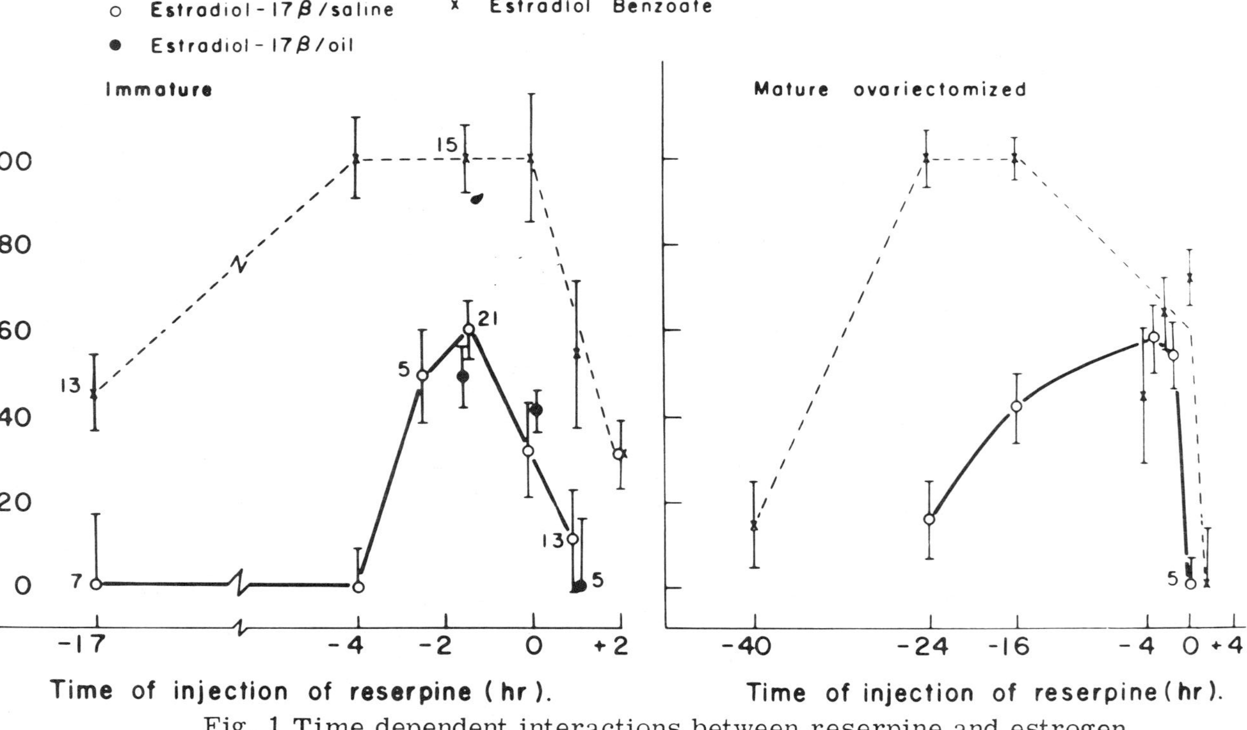


Fig. 1 Time dependent interactions between reserpine and estrogen.

R.W. Schayer: Reserpine will also liberate 5-hydroxytryptamine and the possibility of 5-HT acting like histamine must be considered.

P.F. Kraicer: What's the effect of catecholamines on the vascular nerves of the uterus? I am wondering what effect the reserpine might have had, via the adrenergic system, on the blood supply of the uterus and hence on the potentiality of the uterus to respond to estrogen.

A. Barnea: I think Prof. von Euler, in his lecture, has already answered your question. Since reserpine is not sympathomimetic it doesn't, for example, cause vasoconstriction. I don't think the inhibition I've found is the result of an insufficient or reduced blood supply to the uterus. When I examined the uteri of animals after treatment with reserpine and estrogen (free or as the benzoate) they were hyperemic.

H.R. Lindner: In your reference to Breuer's work you mentioned only methylation of the 2, 3-hydroxylated estrogens. As these are themselves very weak estrogens, I'm not sure that involvement of this pathway would be of any account.

A. Barnea: I don't know whether the O-methylation is related to what we have found. There have been some reports recently of the effects of drugs on the metabolism of progesterone and estrogen. Drugs such as barbiturates, given daily for three days shift the metabolism of these steroids toward the formation of more polar metabolites, which are less active [A.H. Conney, M. Jacobson, W. Levin, K. Schneidman and R. Kuntzman, J. Pharmacol. Exp. Ther. 154, 310, 1966; W. Levin, R. M. Welch and A.H. Conney, Endocrinology, 80, 135, 1967]. This happens in the liver. Perhaps something similar happens with the catecholamines, in the liver or in other organs. Don't forget that all we set out to do, initially, was to see whether catecholamines influence estrogen action. Now that there appears to be some influence of the sympathetic blocking drug, we can look into what's really happening, but possibly there is no relationship to the scheme we've been discussing.

G.J. Marcus: How significant a pathway for inactivation of estrogen is the hydroxylation and O-methylation?

A. Barnea: This hasn't been studied well in the rat. In the human, for example, it is quite an important pathway. In the golden hamster, the major metabolites appearing in the urine after the injection of estrogen, are the 2-hydroxy-and-2-methoxy derivatives [D.C. Collins, K.I.H. Williams and D.S. Layne, Endocrinology, 80, 893, 1967]. Gallagher's group, in New York, claims that the glucuronides appearing in the urine of women after injection of estrogen are mostly the 2-hydroxy, 2-methoxy estrogens or estriol [T.F. Gallagher, D.K. Fukushime, S. Noguchi, J. Fishman, H.L. Bradlow, J. Cassouto, B. Zumoff and L. Hellmann, Recent Progr. Hormone Res. 22, 283, 1966]. This group suggested that there is competition between the 2-hydroxylation and the 16-hydroxylation reactions and that the total of the 2- and 16-hydroxy derivatives is constant. Under certain physiological conditions, the relative amounts of the different hydroxylated estrogens vary. They found variation with different conditions of thyroid activity—this may interest Dr. Schayer—obtaining more of the 2-hydroxy and methoxy derivatives and less estriol in hyperthyroidism and the converse in hypothyroidism.

At any rate, the study of 2-hydroxylation of estrogen and its physiological significance is rather new so I'm not qualified to comment on any relationship to what is taking place in the uterus or any other organ. Now, with regard to the action of barbiturates, Conney and his co-workers found large amounts of polar metabolites of progestrone and estrogen in blood after injection of these drugs and the activity of progestins and estrogens was much reduced. They observed, for example, a 60 per cent inhibition of the estrogen-induced increase in uterine weight in animals pretreated with barbiturates, and the anesthetic effect of progesterone was much reduced.

In our system, the inhibitory action of reserpine may, in part, be due to some effect on the hydrolysis of estradiol benzoate and may be entirely unrelated to O-methylation.

H.R. Lindner: Although with reserpine one obviously thinks first of interaction with catecholamines, reserpine is also known to act on the central nervous system, possibly at sites having receptors for estrogen. For example, it may block gonadotrophin-release or stimulate prolactin secretion. Therefore, one shouldn't lose sight of the possibility that reserpine interacts directly with estrogen receptors in the uterus and may block these receptors. This may be a remote possibility, but worth examining. Also you haven't examined the dose relationship between inhibitor and estrogen to see whether the effect is competitive or not. It would also be valuable to examine the effects on different parameters of the response to estrogen over a longer period.

J. Gorski: What happens to the adrenal steroids under the conditions of these experiments?

A. Barnea: I don't know but I would expect some increase in corticoid secretion.

J. Gorski: What do the corticoids do to wet weight?

H.R. Lindner: Corticoids would inhibit the Astwood type of response.

J. Gorski: Yes, the water uptake would be blocked pretty nicely and if the timing were critical as seems to be the case here, corticoid release could explain the effects observed. You could check that by adrenalectomy.

A. Barnea: We're doing that now.

U.S. von Euler: I wanted to ask you if you had any idea or opinion about the mode of binding of adrenalin in the uterus. I understand from what Axelrod and Wurtman have published that they are not prepared to ascribe the occurrence of adrenalin to chromaffin cells, so it must be bound in some other way. Do you have any idea how adrenalin is bound to the uterus?

A. Barnea: I had intended to ask you the same question.

M.C. Shelesnyak: It's true that Axelrod and Wurtman have done some work similar to ours. We don't quite agree in our findings in certain ways nor are we entirely happy about some of their technical approaches, particularly in the selection of the stage of the estrous cycle. When we say that an animal is in proestrus or estrus, we refer to an animal which we have been smearing for at least two cycles beforehand and so on the basis of the observed pattern we can assume with a certain degree of validity that the animal is in that state. Wurtman and Axelrod's technique was to take a group of animals from their colony, carry out the catecholamine assays and then, later, look at the smears recorded earlier. If they find a vaginal smear containing cornified cells, they say the animal is in estrus, if the smear contains leucocytes, the animal is in diestrus. This is an unsound approach because a leucocytic smear can be obtained from a spayed animal or one lacking gonads, a pseudopregnant animal or an ailing one. A cornified smear may be due to a persistent follicular cyst or even from a type of infection, but does not necessarily reflect a stage of the normal estrous cycle.

J. W. Everett: You can get a cornified smear from a proestrous animal.

A. Barnea: When we assayed the catecholamine content of the uterus during the estrous cycle, the pattern of changes in the adrenalin content was similar to that reported by Wurtman [R.J. Wurtman, E.W. Chu and J. Axelrod, Nature, 198, 547, 1963]. Our findings with respect to noradrenalin, however, were different from those of Wurtman's group. They found no significant changes in the noradrenalin level during the cycle, but we found high levels during metestrus, diestrus and proestrus and a marked drop during estrus (Fig. 2).

Whether or not adrenalin and noradrenalin compete for the same binding sites, as suggested by Green and Miller [R.D. Green and J.W. Miller, J. Pharmacol. Exp. Ther. 152, 42, 1966] isn't clear. Attempts to demonstrate localization of $^3$H-adrenalin in the uterus have, so far, been unsuccessful. Falck was able to show the existence of noradrenalin-containing vasomotor nerves in the uterus, using a very specific histochemical technique, but he couldn't demonstrate localized distribution of adrenalin [personal communication]. We also have tried some autoradiographic work and we were able to demonstrate uptake of labelled noradrenalin by vasomotor nerves, giving a distribution pattern similar to that found by Falck, but we haven't demonstrated localization of adrenalin, so we still have no evidence for a reciprocal relationship between adrenalin and noradrenalin based on competition for the same binding sites.

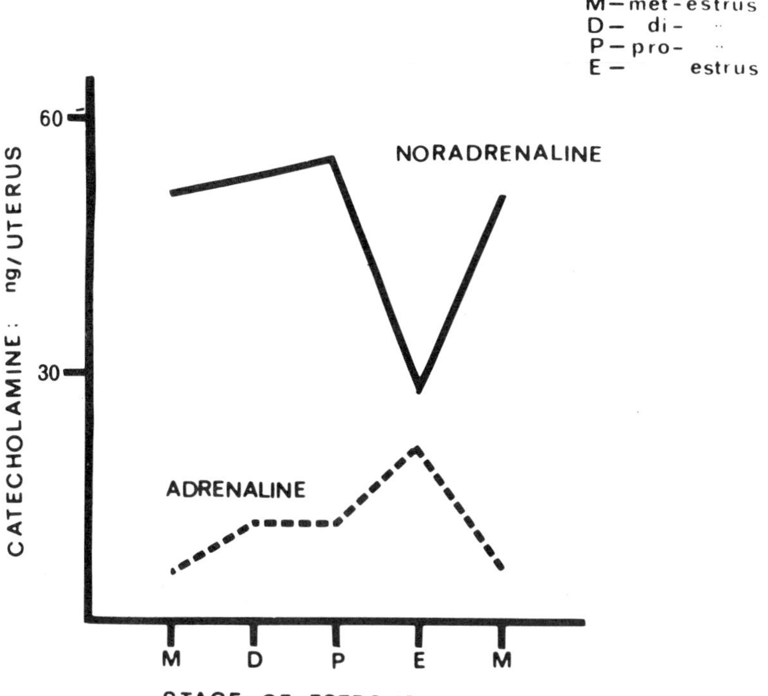


Fig. 2. Changes in the catecholamine content during the estrous cycles.

U.S. von Euler: Have you tried to make different kinds of extracts of the uterus and looked for binding in some particular biochemical fraction?

A. Barnea: I haven't, but I think Wurtman and his co-workers tried something like this and found a high proportion of the adrenalin in the supernatant fraction of the uterus whereas in heart, the adrenalin is concentrated in the particulate fraction.

U.S. von Euler: I meant biochemical rather than structural fractionation, because I think that the approach must be to see whether adrenalin is bound by some particular chemical fraction—lipids or proteins and so on. I think this should be done.

P.F. Kraicer: Harking back to something that was said before about the possibility that your results are due to reserpine inhibiting the estrogen receptor, I seriously doubt that this is the case, at least in our colony. You know that reserpine has been reported to induce delayed nidation when you administer it to an otherwise unoperated rat. And by everything we know induction of delayed nidation must be due to blockage of estrogen action. Reserpine does not do this in our colony. I remember several years ago Prof. Shelesnyak carried out extensive studies with high, low, medium doses injected for one day, for several days. Aside from getting terribly sick animals, we got apparently perfectly normal nidation. This was done in pregnant animals, and as a matter of fact, in another study, an antagonism between reserpine and ergocornine was demonstrated. The reserpine assured a normal progress of pregnancy again.

In Bordeaux, where reserpine was first used for this technique, Mayer [J.M. Meunier and G. Mayer, Bull. Soc. Roy. Belge Gyn. Obstet. 30, 529, 1960] succeeded in inducing delayed nidation with reserpine. With very small doses of estrogen in addition to the reserpine he got some of the ova to implant, then the reserpine was withdrawn and the rest of the ova implanted so that dissociated nidation in one pregnancy were obtained. The reserpine here was obviously blocking gonadotrophin release, but not interfering with the action of exogenous estrogen so that the argument of reserpine blocking estrogen receptors, at least by this criterion, doesn't hold.

H.R. Lindner: I would prefer to test the argument more directly.

Prof. von Euler stressed the remarkable constancy of noradrenalin content in the various organs and the high repeatability of such determinations; but, in the uterus, Dr. Barnea finds a twofold change within 24 to 48 hours. This being so, would Dr. Barnea or Prof. von Euler care to speculate the functional significance of this change, and whether it might explain cyclic changes in uterine blood flow or the state of the microcirculation in the uterus? There certainly are marked changes in the circulation at the time of estrus. But how do you interpret the fall in the content of noradrenalin in the uterus?

U.S. von Euler: It would be hard to believe that the number of active nerve fibers changes in such a short time, at least, I doubt that that is the case.

One has to, I suppose, consider the possibility of altered activity of the synthesizing system. After all, there are three steps and each of them could be influenced by various means. It doesn't take much to block the first step, the hydroxylation of tyrosine, which is fairly sensitive and a rate-limiting reaction, and if that were blocked by some change in the environment, it could be shown. The activity of the tyrosine hydroxylase would be open to an experimental study.

H.R. Lindner: But changes in the stored noradrenalin need not reflect, in your opinion, the changes in the physiologically active or free moiety of noradrenalin?

J. Gorski: Couldn't increased release explain the change? There is more uterine motility at this time.

U.S. von Euler: If the synthesizing system is working properly, even very large differences in the release-rate should be compensated for, but on the other hand, a change in pH might be of importance.

J. Gorski: So you would guess that a block in synthesis would be the most likely?

U.S. von Euler: I think it's a possibility, and it could be tested.

R. Zmigrod: Haven't you measured the uptake of adrenalin and noradrenalin in uterine sections?

A. Barnea: We did measure uptake by assaying the radioactivity of paraffin sections prepared from uteri of animals given the labelled catecholamine in vivo. We found that the uptake of $^3$H-noradrenalin depended on the stage of the cycle: it was high in diestrus and proestrus but low in estrus, in other words, uptake paralleled content. But this was not the case with adrenalin.

These changes in the total noradrenalin content of the uterus tell us little about physiological significance since we don't know whether the noradrenalin is released in inactive form, as induced by reserpine, for example, as you have just heard, and so would produce no vasoconstriction. The noradrenalin may be inactivated by monoamine oxidase or may be released as the active amine as in the case of nervous stimulation. We haven't looked for the catecholamine metabolites produced.

U.S. von Euler: Have you tried monoamine oxidase inhibitors?

A. Barnea: No, not yet.

U.S. von Euler: I will put in one word. Sometimes it is stated in the literature that a monoamine oxidase inhibitor was used, but practically all of them have additional actions. The only one so far that we think is pretty inert in other respects is nialamide.

C. Tachi: Is it possible that the catecholamine changes are directly related to changes in carbohydrate metabolism such as glycogen deposition in the uterus?

A. Barnea: It is possible, but I don't know. It is known of course, that adrenalin will increase phosphorylase activity in the uterus in vivo and in vitro, but whether the catecholamines are involved in the mediation of the action of estrogen on phosphorylase activity isn't known.

P.F. Kraicer: When you checked for binding of radio-labelled material essentially the amount of radio-activity bound would seem to be directly proportional to the content of the tissue of the amines as otherwise assayed. In other words, in a place where you find a lot of noradrenalin, say, in proestrus, you also found a lot of radioactivity. In estrus, where you find less noradrenalin, there was less of the radioactivity taken up. Surely this must mean that there is change in binding capacity rather than in secretory capacity. If the uterus, (A), doesn't contain very much, and (B), doesn't take up very much when you present it with labelled material, then surely it doesn't contain very much because it can't.

U.S. von Euler: I was thinking much the same thing, but, on the other hand, the uptake is very dependent on the perfusion of the organ. This is really quite important. The perfusion of the uterus may be superior during proestrus.

P.F. Kraicer: But the blood supply during the day of estrus, the day of the cornified vaginal smear, is excellent. The blood vessels are very large and the blood flow, as far as one can gauge from histological sections, at any rate, the drainage and the irrigation of the uterus should be fine.

A. Barnea: I just wanted to add to what Perry said, that when Wurtmann and his group measured the content of catecholamines in the uterus, they also did studies on the uptake of tritiated catecholamines, and found a parallelism between the uptake of tritiated adrenalin and the adrenalin content. The curves were practically identical. Green and Miller [J. Pharmacol. Exp. Ther. 152, 42, 1966] in studies with uterine slices or homogenates found that adrenalin does compete with noradrenalin for uptake. They suggested that in the uterus there is competition between adrenalin and noradrenalin taken up from blood. In another study they found that the ratio of adrenalin to noradrenalin in blood changes during the estrous cycle and the changes they observed parallel those we found with respect to content in the uterus.

U.S. von Euler: If the uterine content reflects the blood concentration, this would imply that the synthesizing system is out of action. As long as synthesis is going on in the normal way, uptake from the blood wouldn't contribute very much.

B.L. Lobel: I would like to ask Prof. von Euler a few questions regarding the granules. What kind of membrane surrounds the granules? Do the granules store anything other than noradrenalin?

U.S. von Euler: I don't think there are any complete chemical analyses of the purified nerve granule sediment, but Hillarp [N.A. Hillarp, Acta Physiol. Scand., 47, 271, 1959] has done some studies on the adrenal medullary granules and although they are different in many respects, they might have the same sort of general chemical set up. He finds besides the catecholamines and ATP, of course, a fairly high percentage of phospholipids which bind amines quite effectively, and proteins.

B.L. Lobel: You described the effect of ATP on the reuptake of noradrenalin by the granules. Have you looked at the granules by electron microscopy after incubation with ATP, to see whether the ATP affects the membrane as it does, for example, in the case of mitochondria?

U.S. von Euler: We have tried to look at these with the electronmicroscope, but it's very hard to get any idea of the fine structure of the membrane. I don't think it's possible at present to say anything about whether a change occurs after addition of ATP. Certainly after depletion they can take up amines again and also release at the original rate.

B.L. Lobel: Is there any relation between lysosomes within axons and the granules? You stated that the rate of release of noradrenalin differs in different tissues. Is it possible that there is some relation between lysosomal enzyme and noradrenalin release? This might be so in view of the fact that incubation at higher temperatures and lower pH's gives faster noradrenalin release and this is also true for enzyme-release from lysosomes.

U.S. von Euler: Perhaps I should mention our fractionation procedure first. We homogenize the nerves with the Ultra Turrax apparatus which produces a somewhat larger sediment, that is to say, less catecholamine per milligram of protein, than the squeezing technique which we used earlier, with similar results. If we squeeze the nerves between rollers we get a juice which is centrifuged at about 10,000 G for 10 minutes which sediments a small amount of heavier or larger particles. A section of the granule pellet obtained after spinning down at 50,000 G for half an hour looks rather uniform. There seem to be very few larger or different looking particles. The results are very reproducible with regard to the noradrenalin release-rate from the granules. The lysosomes are fairly large, although they do vary in shape and of course it is difficult to be quite sure that the last lysosomes have disappeared. Single lysosomes would be very hard to exclude and the same holds for the small mitochondria, too.

A. Barnea: With regard to the release of noradrenalin from different tissues, is it possible that the size of the labile pool is higher in, for example, nerves, than in the adrenal medulla so that the release is quicker in the nerves due to higher concentrations of noradrenalin in the labile pool?

U. S. von Euler: The granules seem to have an intrinsic or basic release-rate, which is much higher for the nerve granules than for adrenal medullary granules. It may also be that the release mechanisms differ in the adrenal cell membranes and in the nerve endings.

C. Tachi: Is the ATP added to the incubation medium used up, that is, does the particle have ATPase activity? Does the ATP serve as an energy source during the reaccumulation?

U.S. von Euler: In the homogenate or even in the washed particles there is a certain ATPase activity, so added ATP will be broken down at a fairly high rate. In order to obtain a steady reuptake at a high level, one has to add ATP repeatedly, about 3 millimolar concentration, replenished every half hour at 20°C; so there is ATPase activity.

C. Tachi: Is the effect specific for ATP or can other nucleotide triphosphates do the same thing?

U.S. von Euler: CTP, UTP and GTP are all active but only half as active as ATP, judging from the slope of the reuptake curve. ADP is active also. We don't think this can be due to contamination with ATP. AMP is not active.

G. J. Marcus: Can the ATP be replaced by a non-phosphorylated energy source, for example, an oxidizable substrate? As a corollary to this question, is there any evidence for some components of an oxidizing system such as you have in mitochondria present in these particles? Any of the members of the electronic transport system? You indicated that some of the inhibitors of the electron transport system stimulate release. Was this *in vitro*?

U.S. von Euler: Yes, uncoupling substances like DNP prevent the reuptake.

G.J. Marcus: Have you tested cyanide?

U.S. von Euler: Yes, it has no effect. Azide has some effect, but very little.

G.J. Marcus: By analogy with the behavior of mitochondrial membranes, have you looked for changes in the volume of the granules in the presence of ATP, for example, by light-scattering measurements?

U.S. von Euler: We have observed that in the presence of ATP the volume of the pellet after centrifugation is reduced. Also we tried adding oligomycin and it did retard the noradrenalin-release.

E. Nuriel: It has been claimed that when these granules reach receptors in the membrane, for instance, in the synapse, they explode and release their substance. What kind of receptors are those in the membrane that make the vesicles release their substance?

U.S. von Euler: I don't believe this is true in the case of the nerve granules which we have been discussing today. This may be the case, however, I am not competent to say, for the chromaffin cells. There is no evidence, whatsoever, as far as I know, that the granules in the nerve endings should be displaced or fused with the membranes or explode or anything like that. The nerve granules seem to be in a kind of equilibrium with the extragranular pool from which the transmitter is released directly.

# HORMONE RECEPTORS: STUDIES ON ESTROGEN BINDING TO THE UTERUS

# HORMONE RECEPTORS: STUDIES ON ESTROGEN BINDING TO THE UTERUS[1]

Jack Gorski, David Toft,[2]
G. Shyamala,[3] and Donald E. Smith[4]
Department of Physiology and Biophysics
University of Illinois, Urbana, Illinois

Reproduction is a highly ordered process involving the careful sequencing of a number of biological control systems. In order to fully understand this process it is necessary to investigate its various aspects at all levels of organization and complexity. One important component of this system, the estrogenic hormone, has proven particularly amenable to studies at the molecular level. Work on the molecular action of estrogens is represented by several approaches but we will restrict this discussion to studies concerning the initial interaction

[1] Supported by grant no. AM-06327 from the U.S. Public Health Service.

[2] Present address: McArdle Laboratory for Cancer Research, University of Wisconsin, Madison.

[3] Present address: Department of Biological Sciences, Northwestern University, Evanston, Illinois.

[4] Present address: Department of Zoology, North Carolina State University, Raleigh, North Carolina.

of the estrogens with their target tissues.

It has been suggested for a long time that various pharmacological agents, including hormones, initiate their effects by first interacting with some component in their respective target tissues. The term "receptors" has been given to these components of the target tissues which interact with hormones or other pharmacological compounds.

What then is a hormone receptor? In a general sense there can be no further definition beyond what has been noted above. No one has isolated, let alone characterized, any hormone receptor. However, there are a number of criteria that must be met when discussing a specific pharmacologic or endocrine compound. These criteria are based on the specific biological characteristics of the particular material under discussion. In the case of the estrogens there are a number of unique biological characteristics which dictate the criteria which an estrogen receptor must meet. Such a criterion is chemical specificity. Only certain phenolic compounds show biological activity whereas other compounds with very similar chemical properties may differ greatly in biological activity. One would therefore expect an estrogen receptor to show some specificity in its interaction with estrogens.

Another criteria concerns tissue specificity. Although the term target tissue is not universally accepted, in the case of the estrogens it can be usefully used to designate those tissues which show marked and early responses to the estrogenic hormones. Other tissues may be influenced but the quantitative response is different. The reproductive tract of the female represents such a target tissue and one would expect to find estrogen receptors here but not necessarily in other tissues.

It is also known that the response of the target tissue to increasing quantities of estrogen rises to a certain point and then remains on a plateau with additional estrogen having no effect. One interpretation of these observations is that the quantity of receptor sites is limited to a finite number.

It is obvious that limiting factors other than the receptor could explain the biological observations noted above. However, the receptor hypothesis must be examined in terms of such biological criteria and at least should not contradict them.

Attempts to find evidence for hormone receptors have been numerous and have given much impetus to studies on hormone metabolism. However, these studies generally yielded only negative evidence as to the presence of hormone receptors until the late '50's when Glasscock and Hoekstra (1959) in England and Jensen and Jacobson (1960) in the United States reported on experiments in which they used tritiated estrogens of very high specific-activity.

This highly labeled estrogen enabled these investigators to inject physiological doses of estrogens into animals and then to look for and detect small quantities of hormone in the various tissues. As a result of these studies Jensen and Jacobson (1962) convincingly demonstrated that the female reproductive tract had a different pattern of estrogen uptake than non-target tissues such as liver, muscle, etc.

They showed that when physiological quantities [0.1 μg or less of estradiol-17β per immature (50 gm) rat] were administered, the uterus and vagina showed a high uptake of estrogen which reached a peak one or two hours after injection. Other tissues showed lower uptakes, the peak of uptake occurred within 15 minutes and there was an exponential decline in radioactive estrogen similar to that found in the blood. It was apparent that the equilibrium of estrogen between the blood and the target tissues was not the same as it was with liver, muscle and other tissues. Further more, Jensen and Jacobson (1962) could not find any evidence for the metabolism of estradiol - 17β in the uterus and most of the estrogen was present in a non-covalent bound form. These and other studies suggested that there was binding of the estrogens to target tissues and that this binding was due to receptors specific for estrogens.

## SUBCELLULAR DISTRIBUTION

These findings raised a number of interesting questions and we therefore set out to explore what seemed to us to be an exciting development in the study of the initial step in estrogen action.

We first addressed ourselves to the question of where the estrogen was located in the uterine cell. As shown in Figure 1, the distribution of radioactive estrogen in the various subcellular fractions is similar at both low and high physiologic doses of estrogen (Noteboom and Gorski, 1964, 1965). Over 50% of the estrogen is present in the nuclear-myofibrillar fraction. As will be discussed later there is good evidence that this estrogen is in the nucleus and is not associated

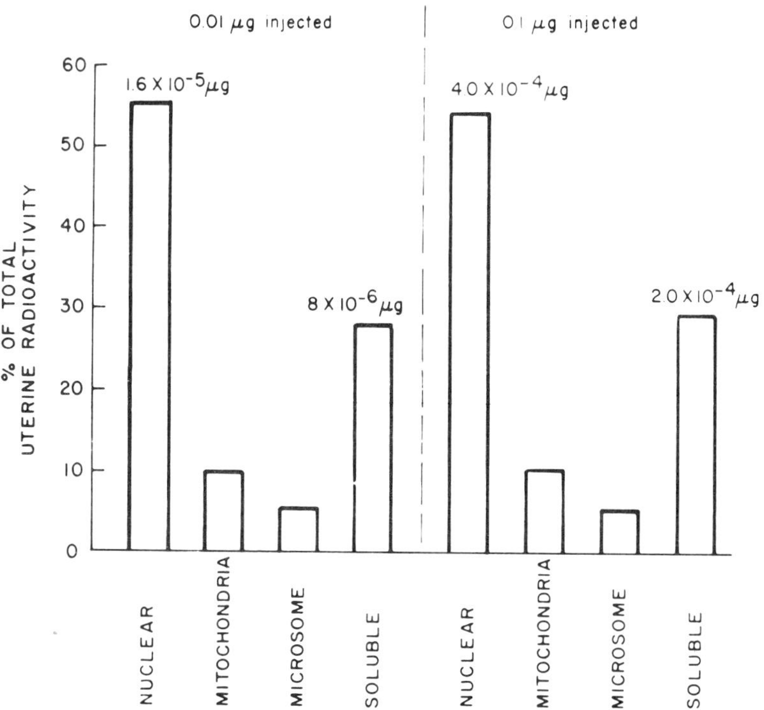


Fig. 1. The distribution of radioactive estradiol in subcellular fractions of rat uteri. Uteri from 5 immature rats were pooled for each determination. At 0.01 µg injected dose, approximately 0.30% of the injected activity was recovered in the uterus and at 0.1 µg 0.07% was recovered. (From Noteboom and Gorski, 1965.)

with myofibrils or cellular debris. Whether the small quantities of estrogen associated with the mitochondria or microsomal fractions are significant or not, has not been determined at the present time. Another large quantity of estrogen was associated with the 105,000 X g supernatant or cytosol fraction. The work we will discuss in this paper will be concerned principally with the nuclear and the cytosol fractions.

## NUCLEAR RECEPTOR

We next directed our attention to the related questions of the specifity of the binding and of the numbers of binding sites. If one hypothesizes that there is a finite number of specific binding sites in each uterus, then one would predict a limited uptake of total estrogen and, in addition, inhibition of uptake of labeled estrogens by unlabeled estrogens because of competition for these binding sites. Such an experiment is shown in Figure 2. (Noteboom and Gorski, 1964, 1965). In this experiment unlabeled steroids and estrogens were injected two hours prior to the injection of labeled estradiol-17$\beta$ to allow the blood levels of steroid to decline and thereby eliminate as much as possible competition for serum transport protein. It can be seen that diethylstilbestrol (DES) markedly reduced the uptake of $^{3}$H-estradiol-17$\beta$ whereas the other compounds had little or no effect. It is of particular interest to compare estradiol-17$\alpha$ and DES. The former is chemically a stereoisomer of estradiol-17$\beta$ but of low biological potency as an estrogen whereas DES is not even a steroid but has a high estrogenic activity. Similar results were seen when the different compounds were

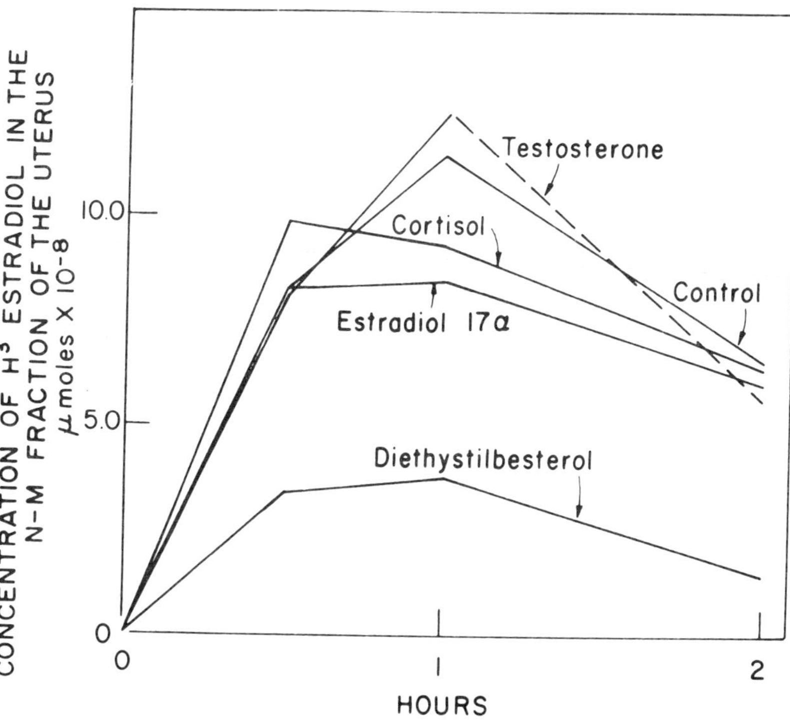


Fig. 2. Effect of 2-hr. pretreatment with testosterone, cortisol, diethylstilbestrol, and estradiol-17$\alpha$ on the incorporation of $^3$H-estradiol-17$\beta$ into the nuclear-myofibrillar fraction of the rat uterus. The amount of hormone injected as the pretreatment was 1.0 $\mu$g, and the amount of $^3$H-estradiol injected was 0.01 $\mu$g. Each point represents the mean of values from 4 individual uteri expressed as $\mu$m x $10^{-8}$ per N-M fraction of one uterus. Estradiol was extracted with ethanol, ethanol-chloroform (1:2) and ether. (From Noteboom and Gorski, 1965.)

administered simultaneously in the same vehicle. It was of some importance to prove whether the interference of binding was due to competition for the same sites or whether some other type of inhibition of $^{3}$H-estradiol uptake was occurring. In Figure 3 is a reciprocal plot of concentration of bound $^{3}$H-estradiol versus the quantity of injected estradiol at different levels of inhibitor (DES). The data fall on lines passing through a common origin on the ordinate and therefore support the thesis that the estrogens are competing for the same sites on the binding agents.

It would appear that the number of binding sites in the nucleus is limited and, when occupied by an active estrogen such as DES, additional estrogen such as the $^{3}$H-estradiol cannot be readily bound. It also appears that the nuclear binding agent is quite specific and can recognize the difference between stereoisomers and between estrogens and non-estrogens.

This binding agent was showing a number of attributes one would expect of a hormone receptor, and we shall hereafter use the term estrogen receptor to designate this binding agent.

Other studies on the nuclear receptor such as those shown in Figure 4 (Noteboom and Gorski, 1965) in which the receptor is shown to be sensitive to proteolytic enzymes but not to nucleases strongly suggested that the nuclear receptor is principally protein. While this in itself is not surprising it did not support suggestions that nucleic acids (T'so and Lu, 1964) or even nucleotides (Engel and Scott, 1961) might be directly linked to estrogens. Our studies, on the other hand, did not rule out the possibility that the receptor contained other components besides protein. If present, however, these constituents probably do not directly bind with the estrogen.

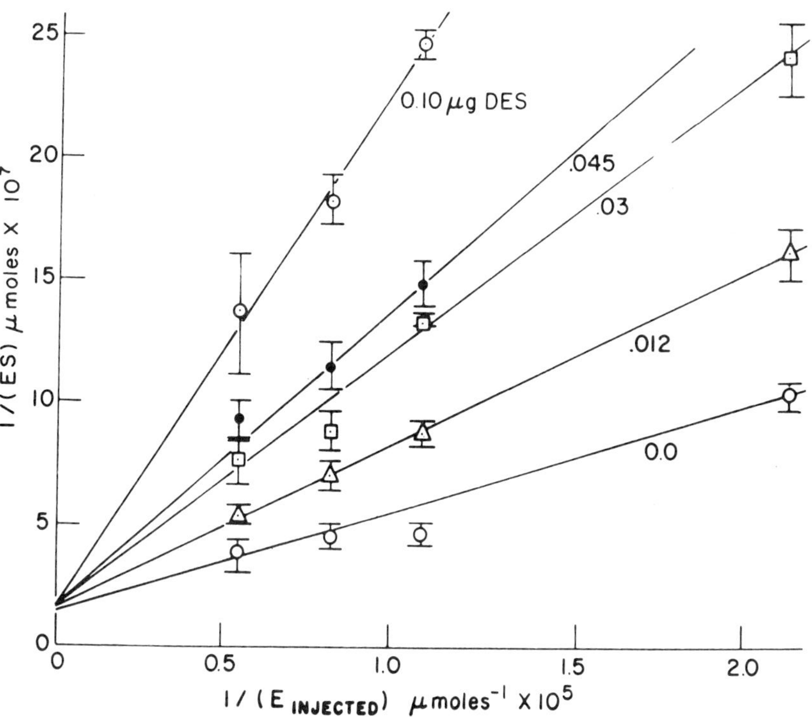


Fig. 3. Inhibition of the incorporation of $^3$H-estradiol by diethylstilbestrol in the nuclear-myofibrillar fraction of the rat uterus. Each point represents the mean values of 4 determinations of individual uteri. The brackets indicate standard errors. Various levels of the estrogens were injected ip simultaneously, uteri removed after 3 hr, and the estradiol extracted as described in Figure 2. Radioactivity extracted from the uterus was converted to [ES] per uterus by using the specific activity of the $^3$H-estradiol of 125 μc/μg. [$E_{injected}$] refers to the concentration of injected $^3$H-estradiol. (From Note-

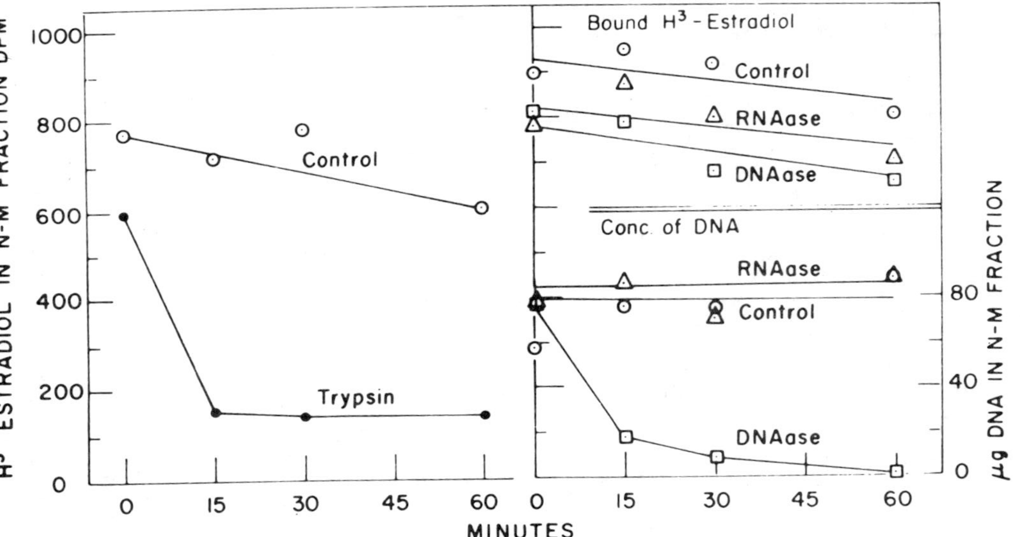


Fig. 4. Effect of enzyme degradation on the release of $^3$H-estradiol from the nuclear-myofibrillar fraction of the rat uterus. Each point represents the mean value of two determinations on the equivalent of one half of a uterus. The lower curves on the right side of the figure show the amount of DNA remaining in the N-M fraction after incubation with the enzyme. Incubations with 500 $\mu$g of RNase or DNase were at 31°C. Incubation with 5 $\mu$g trypsin was at 10°C. (From Noteboom and Gorski, 1965).

## CYTOSOL RECEPTOR

Our attention was now diverted for a time to studying the nature of the estrogen found in the cytosol. This fraction which consistently amounted to 30% of the total radioactive estrogen found in the uterus could have been free estrogen released from the nucleus or perhaps it was another unrelated receptor.

Noteboom (1965) in our laboratory, attempted to fractionate the cytosol by means of molecular sieving chromatography. As shown in Figure 5, and as has been reported by Talwar, Segal, Evans and Davidson (1964), this procedure does not resolve to any great extent the uterine proteins which come off the column together in the void volume. This work did show that much of the estradiol in the cytosol after in vivo administration was bound to some macromolecular component. When competition studies were carried out, however, the estrogen associated with the void volume appeared to be influenced to only a small extent and therefore was not behaving as expected of a receptor.

Other fractionation techniques were explored and Figure 6 shows the results of fractionating the cytosol by centrifugation through sucrose density gradients (Toft and Gorski, 1965, 1966). It is apparent that only a single peak of radioactivity is present on the gradient when 0.1 $\mu$g or less of $^3$H-estradiol-17$\beta$ was administered in vivo. When higher concentrations were injected a second peak of radioactivity appeared. The single peak occurring after injecting low doses of estrogen has a sedimentation constant of 9.5 S which would indicate a large molecule of about 200,000 M. W. Figure 7 shows that when DES at 10 times the concentration of the $^3$H-estradiol-17$\beta$ is injected simultaneously

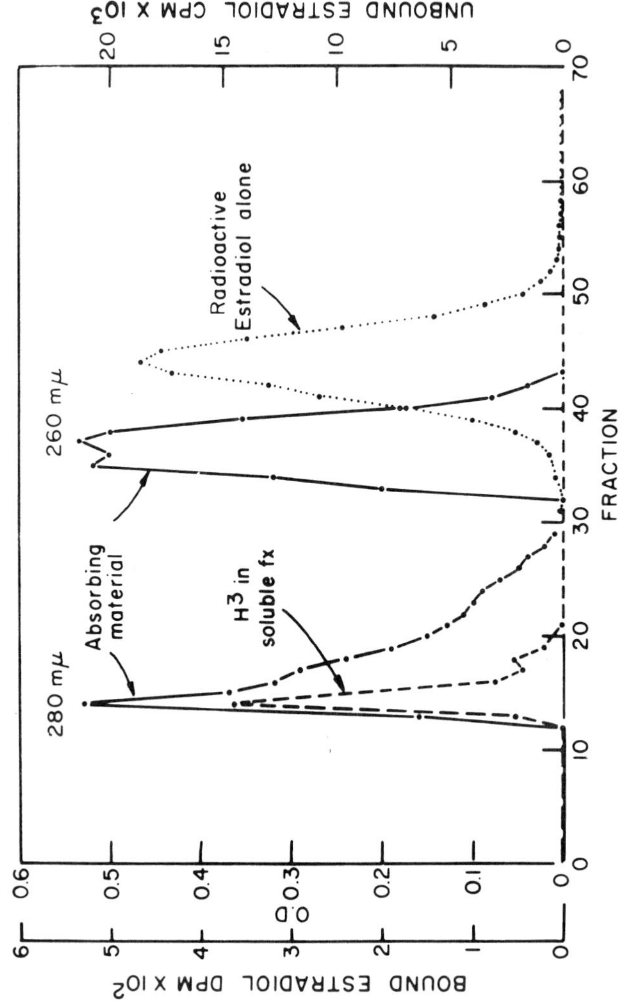
UNBOUND ESTRADIOL CPM X 10³
280 mμ
Absorbing material
H³ in soluble fx
260 mμ
Radioactive Estradiol alone
FRACTION
O.D
BOUND ESTRADIOL DPM X 10²

the 9.5 S peak is obliterated whereas the effect on the 4-6 S peak is questionable. When a similar experiment with lower concentrations of $^3$H-estradiol was tried, no 4-5 peak was found in the controls but the DES caused the $^3$H-estradiol in the 9.5 S peak to disappear and the radioactivity now appeared in the 4-6 S area. The 9.5 S peak of estrogen binding does not occur in blood serum or in the small intestine as shown in Figure 8. Other experiments indicated that the radioactivity associated with the 9.5 S peak after *in vivo* injection of $^3$H-estradiol was also sensitive to proteolytic enzymes and extremes of pH, suggesting that this component was at least partially composed of protein. These studies all strongly supported the notion that after *in vivo* in-

(LEFT)

Fig. 5. Gel filtration on G-75 Sephadex of the soluble fraction of uteri from 10 rats treated with .01 $\mu$g of $^3$H-estradiol for 2 hours. The uteri were homogenized in 2 ml of homogenization medium and centrifuged at 105,000 X g for 1 hour. One milliliter of the supernate was filtered on a column 15 mm by 150mm. Volume of the fractions was 0.5 ml. After optical density determinations at 260 m$\mu$ and 280 m$\mu$ 0.2 ml aliquots were counted in 4 ml of absolute ethanol and 15 ml of scintillation solvent. The dotted line represents the radioactivity of fractions when $^3$H-estradiol was filtered alone. The solid lines represent optical density and the dashed line, the radio-activity of the fractions when the soluble material was resolved on the column. (From Noteboom, 1965).

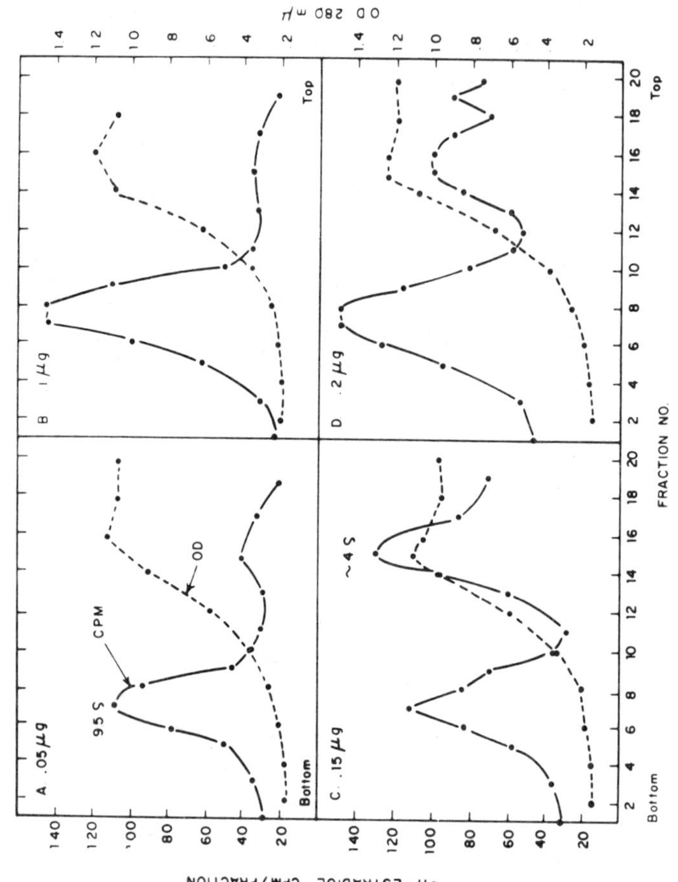
A .05 μg
9.5 S
CPM
OD
B 1 μg
C .15 μg
~4 S
D .2 μg
Bottom
Top
FRACTION NO.
3H-ESTRADIOL CPM/FRACTION
OD 280 mμ

jection at least part of the estrogen was specifically associated with a large protein of approximately 200,000 molecular weight which was present in the cytosol.

## BINDING IN A CELL FREE SYSTEM

The affinity of the estrogen for this receptor was obviously high in order to permit the long centrifugation (10-14 hours) necessary to isolate it. This apparent high affinity suggested that the binding might occur in a cell free system. When various levels of $^3$H-estradiol-17$\beta$ are added directly to uterine cytosol fractions which are then centrifuged, the results shown in Figure 9 are obtained. (Toft, Shyamala, and Gorski, 1967). Again it is apparent that the 9.5 S peak is present at low concentrations and that the 4-6 S peak picks up radioactivity only as the 9.5 S peak becomes saturated. Figure 10 shows that the oviducts and the

(LEFT)

Fig. 6. Density gradient patterns of the soluble fraction 3.5 hr after injection of various amounts of $^3$H-estradiol. Each soluble fraction is from five uteri homogenized in 0.5 ml of medium (Tris, $MgCl_2$, KCl); 0.2 ml was layered on 5-20% sucrose gradient and centrifuged for 9.5 hr at 39,000 rpm, 10 °C. Estradiol injections: (A) 0.05 μg/rat; (B) 0.1 μg; (C) 0.15 μg; (D) 0.2 μg. Counting efficiency, 13-14% Sedimentation is from right to left. (From Toft and Gorski, 1966.)

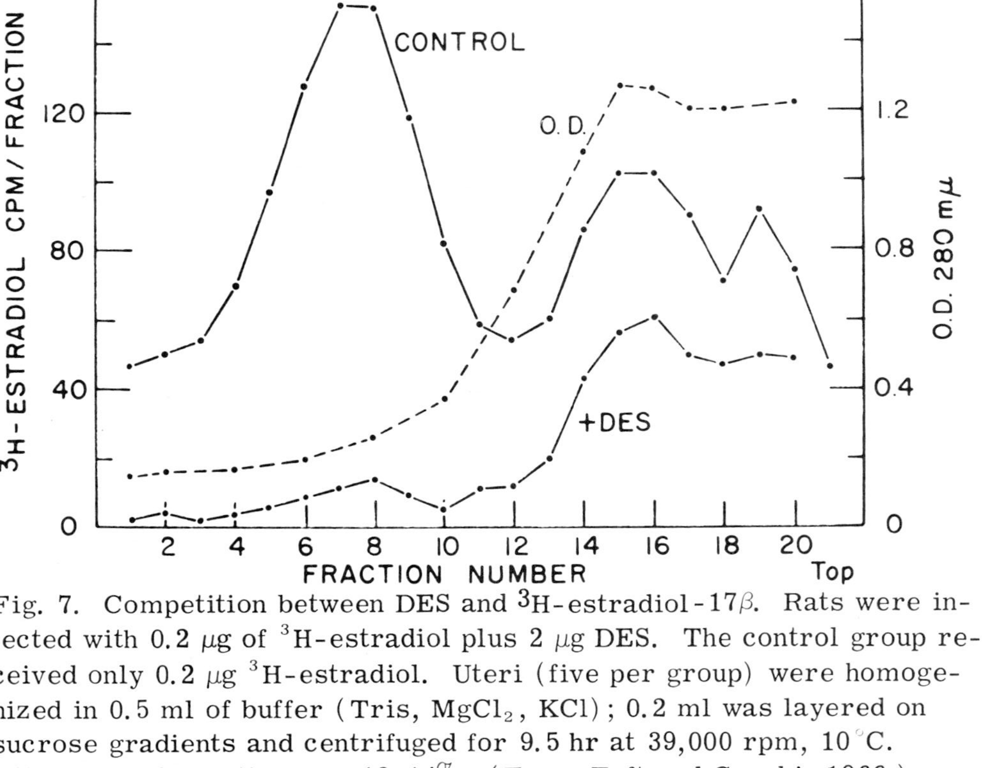


Fig. 7. Competition between DES and $^{3}$H-estradiol-17β. Rats were injected with 0.2 μg of $^{3}$H-estradiol plus 2 μg DES. The control group received only 0.2 μg $^{3}$H-estradiol. Uteri (five per group) were homogenized in 0.5 ml of buffer (Tris, $MgCl_2$, KCl); 0.2 ml was layered on sucrose gradients and centrifuged for 9.5 hr at 39,000 rpm, 10°C. Efficiency of counting was 13-14%. (From Toft and Gorski, 1966.)

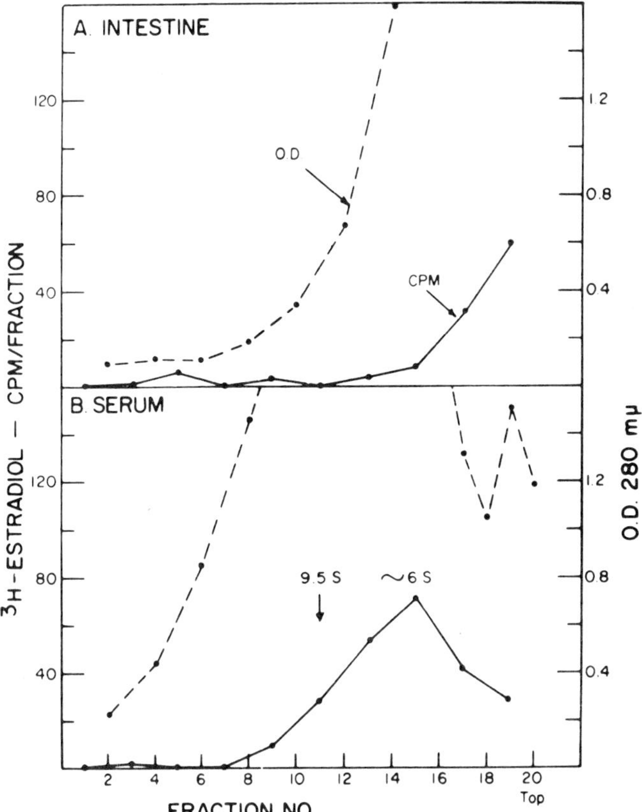


Fig. 8. Density gradient pattern of rat intestine soluble fraction (A), and of rat serum (B). Five rats were injected with 0.02 μg of $^3$H-estradiol and sacrificed after 1 hr. Intestine was homogenized in tris-EDTA buffer, and the soluble fraction was obtained as with uteri. Serum was obtained by bleeding the rats after decapitation. The blood was allowed to clot, and clear serum was obtained by centrifugation; 0.2 ml of sample was layered on 5-20% sucrose gradients and centrifuged for 10 hr at 39,000 rpm, 3°C. Counting efficiency was 13-14%. (From Toft and Gorski, 1966).

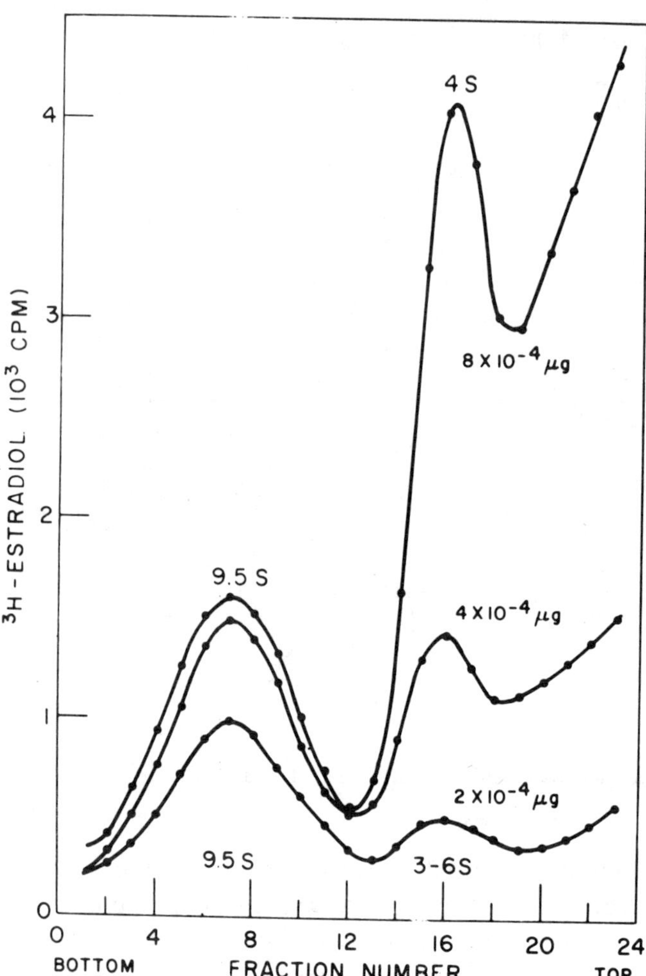


Fig. 9. Density gradient patterns of uterine soluble fraction after the addition of increasing concentrations of $H^3$-estradiol-17$\beta$. One tenth ml of soluble fraction containing the amount of estradiol designated in figure was layered on 5-20% sucrose gradients and centrifuged for 13 hr at 200,000 x g, 3 °C. Counting efficiency was 19%. (From Toft, Shyamala, and Gorski, 1967)

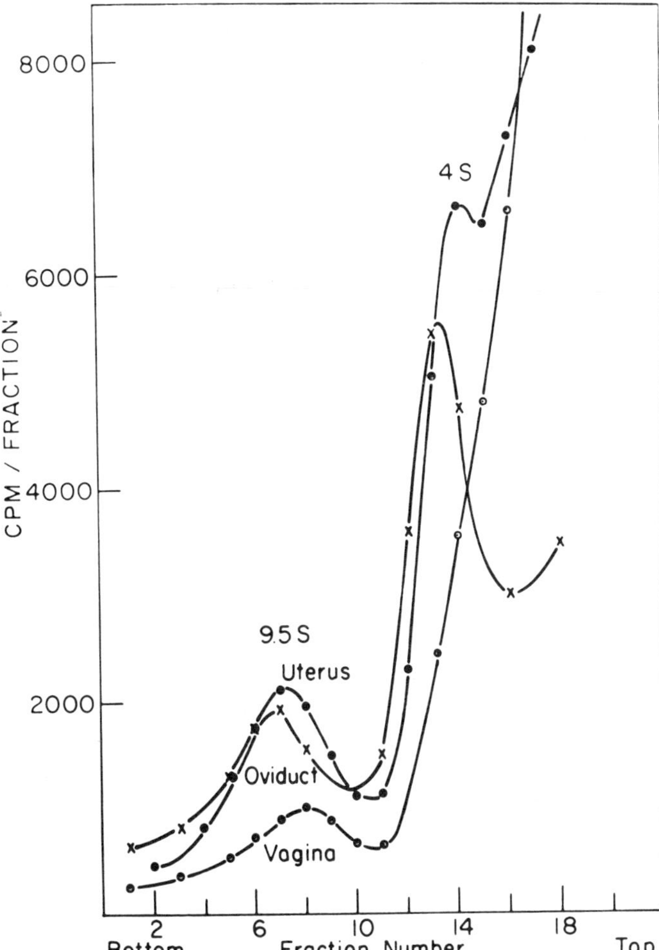


Fig. 10. Density gradient pattern of the binding of $H^3$-estradiol in the soluble fraction from the uterus, vagina and oviduct. $H^3$-estradiol was added to the soluble fractions of each tissue and 0.2 ml samples were layered on 5-20% sucrose gradients. These were centrifuged for 12 hr at 200,000 x g, 3 °C. Counting efficiency was 19-20%.

vagina also have a similar receptor which binds estrogen in a cell free system.

The 4-6 S peak of the uterus has a distribution pattern on sucrose density gradients similar to the albumin and hemoglobin peak of rat serum as shown in Figure 11. Electrophoreis of uterine extracts also indicates that serum albumin is present in this region of the gradients and may be involved in the 4-6 S binding. That the binding to the 9.5 S peak is not a non-specific association of hydrophobic steroids to proteins is shown by the data in Figure 12 in which progesterone and testosterone do not bind to the 9.5 S peak while progesterone does bind to the 4-6 S region. We have looked at a number of other steroids in this system and so far only estrogenic compounds appear to bind to the 9.5 S peak receptor and their relative affinities appear to bear some relationship to their relative biological potencies.

With the cell free system one can now obtain some quantitative data which are not possible in whole animal studies. Figure 13 shows that the 9.5 S peak is saturated at relatively low levels of estrogen, indicating a limited number of these specific sites. The 4-6 S area is not saturated at even the highest dose used in this study. These data can be plotted in a Scatchard plot as in Figure 14 and one gets a straight line whose slope is an estimate of the dissociation constant. This $K_{dis}$ for estradiol-17$\beta$ is approximately $7 \times 10^{-10}$ M and is somewhat comparable to the Michaelis constant ($K_m$) used to describe enzyme-substrate associations. It is apparent that estradiol-17$\beta$ has a much higher affinity for the receptor than estriol and this again indicates a relationship between affinity for the receptor and the relative biological potencies of estrogenic compounds.

From the Scatchard plot one also gets an estimate of the number of binding sites. In this case we estimated

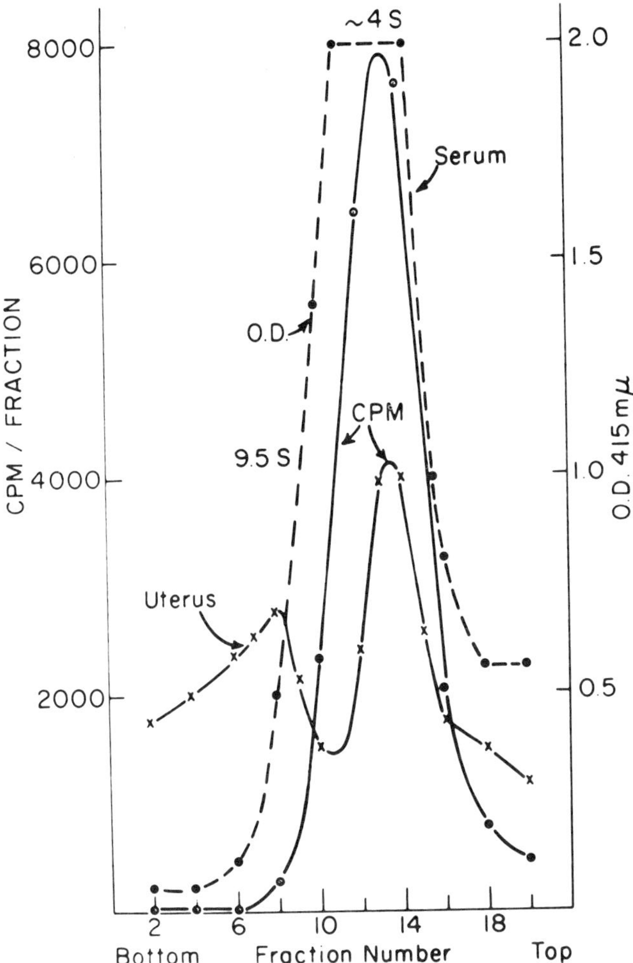


Fig. 11. Density gradient pattern showing the binding of $H^3$-estradiol to rat serum as compared to estrogen binding in the uterine soluble fraction. After the addition of $H^3$-estradiol, 0.2 ml samples were layered on 5-20% sucrose gradients and centrifuged for 12 hr at 200,000 x g, 3°C. The optical density at 415 mμ was used as a measure of hemoglobin content. Counting efifciency was 19%.

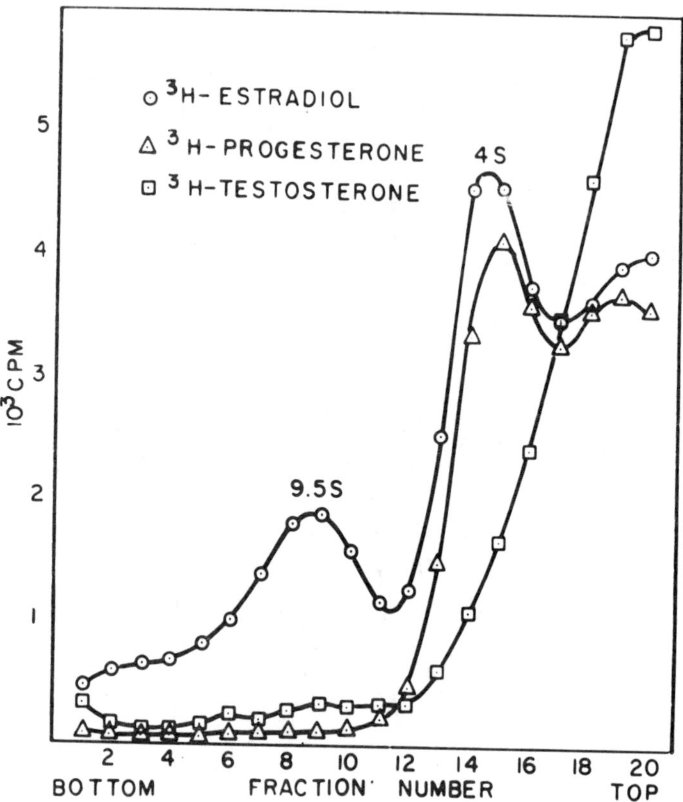


Fig. 12. Density gradient patterns showing uterine binding of estradiol, progesterone, and testosterone. An equal number of microcuries of each steroid was added to uterine soluble fractions and 0.2 ml samples were layered on 5-20% sucrose gradients. These were centrifuged for 12 hr at 200,000 x g, 3 °C. Counting efficiency was 19-20%. The specific activities used were: estradiol, 166.7 $\mu$c per $\mu$g; progesterone, 32.3 $\mu$c per $\mu$g; testosterone, 166.7 $\mu$c per $\mu$g. (From Toft, Shyamala, and Gorski, 1967).

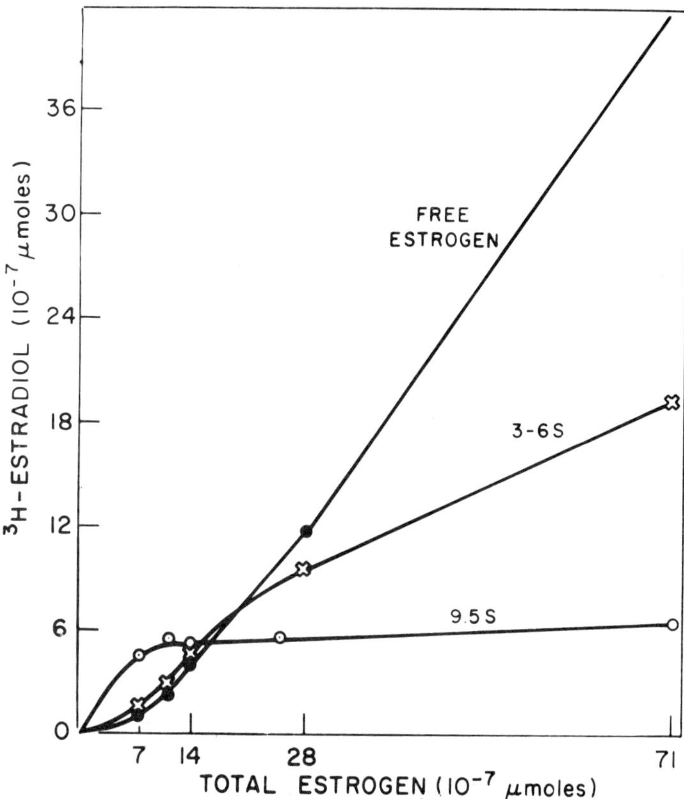


Fig. 13. Titration plot from the density gradient analysis of estradiol binding in the uterine soluble fraction. The sucrose gradient techniques were as described in the methods, using 0.1 ml samples of the soluble fraction. The amount of $H^3$-estradiol in the 9.5 S region, 3-6 S region and free estradiol were determined and plotted versus total estradiol concentration. For these determinations, the radioactivity was measured and converted to μmoles of estradiol. The counting efficiency was 19% and the specific activity of estradiol was 140 μc per μg. (From Toft and Gorski, 1967).

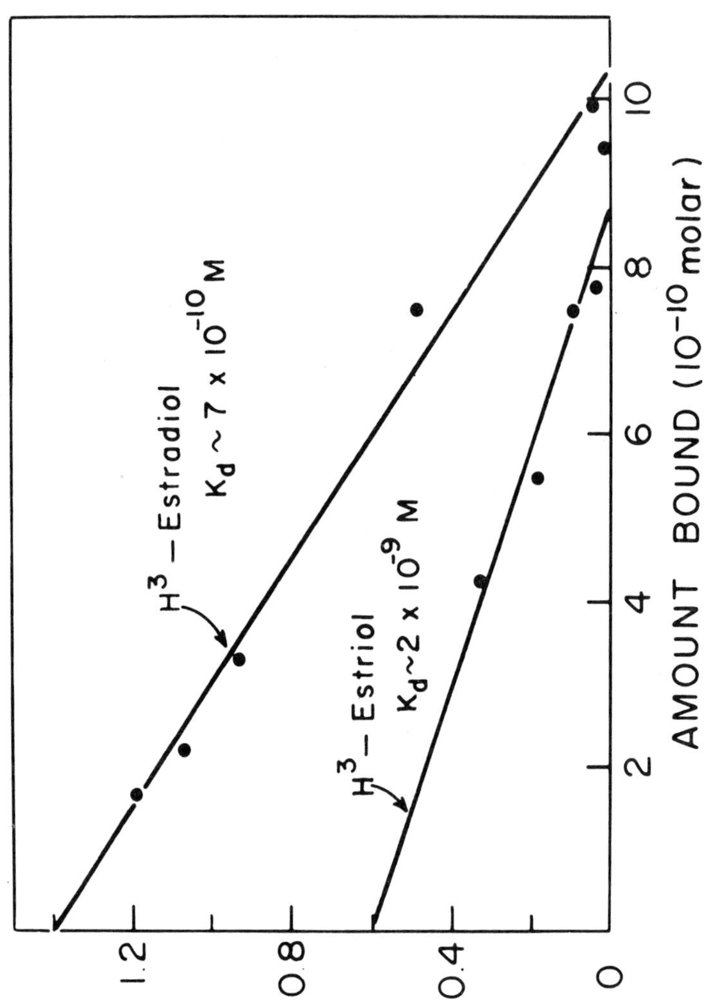
H³ — Estradiol
Kd ~ 7 x 10⁻¹⁰ M
H³ — Estriol
Kd ~ 2 x 10⁻⁹ M
AMOUNT BOUND (10⁻¹⁰ molar)
2
4
6
8
10
0
0.4
0.8
1.2

that 8 to 9 x $10^{-13}$ moles of estrogen were bound in the cytosol of one uterus or approximately 20,000 sites per cell. Previous in vivo studies by Noteboom and Gorski (1965) and Toft and Gorski (1966) were in close agreement that 4 - 5 x $10^{-14}$ moles of estrogen were bound in the cytosol of one uterus. This difference of 20 fold between these two estimates could be rationalized as due to the marked difference between the open-ended system found in vivo and the closed system studied in the cell free system. Also, the cell free system was studied at 0°C compared to the 37°C in vivo system. The difference, however, still appeared surprisingly great and raised the question whether subcellular distribution might be playing a role in these estimates of the numbers of binding sites.

(LEFT)

Fig. 14. Determination of the dissociation constants and the number of binding sites. Using sucrose gradient analysis, measurements were made of the amount of estradiol bound to the 9.5 S component and the amount of "free" estradiol (total - 9.5 S bound estradiol). These values are adjusted to correspond to a protein concentration of 1 mg per ml. The actual protein concentration was 8.6 mg per ml. The relationship used is:

(Bound)/(Free) = 1/K (Binding sites) - (Bound)

K = 1/slope

(Binding sites) = X-intercept

(From Toft, Shyamala, and Gorski, 1967).

TABLE I: Effect of Homogenization and Addition of Nonlabeled Estradiol on the Extraction of $^{3}$H-estradiol from the Nuclear-Myofibrillar Fraction

| Experiment | Radioactivity extracted from N-M fraction (cpm) |
|---|---|
| In vivo[a] | |
| 0.01 μg $^{3}$H-estradiol (2 hours) | 1050<br>736 |
| 0.01 μg $^{3}$H-estradiol (2 hours) Homogenized with 10 μg unlabeled estradiol | 1010<br>797 |
| In vitro[b] | |
| 1000 cpm $^{3}$H-estradiol before homogenization | 134<br>106 |
| 1000 cpm $^{3}$H-estradiol + 10 μg unlabeled estradiol before homogenization | 69<br>67 |
| 1000 cpm $^{3}$H-estradiol after homogenization | 122<br>97 |

[a]*In vivo* experiments were carried out by intraperitoneal injection of $^{3}$H-estradiol 2 hours prior to killing. Where noted, 10 μg estradiol-17β was added to homogenization medium prior to tissue homogenization.

[b]The *in vitro* studies were with uteri from rats which had not been previously injected. These uteri were homogenized with 1000 cpm of $^{3}$H-estradiol-17β or homogenized and then 1000 cpm of $^{3}$H-estradiol-17β was added. Where it is indicated, 10 μg of unlabeled estradiol-17β was added before homogenization.

TABLE II: Incorporation of $^{3}H$-estradiol into Homogenate and Nuclear Fractions of the Immature Rat Uterus

| | Bound Estradiol | DNA | Protein | Specific Activity | |
|---|---|---|---|---|---|
| Cell Preparation | CPM/uterus | ug/uterus | ug/uterus | CPM/ug DNA | CPM/ug Protein |
| Homogenate | 5082 | 219 | 2448 | 23.2 | 2.07 |
| Nuclei | 800 | 72 | 228 | 11.1 | 3.50 |
| Purified Chromatin | 559 | 47 | 100 | 11.8 | 5.59 |

The $^{3}H$-estradiol-17$\beta$ (0.05 ug/rat) was injected intraperitoneally three hours prior to killing, 15 rats were used in this study.

## CYSTOSOL-NUCLEAR INTERACTION

Table I shows some earlier data (Noteboom and Gorski, 1965) that indicates the nuclear fraction does not take up estrogen under cell free conditions as contrasted to the data we have just discussed concerning the cytosol fraction. Again there are several rationalizations for this data but it reinforced our interest in further testing the possibility that in the uterus there exists only one type of estrogen receptor which at the outset is present exclusively in the cytosol.

Table II shows the distribution of radioactive estrogen in nuclear fractions of the uterus after in vivo administration of the hormone. A new procedure for isolating nuclei relatively free of contaminating material, was developed based on a procedure of Kostyo (1966). The nuclei prepared by this procedure are capable of synthesizing RNA and microscopically appear normal (Barry and Gorski, 1966). Preparation of chromatin from these nuclei results in some purification of protein and recovery of the DNA and of the estrogen. The chromatin prepared by this procedure, however, is still a very crude preparation with a host of proteins including both histones and non-histones. King, Gordon and Martin (1965) in a short abstract also suggested that nuclear chromatin contained bound estrogen. When these relatively purified nuclei and the chromatin were tested directly for estrogen binding in cell free preparations we obtained data similar to that discussed and shown above in Table I. There again was no evidence of specific binding to these nuclear fractions under cell free conditions (Shyamala and Gorski, 1967).

In order to look at the distribution of estrogen in subcellular fractions under more closely controlled conditions, we turned to the use of in vitro incubations of whole uteri which had been demonstrated by Stone and Bagget (1965) to meet many of the same criteria for specific binding as in vivo systems.

Figure 15 shows the distribution of estradiol-17$\beta$ between nuclear and cytoplasmic fractions at various times of incubation at 0°C and 37°C (Shyamala and Gorski, 1967). After incubation for 1 hour at 37°C the distribution was not too dissimilar to that found after in vivo administration of this hormone. In contrast, at 0°C there was very little uptake of estrogen by the nucleus and a disproportionate amount by the cytosol. Subsequent analysis of the cytosol on sucrose gradients indicated that the estradiol was mainly associated with the 9.5 S peak.

Figure 16 shows the results of incubating uteri first at 0°C with radioactive estrogen followed by incubating at 37°C in a medium free of estrogen. It is apparent that the estrogen moves from the cytosol to the nuclei under these conditions. Sucrose density gradient analysis (Figure 17) shows that corresponding to the movement of the estrogen into the nucleus there is a drop in the estrogen bound to the 9.5 S peak. The loss of radioactivity from the 9.5 S receptor could be due to estrogen coming off the receptor or to the movement of an estrogen-receptor complex into the nucleus. In order to test these alternative hypotheses, uteri were incubated with or without estrogen and then cytosol fractions prepared, treated with labeled estrogen and analyzed on sucrose density gradients. The results of such an experiment are shown in Figure 18. The cytosol obtained from uteri incubated at 37°C with estrogen was unable to bind estrogen added under cell free conditions and indicates that the 9.5 S receptor has disappeared from the cytosol. If estrogen is not present during the 37 C incubation, the receptor remains in the cytosol.

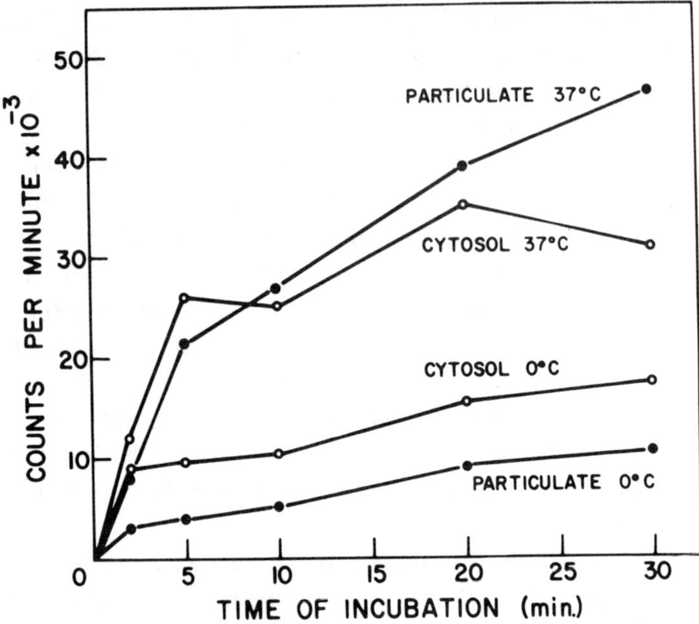


Fig. 15. The distribution of radioactive estradiol between cytosol and particulate fraction. In each group two uteri from immature rats were incubated in 2 ml Eagle's medium containing 0.005 $\mu$g $^3$H-estradiol-17$\beta$ at 0 °C or 37 °C for various times as indicated. (From Shyamala, and Gorski, 1967).

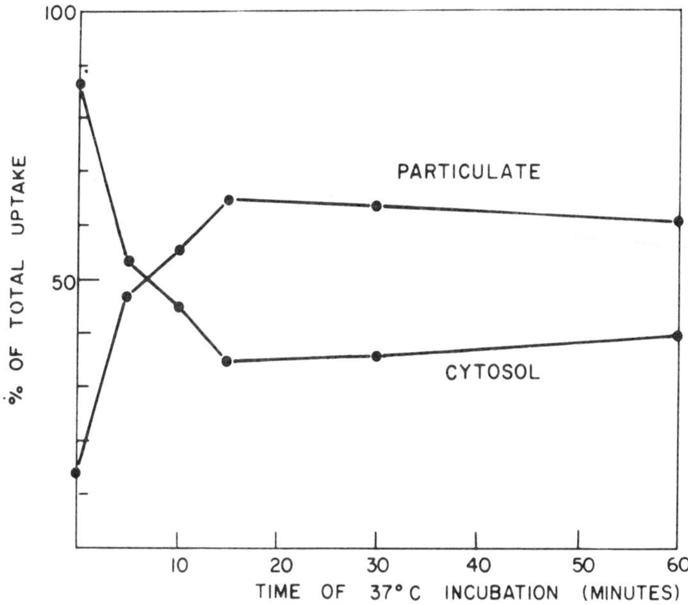


Fig. 16. The release of radioactive estradiol from cytosol into particulate fraction upon incubation at 37°C. In each group two uteri were incubated at 0°C for 1 minute in 2 ml of Eagle's medium containing 0.02 μg $^3$H-estradiol-17β. The uteri were then transferred to fresh medium without any estradiol and incubated at 37°C for various times as indicated. (From Shyamala and Gorski, 1967).

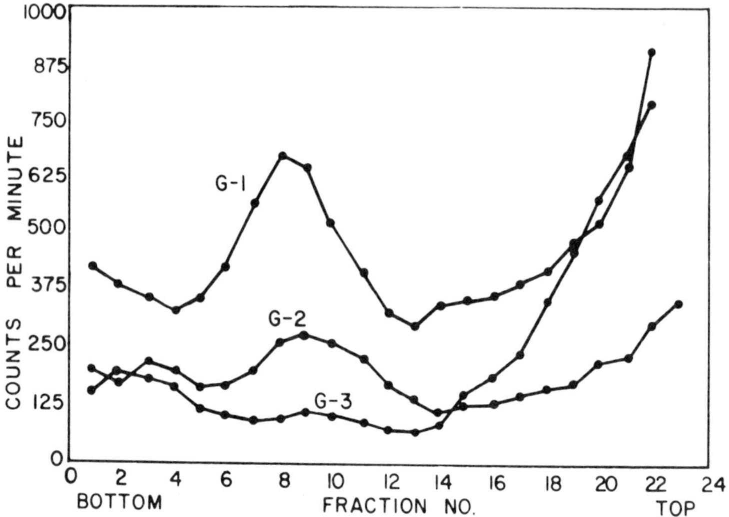


Fig. 17. Sucrose density gradient patterns of uterine cytosol. In each group four uteri were incubated at 0 °C for 1 minute, in 2 ml Eagle's medium containing 0.05 μg $^{3}$H-estradiol-17β. The uteri were then transferred to fresh medium without any estradiol and treated as follows: G-1 had no 37 °C incubation, G-2 the uteri were incubated at 37 °C for 15 minutes, G-3 the uteri were incubated at 37 °C for 1 hour. 0.2 ml samples of cytosol from each group were layered on 5-20% sucrose gradients and centrifuged at 45,000 rpm for 15 hours at 4 °C. Counting efficiency was 19-20%. Data are adjusted to represent one uterus. (Shyamala and Gorski, 1967)

## SPECULATIONS

The above data strongly supports the following model which is also illustrated in Figure 19. Estrogen administered *in vivo* likely comes to the target cells mounted on a serum albumin molecule (Westphal, U., 1961). It can readily come off this molecule and move through the cell membrane to be bound to the 9.5 S receptor. It is possible that the 9.5 S receptor is associated with the cell membranes and aids in this transport process but no evidence for such a mechanism has been obtained so far. The high affinity for estrogens of the 9.5 S receptor as compared to that of serum albumin facilitates the transfer described above. The 9.5 S receptor-estrogen complex now assumes a form which permits it to move through the nuclear membrane into the nucleus. Apparently some changes occur in the receptor at this time such that one cannot isolate from the nuclei a 9.5 S protein bound to estrogen. Salt extraction of the nuclei releases a 4-6 S protein which is bound to estrogen according to Jensen and colleagues (De Sombre *et al.*, 1967), and confirmed recently by us. This 4-6 S material is present in the clean nuclei as well as in the chromatin preparations discussed above. The high affinity of estrogen for the 9.5 S receptor, its apparent movement into the nucleus and the failure of 4-6 S fractions from untreated nuclei to bind estrogen, make us believe that the 4-6 S nuclear receptor is a product of the 9.5 S receptor. More direct proof for this model is necessary but it should prove useful as a working hypothesis for further experimentation.

The function of the 9.5 receptor in the nucleus is still open to question. It would appear that estrogen, in this case, facilitates the intracellular movement of a

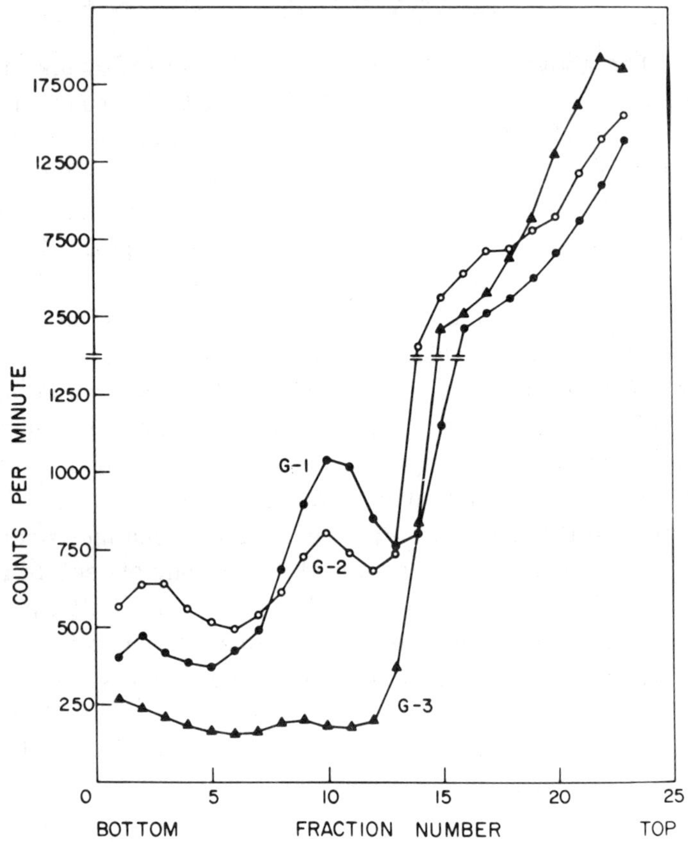
17500
12500
7500
2500
1250
1000
750
500
250
COUNTS PER MINUTE
G-1
G-2
G-3
0
5
10
15
20
25
BOTTOM
FRACTION NUMBER
TOP

complex protein. The apparent unidirectional movement into the nucleus infers some relationship of estrogen action to nuclear function. The rather constant proportion bound estrogens (30%) which remains in the cytosol may also have some specific function outside of the nucleus.

Our model is based on a single receptor but does not rule out the possibility of this receptor having more than one function. Cline and Bock (1967) have suggested that a single protein might be involved in regulation of specific gene expression, translation and enzyme activity. Such a role for the estrogen receptor is purely speculative but does represent a possibility which should be considered.

(LEFT)

Fig. 18. Sucrose density gradient patterns of uterine cytosol. Treatment of the uteri were as follows: G-1 four uteri were incubated at 37°C for 1 hour in 2 ml Eagle's medium, G-2 four uteri were incubated at 0°C for 1 minute in 2 ml Eagle's medium containing 0.05 μg $^3$H-estradiol-17β, G-3 four uteri were incubated at 0°C for 1 minute in 2 ml Eagle's medium containing 0.05 μg $^3$H-estradiol-17β and then transferred to fresh medium without estrogen and incubated for 1 hour at 37°C. In each case 0.005 μg $^3$H-estradiol-17β was added directly to 0.4 ml of cytosol. 0.2 ml samples were layered on 5-20% sucrose gradients and centrifuged at 48,000 rpm for 14 hours at 4°C. Counting efficiency was 19-20%. Data are adjusted to represent one uterus. (Shyamala, and Gorski, 1967).

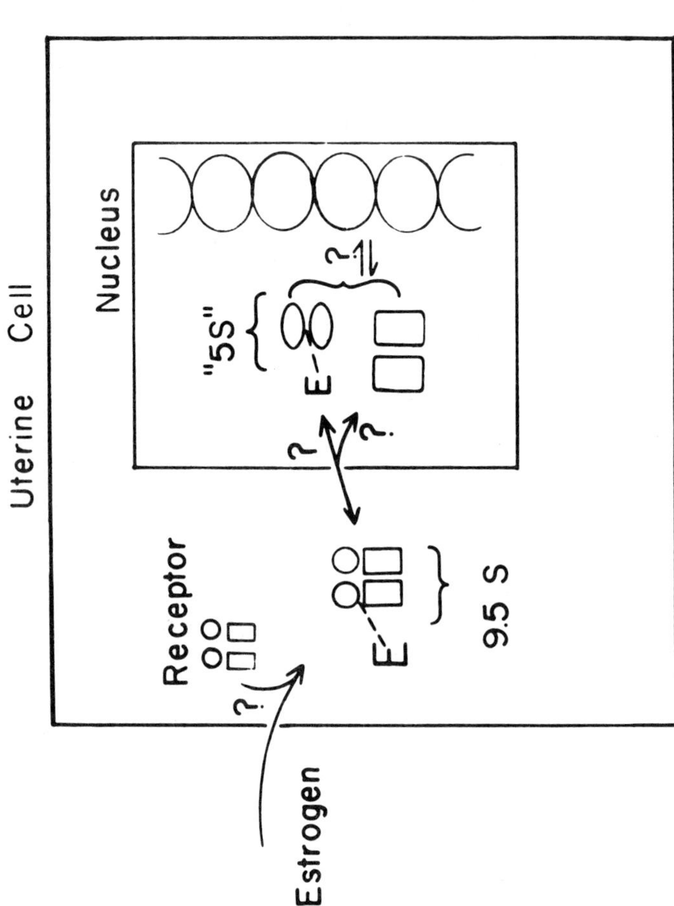


Fig. 19. Hypothetical model for estrogen interaction with uterine cell.

A considerable body of literature from a number of laboratories including own own have suggested an involvement of protein and RNA synthesis in early estrogen action. Tying these observations to the observations reported here on the estrogen receptor may result in our understanding the initial mechanism of action of estrogen. Such an understanding will then provide one foundation stone out of the many needed for the assembly of a comprehensive knowledge of the reproductive process.

## REFERENCES

1. Barry, J. and Gorski, J. (1966). Unpublished data.

2. Cline, A. L. and Bock, R. M. (1966). Translational control of gene activity. Cold Spring Harbor Symp. Quant. Biol. 31: 321-333.

3. De Sombre, E., Hurst, D., Kawashina, T., Jungblut, P., and Jensen E. V. (1967). Sulfhydryl groups and estradiol-receptor interaction. Fed. Proc. 26: 536.

4. Engel, L. L., and Scott, J. F. (1961). Mechanisms of Action of Steroid Hormones, ed. C. Villee, pp. 20-32. Pergamon Press, New York.

5. Glascock, R. F. and Hoekstra, W. G. (1959). Selective accumulation of tritium labeled hexoestrol by the reproductive organs of immature female goats and sheep. Biochem. J. 72: 673-682.

6. Jensen, E. V. and Jacobson, H. I. (1960). Fate of Steriod Estrogens in Target Tissues. In: Biological Activities of Steriods in Relation to Cancer,

ed. by G. Pincus and E. P. Vollmer, pp. 161-178, Academic Press, N. Y.

7. Jensen et al. (1962). Basic guides to the mechanism of estrogen action. Rec. Prog. Horm. Res. 18: 387-414.

8. King, R. J. B., Gordon, J. and Martin, L. (1965). The association of (6, 7-$^3$H) estradiol with nuclear chromatin. Biochem. J. 97: 28P.

9. Kostyo, J. (1966). Private Communications.

10. Noteboom, W. D. (1965). Studies on the interaction of estrogen with the rat uterus. Ph.D. thesis, University of Illinois, Urbana, Ill.

11. Noteboom, W. and Gorski, J. (1964). Sterospecific Binding of Estrogen in the Rat Uterus. Program of the Endocrine Society.

12. Noteboom et al. (1965). Sterospecific Binding of Estrogens in the Rat Uterus. Arch. Biochem. Biophys. 111: 599-568.

13. Shyamala, G. and Gorski, J. (1967). Interrelationships of Nuclear and Cytosol Estrogen Receptors. J. Cell Biol. 35: 125A-126A.

14. Stone, G. M. and Bagget, B. (1965). The in vitro uptake of tritiated-estradiol and estrone by the uterus and vagina of the ovariectomized mouse, Steroids 5: 809-826.

15. Talwar, G. P., Segal, S. J. Evans, A., and Davidson, O. W. (1964). The binding of estradiol in the rat uterus: A mechanism for derepression of RNA synthesis. Proc. Natl. Acad. Sci., U. S. 52: 1059-1066.

16. Toft, D. (1967). The Interaction of Estrogens with a Receptor Molecule from the Rat Uterus. Ph.D. thesis, University of Illinois.

17. Toft, D. and Gorski, J. (1965). A receptor protein for estrogens: Its isolation and preliminary characterization. J. Cell Biol. 27: 107A.

18. Toft et al. (1966). A receptor molecule for estrogens: Isolation from the rat uterus and preliminary characterization. Proc. Natl. Acad. Sci., U. S., 55: 1574.

19. Toft, D., Shyamala, G. and Gorski, J. (1967). A receptor molecule for estrogens: Studies using a cell free system. Proc. Natl. Acad. Sci., U. S. 57: 1740-1743.

20. Ts'o P.O.P. and Lu, P. (1964). Interaction of nucleic acids I. Physical Binding of Thymine, Adenine, Steroids and Aromatic Hydrocarbons to Nucleic Acids Proc. Natl. Acad. Sci., U. S. 51: 17-24.

21. Westphal, U. (1961). Interactions between steroids and proteins. In: Mechanism of Action of Steroid Hormones, ed. by C. A. Villee and L. L. Engel, pp. 33-83, Pergamon Press, N. Y.

## DISCUSSION

H. R. Lindner: I last heard an account of Dr. Gorski's work about three months ago, and again I enjoyed very much hearing his presentation. The story has become infinitely more complex over these three months; this study is progressing really at a tremendous pace.

There is no doubt that Dr. Gorski's group, and Dr. Jensen's, have unequivocally demonstrated the presence of specific receptors for estrogens in uterine tissue. As Dr. Gorski mentioned, we have all been talking for many years about "receptors", but we were always inclined to put these in quotation marks because no one had ever seen a receptor; what Dr. Gorski is actually engaged in is to remove these quotation marks at last, i.e. to characterize these molecules. This work also gives rise to thoughts about the physiological significance of the intracellular estrogen receptor.

We have become used to think of estrogen target tissues, and generally of target organs of hormones, as tissues that respond by increased cell growth and accelerated cell division to the presentation of hormones. It may be more useful, perhaps, to think of them as tissues that atrophy in the absence of the hormone. In other words, the peculiar thing about them is that maybe in the course of differentiation they have either lost a factor essential for growth, or acquired an inhibitor which prevents normal growth except in the continuous presence of a specific hormone; the hormone then, may be assumed either to restore such a growth factor or to block this putative inhibitor or repressor, if you like. Dr. Tausk earlier referred to the longing of the human mind for simplicity, and it is tempting to think that the receptor Dr. Gorski has demonstrated, this 9.5 S component or maybe a derivative thereof, is acting as such an inhibitor, and that the association of the receptor with estrogen might remove this inhibition. Alternatively, the 9.5 S receptor may merely have a transport function; perhaps something analogous to a permease system, facilitating hormone uptake; or perhaps shuttling estrogen from the cytoplasm to the nucleus. At present we can only speculate about these possibilities.

One of the curious things about the biochemical approach is that we have acquired information about the detailed subcellular distribution of estrogen on uterine cells and even the approximate molecular weight of the receptor, before knowing precisely which cells actually take up the estrogen and contain the specific receptors. Some of this information is being filled in now. I can perhaps relate some gossip I acquired on my way back from the States when visiting Jensen's laboratory where they have done some beautiful radioautographic studies [See E. V. Jensen, E. R. De Sombre and P. W. Jungblut in Endogenous Factors Influencing Host-Tumor Balance, R. W. Wissler, T. L. Dao and S. Wood, Jr., eds., University of Chicago Press, 1967, p. 15]. There is some discrepancy between the results of these studies and the *in vitro* results we heard about. The radioactivity due to tritiated estradiol seems to be largely concentrated in the nucleus, particularly near the nuclear membrane, whereas after tissue fractionation, one usually finds almost half of the activity in the soluble fraction. I would like to have Dr. Gorski's opinion on this. Dr. Jensen seemed to feel that this receptor is really associated with the nuclear membrane and that during fractionation, some of it is invariably detached and enters the supernatant fraction. One reason that makes him think this is related to the technical question that Dr. von Euler raised about the method of homogenization. The uterus, being very muscular, requires fairly rough methods for homogenization. Dr. Jensen's group has also been working with mammary tumours induced with dimethylbenzanthracene, and these being of much softer tissue can be homogenized by very mild methods; in this preparation they always get 85 to 90 per cent of the activity associated with the nuclear fraction and very little activity in the soluble fraction. There are other interesting features about these mammary tumours; the estrogen receptor appears to be present in those tumours that are hormone dependent and seems to be lost in those that acquired autonomy. This observation could be useful too for predicting whether tumours are going to respond to surgical hormone deprivation.

This question about the relation between the nuclear receptor and the one in the soluble fraction is still a puzzling one to all concerned. There seem to be points of similarity between the two, for instance, sulfhydryl-blocking agents abolish the affinity to estrogen in either case [E. V. Jensen, D. J. Hurst, E. R. DeSombre and P. W. Jungblut, Science, 158, 385, 1967; L. Terenius, Mol. Pharmacol. 3, 423, 1967], but this may not be a very specific feature. (Note added in proof: In recent reports from two different laboratories, evidence was presented that the 9.5 S receptor plays a role in the nuclear binding of estradiol and may in fact give rise to the 5 S receptor as Dr. Gorski has suggested [P. I. Brecher, R. Vigersky, H. S. Wotiz and H. H. Wotiz, Steroids, 10, 635, 1967; E. V. Jensen, T. Suzuki, T. Kawashima, W. E. Stumpf, P. W. Jungblut and E. R. DeSombre, Proc. Nat. Acad. Sci., 59, 632, 1968]).

Regarding the specificity of these receptors, I might perhaps add one snippet of information from my former laboratory in Sydney. Mr. Shutt recently found that a plant estrogen, genistein is able to displace estradiol from vaginal receptors. This is an isoflavone, not a steroid, but bears some resemblance to the mammalian estrogens in being a phenol, in the special relationship between its free hydroxyl groups, and in stimulating uterine growth.

In any pioneer study, one obviously looks for the simplest system to work with, for example, the castrated or immature animal. There are, however, very important physiological interactions between estrogens and progesterone, and one of the things we would like to examine is the behavior of the uterine estrogen receptor in intact animals, perhaps, during progestation, or in delayed implantation.

R. W. Schayer: I have a bias, so I will get back to microcirculation for a bit. I think the work is perfectly beautiful. The only thing I'd like to point out is, that I've been told that there is hyperemia within

30 to 45 seconds after injection of estrogen. Have you tried to find the evidence for the receptor complex at such an early time?

J. Gorski: Well, you are talking about one minute incubations of estrogen.

R. W. Schayer: Yes, but that's just in vitro. Do you think there would be no decent way to kill an animal almost immediately after injection and working at low temperatures?

J. Gorski: The trouble is you would never really know what happens after an in vivo injection because the binding occurs in a cell-free system. When the tissue is taken out you'd never be able to say whether the steriod is bound or not. Maybe you could say it was bound in nuclei. I don't think we can ignore the microcirculation, but, on the other hand, I question its importance in early estrogen action. A lot of work suggests that estrogen stimulation of uptake doesn't occur as fast as other responses.

R. W. Schayer: It just occurred to me about calling this a receptor, wouldn't it be safer to call this a binding site? I mean, shouldn't the term "receptor" be saved for the point at which estrogen exerts its action?

J. Gorski: I think this is just a matter of semantics, like the term target tissues. I've heard people say we shouldn't call them target tissues. I remember reading about Pincus scolding Jensen because he used the term "target tissue". Well, when I said target tissue, you knew what I meant. When I said receptor, it's obvious I'm defining it in a sense by my own work. I think we have been extremely cautious in what we call receptors, but the binding agent fits all the criteria we can think of. At the present time, the term receptor has no specific meaning. No one really knows what one is and we are trying to use the term as carefully as we can.

R. W. Schayer: We think of a receptor as something at which the drug hits or triggers something, whereas you might be measuring a storage depot or something like this. Maybe, it is desirable for the animal to keep some estrogen around for a while and use a tiny amount at any one time and you've got a specific protein for that.

J. Gorski: I have heard that objection raised before. It's my own feeling that this is not likely and that the binding is to a receptor. I'll take the chance on being wrong.

R. W. Schayer: One more point. I think if I am right in quoting you, you mentioned that the edema caused by estrogen in uterus can be blocked by cortisone but all the rest of the process will go on, and that was cited as evidence against the primary microcirculatory effect.

J. Gorski: Yes, if you are associating water response with microcirculation.

R. W. Schayer: Okay. The point I want to make there is that edema depends on two factors, first relaxation of the sphincters and second, intraendothelial gaps so that protein molecules get out and hold water. Now, if in the uterus, corticoids block the swelling and pulling apart of the endothelial cells, then you would get no edema but you could certainly have expanding microcirculatory system, so these changes could still be secondary to an accumulation of metabolites. I don't think that's good evidence against Clara Szego's theory.

J. Gorski: There is no evidence that really rules it out, but on the other hand, there is no good evidence to rule it in.

R. W. Schayer: In the first place, in the rat, you always have to worry about 5-hydroxytryptamine right along with histamine because it's more potent and does essentially the same thing when released from mast cells. To me the microcirculatory mechanism is extraordinarily attractive because I see no difficulty whatsoever to get 10,000 reactions from one primary action on microcirculation; I do find it very difficult to envisage what a hormone entering the nucleus could possibly do there which would explain all these later changes.

J. Gorski: There are a lot of examples, but a good one is provided by a mutant strain of a certain yeast. All the genetic evidence suggests that a single point mutation with a change in one protein is the only difference from the wild type. If you were to look at pictures of the two strains, you wouldn't even think that they were related. Their gross morphology is completely different. It turns out that glucose-6-phosphate dehydrogenase is the enzyme which differs in the mutant strain. The physical appearance and, apparently much of the physiology is different due to a mutation affecting a single protein.

R. W. Schayer: Is there to your knowledge any primary inducer of enzymes other than a sort of metabolite, in other words, anything else really proven?

J. Gorski: As I said, in the case of hormones, there might be. This is only a possibility. No one really knows what a hormone does, so one cannot say.

R. W. Schayer: I don't know too much of that field, but generally isn't it a response to a normal metabolite?

J. Gorski: But it doesn't have to be a metabolite.

H. R. Lindner: It can be something that the organism has never seen before.

J. Gorski: I think the point about whether all of the estrogen is in the nucleus or associated closely with the nucleus is interesting. There are a couple of different reports suggesting different ratios, and I'm not sure which one is right and which one is wrong, but I'd tend to believe Jensen before I believe conflicting data, in most cases. The fact that he finds a lot of estrogen around the periphery of the nucleus is also interesting.

There is no reason, from what we have seen, why the receptor couldn't be there initially. I don't think it's inside the nucleus, though, because it would be pretty hard to explain the difference between incubation at 0° and at 37° on the basis simply of the 9.5 S receptor coming out during homogenization.

H. R. Linder: There would seem to be two possible interpretations of your results: On the one hand, at zero degrees, estradiol may be so tightly bound to the 9.5 S receptor that it is not readily passed on to the nuclear receptor. On the other hand, the transfer to the intranuclear site may require some metabolic activity [cf. Jensen et al., Proc. Nat. Acad. Sci., 59, 632, 1968].

J. Gorski: I don't know what is going on except that it is apparently unaffected by cyanide or by absence of oxygen and yet it is affected by temperatures. Jensen has some slightly conflicting data, but I don't know quite the whole story. That the receptor is more closely associated with the nuclear membranes is a possibility. Jensen's theory depends a great deal on his radioautographs which I have not seen as yet.

G. J. Marcus: One distinct virtue to the model that you propose, Dr. Gorski, is that it offers a rational explanation to a problem which I suppose many of us have wondered about ever since Jensen showed that estradiol is not used up or transformed in the uterus in any way. That is, if estradiol is not inactivated, how is it that it doesn't go on acting? Why is it, when you give one injection you get a certain response, a response lasting for a limited period? Your model offers an explanation. There wouldn't be any more receptor, the 9.5 S material, to take the hormonal into the place where it really acts. The receptor supply would be exhausted in binding estradiol and thus it may be the primary carrier-receptor which is used up or inactivated rather than the hormone.

J. Gorski: I think that under in vivo conditions this is probably replenished.

G. J. Marcus: Agreed, but the question really is then, how rapidly?

J. Gorski: I have no direct evidence that would answer your question. If one accepts our interpretation of the existing data, it appears that the 9.5 S binding agent moves into the nucleus, where it becomes the 5 S nuclear receptor. The 5 S material cannot bind estrogen by itself. Therefore, the 9.5 S material would have to be regenerated, by synthesis or some other process. We think this regeneration is going on rather continuously under in vivo conditions because there always appears to be some 9.5 S receptor present in the cytosol.

G. J. Marcus: But, in your in vivo work, have you not always used immature rats in which the 9.5 S protein would not have been depleted, or else, ovariectomized rats in which the interval between ovariectomy and experimental treatment would have been sufficient to allow replacement or regeneration?

All that would be necessary in order that there be no perpetually continued response to a single dose of estrogen is that the receptor, the 9.5 S protein be replaced or regenerated more slowly than the estrogen diffuses out of the uterus after being released from its site of action, presumably the chromatin, and is cleared from the circulation by the liver where it is inactivated.

J. Gorski: This seems reasonable. However, *in vivo* we probably never saturate the 9.5 S receptor. This would mean that some 9.5 S receptor should always be present in the cytosol, even after estrogen treatment.

P. F. Kraicer: Surely, one of the most relevant questions concerning the action of estrogen on the uterus relates to the fact that the uterus consists of three tissues, the myometrium, the endometrium, and the epithelium, which, may very well be totally dissimilar in their responses to estrogen. Thus autoradiographic studies with tritiated estradiol are important because they may indicate the cellular and tissue elements which accumulate estrogen. At least one study [A. Attramadel, *Acta Endocr.* (Kbh.) Suppl. *100*, 198 1965] showed by autoradiography abundant labelling of luminal and glandular epithelium, though radioactivity was also found in the stromal cells and in the muscle cells of the myometrium. The labelling was found over the nuclei as well as over the cytoplasm of the cells. The question, therefore, is whether studies like those of Dr. Gorski would not yield even more information if performed on a single uterine tissue.

Recently, Mr. Chikashi Tachi, in our department, has been studying a particular enzyme system of the endometrium. He has found that endometrial tissue can be scraped off very nicely with a semi-sharp scalpel blade after opening the uterus by slitting it lengthwise. The scrapings are so soft that they can almost be homogenized with a glass rod by stirring vigorously in a test tube. Since the endometrial response to estrogen is the one which interests us more than the myometrial, we would be very interested in finding out whether the receptors you have characterized in extracts are exclusively endometrial or otherwise.

J. Gorski: Work along these lines has been done by others and there appears to be some disagreement. We presume that in the uterus of the immature rat, the bulk of myometrium is so large that in comparison the amount of endometrium is negligible. We have read one study in which the endometrium was scraped off and there was a higher concentration of $^3$H estrogen in the endometrium, but the total amount of radioactivity was greater in the myometrium. Jensen has more or less found the same thing. We have found the 9.5 S receptor in both the myometrium and endometrium of sheep uteri, but these were preliminary experiments and we can't really say much about them. We know from electron microscopic studies that myometrium responds to estrogen just as fast as endometrium and, therefore, I would guess that estrogen should be present in both places.

P. F. Kraicer: Nevertheless, the uterus is three distinct organs stuck together. It's an epithelium; it's an endometrium and it's a myometrium, and I don't think it's particularly fair to talk of responses of the uterus to a hormone. You must think of responses of the epithelium, of the endometrium, and of the myometrium. I wonder whether turning them all into mashed meat and extracting from this a component, is going to give the best possible answer from a physiological point of view.

J. Gorski: I agree it's a problem, but I haven't figured out the solution.

M. C. Shelesnyak: Incidentally, the uptake of both progesterone and estrogen by the pituitary is a fascinating bit of confusion.

J. Gorski: Yes, this is really interesting. It would be even more so if this could be used as technique for finding out where these hormones work. Generally, people think the pituitary is not as involved in feedback regulation as much as the hypothalamus, but the pituitary binds estrogens in extremely large amounts. It is all right to suggest storage depots and such, but I feel there must be something more significant to this.

S. Lamprecht: One basic assumption in your work is that for any biochemical effect of estrogen, there must first be estrogen binding to the receptor. What is the earliest time you can demonstrate this binding <u>in vivo</u>?

J. Gorski: As I have said, this is a difficult thing to determine. From all the <u>in vitro</u> work, I'd say it happens as soon as the estrogen gets to the tissue. With the high affinities we find, I can't imagine that it's anything but instantaneous, at least in the cytoplasmic fraction. There seems to be a little delay in getting to the nuclear fraction, but judging from the number of molecules we actually find in vivo, the time for those to get in probably wouldn't be very long. In the whole cell incubations, we are trying to get higher concentrations than you would normally expect to find. In the first five minutes, the uptake is pretty rapid and then it slows down.

S. Lamprecht: I raised this question because there is some work by Means and Hamilton [A. R. Means and A. H. Hamilton, Proc. Nat. Acad. Aci., 56, 1594, 1966] showing that within two minutes there is already RNA synthesis, increased incorporation of radioactive precursors into RNA, so it would be interesting to know whether in this short time you have binding with the receptor.

J. Gorski: All our work presumes that the estrogen response starts immediately. Because of technical problems, the earliest response that we have observed is at 15 minutes. This is the synthesis of a specific protein that, by 15 minutes is just as great as it is by 3 or 4 hours. I mean, synthesis is maximally stimulated by 15 minutes. We have never really done the intervening times, because it's just too difficult to handle enough rats in that kind of experiment. But, if you have a maximum at 15 minutes, it is probable that the induction was initiated about the time the estrogen was reaching the uterus.

S. Lamprecht: You believe that your receptor is a protein in nature, and I think most of your data came from proteolytic enzymes, i.e. in the presence of trypsin or pronase, but if I remember well you didn't determine whether the proteolytic activity of the enzymes parallels the release of the estrogen from the receptor. Is that true? Several studies have shown that estradiol can be bound for proteins such as albumin, hemoglobin, lysozme, ribonuclease and so on, so could there not have just been displacement of estradiol in the presence of the enzymes without the receptors actually being attacked?

J. Gorski: No, we've checked this with trypsin inhibitor and by inactivating trypsin with heat. Trypsin is denatured so that there is very little activity; but, it causes trouble because it starts renaturing as soon as you bring it back to a normal temperature.

S. Lamprecht: What pH did you use, since you point out that the optimum for binding is pH7?

H. Gorski: Right, or in that region. But, we didn"t use trypsin at its optimal pH but rather, near neutrality.

M. C. Shelesnyak: Talking about trypsin, one of my former students, Dr. Varavudhi, observed that in the hypophysectomized, pregnant rat which had intact ovaries, but was in a state of delayed implantation, the administration of trypsin parenterally apparently released enough estrogen, assuming estrogen to be the essential requirement, so that the animal's blastocysts implanted.

J. Gorski: Another point to consider is that even if we didn't have the trypsin data, I would say, because of the binding affinities and the sterospecificity, that a protein is involved. There has been a suggestion that the serotonin receptor is a polysaccharide, but the affinities and specificity reported are nothing like what we find.

H. R. Lindner: According to Jensen, the nuclear estradiol-receptor is a protein containing phosphorus. This is the receptor isolated from an estradiol-aminobenzylcellulose-conjugate column [Jensen et al. in Endogenous Factors Influencing Host-Tumor Balance, R. W. Wissler, T. L. Dao and S. Wood, Jr. eds., University of Chicago Press, 1967, p. 15].

J. Gorski: I am not sure of the relationship of that material to the 9.5 S binding agent. I haven't seen this work so that I cannot comment. But is certainly is possible that other components, such as RNA, are part of the receptor.

S. Lamprecht: Have you tried incubating the complex with urea to check for hydrogen bonding and have you tried incubation with periodate to detect carbohydrate components?

J. Gorski: We've never tried periodate, but urea has been checked out. At high concentrations of urea there is no binding, but that's not really surprising because urea denatures proteins, particularly when there are subunits. Almost anything that denatures pi uteins affects the receptor. The same holds true with respect to the action of sulfhydrul-blocking compounds. I don't feel their action is very informative because sulfhydryl reagents affect very many proteins.

S. Lamprecht: Is there any evidence that the receptor is a histone-like protein?

J. Gorski: That would be interesting but there's no evidence for or against this as far as I know. When we first obtained the trypsin data, we also wondered about this. The real problem, however, is that we don't have enough receptor to analyze. The receptor is susceptible to trypsin attack, but then any protein that has a trypsin sensitive link in a key place would be inactivated.

C. Tachi: If I understood you correctly, you homogenize the uterus in a tris-buffer EDTA solution. If you change the ionic composition or the ionic strength, is the dissociation constant affected?

J. Gorski: Sometimes we used just plain water but in general we use two basic media. One, our old standard medium is Winnek's medium which is more or less a physiological salt solution, KCl, tris and magnesium and that gave essentially the same results as the others. The routine medium is the tris-EDTA. This, if anything, gets rid of a little more protein from the soluble fraction, but leaves essentially the same amount of receptor.

C. Tachi: You have referred to estrogen stimulated synthesis of soluble protein. Is there any correlation between the soluble protein and control of translation?

J. Gorski: This is the synthesis that is maximally stimulated by 15 minutes. We don't know of any relationship although we have considered the possibility of a relationship to the receptor protein. However, the induced protein has been calculated to be roughly one per cent of the soluble proteins and this would be too much for it to be the receptor which we estimate to be only one ten thousandth of the total uterine protein.

H. R. Linder: Since you have mentioned this component, which is really a subject in itself, I am curious to hear your current view of its signficance. This seems to revive the idea that the steroid hormone induces specific depression of a particular cistron and synthesis of one specific protein. Dr. Liao's work [S. Liao, R. W. Barton and A. N. Lin, Proc. Nat. Acad. Sci., 55, 1593, 1966] with testosterone and the prostate seems to suggest that this is not what happens in his system at least. He is getting mainly stimulation of nucleolar synthesis, prooably of ribosomal RNA precursors.

J. Gorski: We have been saying this since 1963, that there is a general increase in RNA synthesis in which, obviously, ribosomal RNA is the one major component. But, no one yet has been able to say anything about specific RNA, because the procedures are not good enough. In other words, if you have a change of one part in a hundred in RNA, it cannot be detected. If you had change of one new segment of RNA on a genome, this won't be only one part in a hundred, but more likely one part in 20,000 to 50,000. You can't eliminate the possibility of a small change. All we can say, at present, is that there is good evidence that RNA synthesis in general and particualrly ribosomal RNA synthesis are turned on. This is fine, because later on there is a big increase in the number of ribosomes, which, by electron microscopy, can be seen moving out of the nucleus after six hours. This is reflected in an increase in general protein synthesis, but as for specific RNA synthesis, we don't have adequate data at the present time. We find synthesis of a specific protein but we are unable to say how the RNA synthesis affects it. It is not affected by actinomycin-D, as other responses are. This is where I think we have to look now in all studies of hormone actions. We have to get down to specifics. Measuring radioisotope incorporation into total RNA or protein is meaningless. One has to fractionate these macromolecules in some way, but it's difficult, particularly in the case of RNA.

R. W. Schayer: You wanted me to do that, the other day, in a rat's paw.

J. Gorski: No, I wanted you to find out whether actinomycin-D really blocked RNA synthesis in your system. We know that when we inject 200 micrograms of actinomycin-D into a 50 g rat, it will not block RNA synthesis in the ovary by more than 50 percent. I don't know about paws.

M. Tausk: Dr. Gorski said something about the controversy regarding the hypothalamus and the pituitary, and which one binds the estrogens. I just wanted to say that although it is usually maintained that the feedback action acts at the hypothalamus, there is the work of Bogdanove [E. M. Bogdanove, _Endocrinology_, _73_, 696, 1963] who says it does act at the pituitary level. The hypothalamus, in his opinion, is such a good site for this action only because from there the estrogen gets into the pituitary so easily. Attramadal, who was just cited here, assumes that the feedback acts both on the pituitary and on the hypothalamus. That's just a side issue.

J. Gorski: Yes, I think there is some other evidence. Everyone has swung so much to the hypothalamus that I think we've forgotten some of the data for the other level.

A. Barnea: Your studies with the _in vitro_ and _in vivo_ binding to the receptor showed similar results. I wonder whether it is really only estradiol 17-beta which will act on the uterus. For example, Mueller [G. C. Mueller, _Nature_, _176_, 127, 1955] reported that when he measured incorporation of $^{14}C$-formate into protein _in vitro_, in tissue slices, he got increased incorporation only with 2-hydroxy or 4-hydroxy estradiol. He didn't get any effects with estradiol or estrone. Would you comment on this?

J. Gorski: I'm good at negatives. We have never been able to duplicate some of these studies, but perhaps our technique was faulty.

U. S. von Euler: Have you ever found any inhibitor which would prevent the formation of the 9.5 S complex that might possibly give some clue about the binding site?

J. Gorski: Other than these things that denature proteins, no. We have tried actinomycin-D and puromycin in the whole tissue incubation and they had no effect. We also tried some metabolic inhibitors and they did not affect it. The only thing that affected the movement of estrogen into the nucleus has been reducing the temperature. Nothing that I know of affects the uptake into the 9.5 S material except other steroids or protein denaturants.

P. F. Kraicer: Why haven't you tried MER-25?

J. Gorski: That's been done, but what good does it do? It's just another competitor. I can do it with unlabelled estradiol-17-beta or DES. It's just another competitive binder. You need some way to follow the receptor other than just by its estrogen binding. We have one idea that we are going to try.

S. Lamprecht: You mean you would like a compound with a covalent bond in order to rule out the reversibility of the reaction?

J. Gorski: No, so that you have an estrogen covalently linked to the receptor to enable you to follow it wherever it goes even if it changes form. If it's a big protein that breaks into sub-units, you could tell. If it really is migrating in to the nucleus, you could also tell. Probably a lot better job could be done in radioautographic experiments if covalently fixed steriods were used.

S. Lamprecht: You don't have any details on the energy involved in the binding of receptors?

J. Gorski: It works in the cold but nothing else is known at present.

M. C. Shelesnyak: I'm curious; whether any of you who work on this problem and use various target tissues, for the study of tissue response, plan to investigate the perineal or facial tissues as tissues responsive to estrogen.

J. Gorski: Well, I don't plan to but I think there are a lot of these things that bear investigation.

M. C. Shelesnyak: I think it would be very revealing because it's a rather different tissue but, nevertheless, shows a marked response, which, I believe, is even evident in lower animal forms. I think such a study would be a very revealing for comparison because these tissues are more uniform in response than the uterus, but nevertheless, are responsive.

J. Gorski: My philosophy in my own research is that there are certain problems we should aim for and that other people who are better set up to handle certain patterns should carry out such studies.

M. C. Shelesnyak: I agree with you on that.

J. Gorski: I think the problem is interesting though, and techniques such as use of the cell-free system may be useful in studying it. A lot of work can now be done in the human, because there are few problems in obtaining biopsy samples of human tissues in order to confirm some of these observations.

M. C. Shelesnyak: When you take scrapings of human endometrium, you should at least be aware that different portions of the uterus, even of endometrium, in the human represent different tissues and you may be complicating your problem.

J. Gorski: What would be interesting would be to compare the distribution of the 9.5 S component in different tissues which respond to estrogen. Is it the same compound?

H. R. Linder: How much is known about this?

J. Gorski: It is the same in vagina and in the immature rat oviduct, so far. We don't find any difference. Also, Jensen reports binding in the mammary tumor.

P. F. Kraicer: I have often wondered why no one ever looked at the biochemistry of one of the curious genital tissues of the rat, namely, the membrane that closes the vagina until puberty. Its response to estrogen, rather than growth, is to wither away and die. It gets white before it perforates, which is never a very healthy sign for a tissue. Exogenous estrogen administration results in its disappearance.

G. J. Marcus: While we are talking about puzzling actions of estradiol, I wonder if Dr. Schayer would comment on a recent report of pharmacological quantities of estradiol conferring protection in the rat against endotoxin shock [J. P. Nolan, Nature, 213, 201, 1967].

R. W. Schayer: I wouldn't particularly want to comment. I hadn't heard about that. But, a lot of things protect against endotoxin on Tuesday and Wednesday but not the rest of the week. I just imagine if you have huge amounts of any steriod that may sit down on the capillaries, it will protect them. I'm just guessing.

M. C. Shelesnyak: I'd like to ask Prof. Gorski if he would be prepared to comment on the nature of what we call priming estrogen in building up uterine responsiveness or sensitivity to subsequent stimulation.

J. Gorski: I would guess that God has done this for more reason than just to entertain you and me. I presume that this response of the estrogen involves the development and formation of structures or components which are available when progesterone comes along. I don't want to put it in a more specific way because I don't know if specific molecules are involved or maybe it's just a matter of preparing the cells in a general way. It's too bad we can't get at progesterone receptors so that one could find the sequence in which these things occur.

M. C. Shelesnyak: I think that one of the reasons is that up to now progesterone hasn't been quite as fashionable, nor apparently, as easy to study as estrogen is.

J. Gorski: Actually, Walter Wiest was doing the same thing with progesterone even before Jensen. He did all the right experiments and looked for progesterone in the uterus. He was one of the few people I know of whom at the time were doing metabolic studies with steroid hormones and didn't stop at the liver. He did look in the uterus at different times, with and without deciduomata in one horn. Unfortunately, he found little evidence for anything different in localization by the uterus as compared to other tissues [D. L. Berliner and W. G. Wiest, J. Biol. Chem., 221, 449, 1956; W. G. Wiest, J. Biol. Chem., 235, 94, 1963].

If you think of the amounts of progesterone needed to produce a response in comparison with estrogen, it is very likely that the affinity for progesterone is very much lower and therefore, biochemically, it's going to be a much tougher problem to work with. I think it may still be able to be done, but it may take some tricks. Or it may be a matter of using different progestational agents, with a much higher affinity. If you can find a progestational agent that is much more effective may be this means it binds with a much higher affinity.

M. C. Shelesnyak: May I suggest that rather than looking for progestational agents, you look at the corpus luteum for a solution. It's probably much easier. Can Prof. Tausk enlighten us a little bit about the future of progesterone?

M. Tausk: I will try to touch on the point tomorrow in my paper.

C. Tachi: There is a lot of speculation and some experimental data that the estrogens and progesterones have an effect on the cellular membrane and active transport. But, in the case of the estrogen, it is very unlikely that the estrogen is so distributed as to affect the cell membrane itself directly, because of the small amounts of estrogen and the low affinity for the membrane. In the case of progesterone, for example, Seeman showed that erythrocytes can be stabilized very nicely by progesterone, rather higher amounts compared to the usual in vivo concentrations, but still, of the steroid hormones, it has a very nice stabilizing effect, reducing hypotonic lysis of the cells [P. Seeman, Int. Rev. Neurobiol, 91, 145, 1966]. I don't know whether this can be interpreted in terms of an effect on uterine cells because Seeman's experiment using the erythrocytes was based on the assumption that the cellular membrane more or less has a similar structure to that of erythrocytes. In the case of the progesterone, I think there is a possibility that progesterone can directly affect the membrane structure itself.

J. Gorski: I worry about that kind of experiment; I'm not familiar with it, but again because of the question of polarity, progesterone is a difficult compound to work with in binding experiments. It may be possible, if you had a control steroid which was very non-polar, to show some specificity for the progestational steroid. I know of nothing that rules out membrane or permeability effects in progesterone action.

We have been studying glucose metabolism in the uterus where the estrogen effect is very dramatic and early. Our present data suggest that estrogen stimulates either glucose transport or phosphorylation. It looks as though it stimulates the synthesis of the rate limiting protein that is involved. Our most recent data suggest that it is probably synthesis of a key transport or phosphorylating molecule.

C. Tachi: In our own experience we have found a fluctuation in the activity of the sodium-potassium dependent transport APTase during the estrous cycle with a maximum at proestrus and a minimum at diestrus. But, in the case of amino acid transport using amino-isobutyrate, it's interesting that _in vivo_ treatment with estrogen stimulates the amine acid uptake _in vitro_, but if you add estrogen to the incubation medium you get conflicting results.

J. Gorski: This is an area which hasn't been explored too well. I don't want to support Dr. Schayer too much, but I don't think we know how to incubate whole tissues properly at the present time and get completely physiological conditions. This may very well be why estrogen or some other hormones do not work under _in vitro_ conditions. As an example, we know that in the uterus estrogen stimulates RNA synthesis. You can measure this _in vivo_ and with isolated nuclei, but if you take whole tissues and incubate them you find no effect of _in vivo_ pretreatment with estrogen on _in vitro_ RNA synthesis. It's odd, but it disappears.

M. C. Shelesnyak: That's one of the acts of God.

S. Katsh: That's the third time that God's name has been invoked here. What are we doing?

G. J. Marcus: About 10 years ago, Hechter reported some experiments, attempts to get some responses to ACTH from isolated, perfused adrenal glands, and found that in general the tissue did not respond to added ACTH during incubation unless the tissue were preincubated with blood or serum. He was able to correlate some of the differences in the behavior of the tissue with degenerative processes which took place in the tissue if serum were not added to the medium [O. Hechter, Cancer Res., 17, 512, 1957; J. Luft and O. Hechter, J. Biophys. Biochem. Cytol., 3, 615, 1957].

J. Gorski: In the case of uterus, this has been done. Cells and whole tissues have been incubated under conditions of cell culture with serum present. We don't routinely add it; however, Mueller did this many times. It's interesting that the longer you incubate the uterus, the greater the rate of RNA and protein synthesis is in the controls. By 12 hours the control is functioning as well as the estrogen-treated.

G. J. Marcus: Well, Hechter's findings could explain this kind of response on the basis of degenerating barriers to nutrients or dissolution of restrictive intracellular organization.

J. Gorski: I think this is a matter of nutrition. In other words, we don't really understand the nutrition and isolated cells in culture.

G. J. Marcus: Or ultimately permeability.

J. Gorski: Or whatever it is.

P. F. Kraicer: Or microcirculation.

G. J. Marcus: No, I wouldn't go that far.

M. C. Shelesnyak: Not with Dick around, at any rate.

B. L. Lobel: We made an observation which I'd like to ask you to comment on. We treated some ovariectomized rats with estrogen about four weeks after ovariectomy and killed them about a week later. Now, in cases where the animals received about 0.2 μg of estrogen, the estrogen effects were gone within a week. In some cases, we gave 10 micrograms, and in these animals estrogen's effects were still apparent in the uterus seven, eight, and nine days later, particularly in the height of the epithelium and the state of the glands. How would you explain this in terms of your hypothesis?

J. Gorski: I can only tell you that what we think occurs there. Remember that when you inject the steroid, a very small percentage gets into the uterus, but it's distributed throughout all the rest of the tissues, particularly in the fat depots. If you look in the fat depots, you'll find at least a certain amount of steroid present there for a little longer period of time than in other places. I don't know of any data in the case of estrogen, but I know there is nice data on this in the case of progesterone. I think that the more you give, obviously, the more will be stored in fat depots to trickle back slowly into the blood stream. This is my rationalization but, obviously, it would have to be verified experimentally.

M. C. Shelesnyak: We are approaching a rather treacherous area. For, in fact, large doses of most hormones, in general, have a tendency to do exactly the opposite of what the small, physiological, doses do. And here if one is proposing that what you really do by administering a large dose is to supply or simply make available a mechanical pool or reservoir as a depot for slow secretion over a period of a time, if large doses did act thus, then all the searching for long or slow-acting hormones would be unnecessary. Just give a massive dose and wait. I don't think history has borne out this approach as an effective method.

J. Gorski: I think there is some evidence for this with progesterone. That would be my rationalization at this point. I have no facts.

M. C. Shelesnyak: Progesterone is a particularly good example against my argument.

M. Tausk: I am not so sure. Certainly there is a difference in the duration of action, say, between progesterone and 17-hydroxy progesterone esters like the enanthate or the other esters with prolonged action. It is certainly not only a matter of dose, and giving a large dose of progesterone is not the same as giving perhaps a smaller dose of long-acting ester.

H. R. Linder: With plant estrogens at least, it is our experience that these do accumulate and may be retained for a long time.

J. Gorski: They are more polar.

H. R. Lindner: Yes, they are more polar. There is the additional problem with plant estrogens that after prolonged exposure you get irreversible changes in the endometrium and infertility for the rest of the life of the animal, even when further contact with these isoflavones is prevented.

J. Gorski: All we really know is that if you give a large dose and look at the tissue response within 6 hours there is no greater response. There is little doubt about these plateaus of response. There is a lot of data in the literature on plateaus which says that it does give a response for a longer period of time. The times you have mentioned are much longer and I just don't know the answer. The fact is if you give a very large dose, a certain percentage will be stored. If it is returned to the blood stream, at a rate of only .01 micrograms per day, it would maintain the tissue response. This is a possibility.

M. Tausk: Particularly from the site of the injection. There is lots of data available on the speed with which certain preparations are removed from the site of injection.

# DIENCEPHALIC REGULATION OF CORPUS LUTEUM FORMATION AND SECRETORY ACTIVITY

# DIENCEPHALIC REGULATION OF CORPUS LUTEUM FORMATION AND SECRETORY ACTIVITY

John W. Everett, Ph.D.
Department of Anatomy
Duke University School of Medicine
Durham, North Carolina

Hohlweg and Junkmann (1932) are credited with the concept that gonadotropic functions of the adenohypophysis are governed by a "sex center" in the hypothalamus. Useful as this hypothesis has been as a first approximation, the idea that one specialized and circumscribed "center" controls all gonadotropic secretions is becoming inadequate. One may grant that the complex comprising the hypophysiotropic area (HA) of Halász, Pupp, and Uhlarik (1962), the median eminence and stalk (MEm), and the hypophysial portal vessels (PV) constitutes the final path through which all hypothalamic control of the adenohypophysis is exerted. It is a moot question, however, to what extent various functions are differentially localized within this complex. It is reasonable to assume that patterns of functional localization in the HA are approximated by patterns in the median eminence, especially in the anteroposterior dimension. Tubero-hypophysial fibers, which seemingly originate from HA cells, enter the palisade zone of the MEm transversely (Szentágothai, 1964), there coming into close relationship with the primary plexus of the portal system. On account of the small size of the HA and MEm, attempts to discern functional patterns therein by means of lesioning and stimulation techniques have led to ambiguous results. Even when there is general agreement among various workers (for example, that lesions including the anterior hypothalamic area between the paraventricular nuclei and the median eminence impair TSH secretion (Reichlin, 1966), this usually tells little about the HA and MEm, for much of the surrounding hypothalamus is also involved in the lesioning or stimulation. Perhaps the strongest evidence for a patterning of function in the MEm comes from an experiment by Pasteels (1960), who disconnected the adenohypophysis of Pleurodeles and replaced it after rotation of 180° in the transverse axis. Subsequently the pattern of cell types became rearranged roughly according to the original pattern in the animal. On the basis that the pars distalis is connected to the MEm through an orderly array of portal vessels (Daniel, 1966), it should follow that the cell pattern in the gland reflects a functional pattern in the MEm and HA.

Application of lesioning or stimulation methods to hypothalamic or other brain areas at a considerable distance from the HA and MEm may at times disclose geographic dissociations of function more satisfactorily than in the basal tuberal region. I shall illustrate this with respect to the differential control in rats of the discharge of LH expressed in ovulation and of prolactin secretion expressed in pseudopreganancy. By a particular type of brain stimulation it is possible to stimulate ovulation in rats without at the same time inducing pseudopregnancy. By a different method, not appropriate for ovulation, pseudopregnancy can readily be provoked.

While the HA-MEm-PV complex suffices for the day-to-day (tonic) secretion of gonadotropin, incitement of the ovulatory "surge" of LH involves a neuronal system operating through the medial preoptic area (mPOA) and the anterior hypothalamic area (AHA), playing upon the HA. We have proposed that this neuronal system originates diffusely throughout the septal region, that it remains diffuse in passing through the POA and AHA, and that is converges sharply to the base upon entering the medial basal tuber. Here would be its connection with the HA. Our evidence for this diffuse septal-preoptic-tuberal system in control of ovulation has been recited elsewhere (Everett, 1964a) at length and needs only brief outline here.

First was the observation that pentobarbital will block spontaneous ovulation when injection is suitably timed on the afternoon of proestrus (Everett and Sawyer, 1950). Critchlow (1958) later noted that stimulation of the basal tuber in pentobarbital-blocked rats will induce ovulation in spite of the blockade. Our attempts to repeat this disclosed that, in contrast to basal tuberal positions of stimulating electrodes, electrode localization in the AHA and mPOA is not critical (Everett, Radford and Holsinger, 1964). The "electrical" stimulus used in much of that mapping work proved to be actually electrochemical, the result of an irritative focus produced by the anodic deposition of iron from the stainless steel electrode, the irritation continuing to act long after the passage of current (Everett and Radford, 1961). The size of focus was important as well as its location. Throughout the mPOA a unilateral focus approximately 0.5 mm in diameter was adequate, but in the septal complex a much larger focus was needed and, consequently, a larger amount of electricity.

The amount of LH released from the hypophysis per unit time seems to depend on the size of the stimulating focus (Everett, 1964a), suggesting strongly that the greater the number of fibers activated in the preoptictuberal pathway, the greater the amount of LH-RF delivered from the MEm through the PV and, hence, the greater the amount of LH discharged.

Comparisons between proestrous rats and those in diestrus day 3 of the 5-day cycle showed a need for a larger preoptic focus in the latter animals. They required about twice the amount of anodic electrolysis needed in proestrus. By means of hypophysectomies performed at various intervals after introduction of standard irritative POA foci, it was demonstrated that the release of an ovulation quota of LH on diestrus day 3 takes significantly longer than on the day of proestrus. Greatly enlarged stimulating foci placed bilaterally shortened the time of release. The ovulation quota for LH (Table 1) is apparently somewhat larger (about 30%) on diestrus day 3 than during proestrus as indicated by injection experiments (Everett, 1964a), Hence, the diestrus rat requires a larger minimal stimulus than the proestrous rat or, on the other hand, a longer time for hormone release in response to a standard stimulus.

Indirect evidence (Everett, 1956) indicated strongly that both the atropine-sensitive phase of spontaneous neurogenous stimulation of the pituitary and resulting discharge of LH proceed in concert. Other implications of parallel temporal relationship between stimulus and hormone release were seen after electrical stimulation by the platinum electrodes. The current was deliberately spread between two unipolar electrodes spanning 2 mm across the midline in the preoptic (Everett, 1965) or tuberal regions (Quinn and Everett, unpublished).

TABLE I: Comparative Ovulatory Potency of Bovine LH Administered to Pentobarbital-Blocked Rats in Proestrus (4-day cycle) and Diestrus Day 3 (5-day cycle).

| Dose of LH $\mu g$/100 g body wt | Proestrus No. of rats | No. of ova per rat 8-11 | 2-7 | 1 | 0 | Mean + S. E.* | Diestrus day 3 No. of rats | No. of ova per rat 8-11 | 2-7 | 1 | 0 | Mean + S. E.* |
|---|---|---|---|---|---|---|---|---|---|---|---|---|
| 2.0 | 8 | 1 | 1 | 1 | 5 | 2.4 ± 1.2 | 4 | 0 | 0 | 0 | 4 | 0 |
| 2.5 | 6 | 1 | 0 | 1 | 4 | 1.5 ± 1.3 | | | | | | |
| 3.0† | 8 | 3 | 3 | 1 | 0 | 5.2 ± 1.5 | 8 | 0 | 0 | 2 | 6 | 0.5 ± 0.6 |
| 3.5† | 11 | 5 | 4 | 2 | 0 | 6.7 ± 1.2 | 7 | 0 | 3 | 0 | 4 | 1.7 ± 0.8 |
| 4.0 | 5 | 3 | 1 | 0 | 1 | 6.4 ± 2.1 | 10 | 5 | 2 | 1 | 2 | 5.8 ± 1.4 |

*Standard error

†At these dose levels the differences between proestrus and diestrus day 3 are highly significant ($P < 0.01$).

With matched pairs of biphasic, 1 msec pulses, 30/sec. 30/sec/min, 1000 μamp peak-to-peak, pentobarbital-blocked proestrous rats were stimulated for periods ranging from 5 to 60 minutes. The average number of tubal ova present on the next morning was the measure of the amount of LH released. Effectiveness of stimulation increased progressively with length of stimulation, reaching a maximum at 45 minutes. It is noteworthy that while this length of stimulus was necessary to produce full ovulation in all rats, a few of them ovulated completely after stimulation for only 15 minutes in either the POA or the tuber (2/8 and 2/5 rats, respectively). Tuberal stimulation for only 30 minutes produced full ovulation in only 4/11 rats and failed to produce any tubal ova in 4 others of the group. This implies a fairly wide scatter of individual ovulation quotas of LH. A similar indication can be found in the data from LH injection. For example, subcutaneous injection of 2 μg/100 g body weight of NIH-LH-B1 produced 7 and 11 ova, respectively, in two pentobarbital-blocked proestrous rats, while 4 failed to ovulate at all (Table 1). Dosage increased to 4 μg/100 g gave 8 to 10 ova in 3 rats, 3 ova in 1 rat and none in 2 rats. These variations of response will be referred to again in another context.

In addition to our stimulation studies, several other lines of evidence support the conclusion that control of ovulation, in rats at least, involves a neurónal system that is highly dispersed in its passage through the anterior hypothalamus. Hillarp (1949) produced constant estrus by placing bilateral lesions in the AHA, provided they were sufficiently large, by contrast with smaller effective lesions in the tuber near the arcuate nuclei. The recent observations by Halász and Gorski (1967), on the basis of various partial disconnections of the median eminence region and the effect on spontaneous cyclic ovulation, indicate a wide lateral dispersion of fibers at the caudal margin of the optic chiasma, whence they converge toward the MEm. I should point out that this agrees with our data from the mapping studies with respect to stimulations in suprachiasmatic planes. When electrode positions are plotted on a frontal section instead of a parasagittal section (Fig. 1) the extent of the lateral dispersion is strikingly apparent. These stimulations were electrochemical, made with the concentric stainless steel electodes and monophasic 1 msec pulses, 100/sec for 60 sec. Note the many positive cases with electrode tips in the lateral hypothalamus.

In a recent study, Tejasen (Tejasen and Everett, 1967) made transverse cuts unilaterally or bilaterally, in suprachiasmatic or tuberal planes, with or without subsequent POA stimulation (electrochemical, unilateral). The operations were usually performed on the afternoon of proestrus under pentobarbital, otherwise on diestrus day 3. The preoptic stimulation was administered immediately after the cut, with the exception of certain long-term experiments. In the animals receiving the stimulus, its effect was uniformly blocked by ipsilateral cuts in suprachiasmatic planes extending ventrally to the optic chiasma, laterally 1.4 mm and to at least 0.3 mm of the midline. In the tuberal region, however, ipsilateral cuts to the midline through the middle of the ventromedial (VMH) nucleus did not prevent ovulation, unless a midsagittal cut had also been made. The midsagittal cut by itself did not block. For technical reasons the combined mid-VMH transection and midsagittal section had to be made several weeks before the preoptic stimulation instead of immediately beforehand. This favored regeneration of portal vessels originating in the

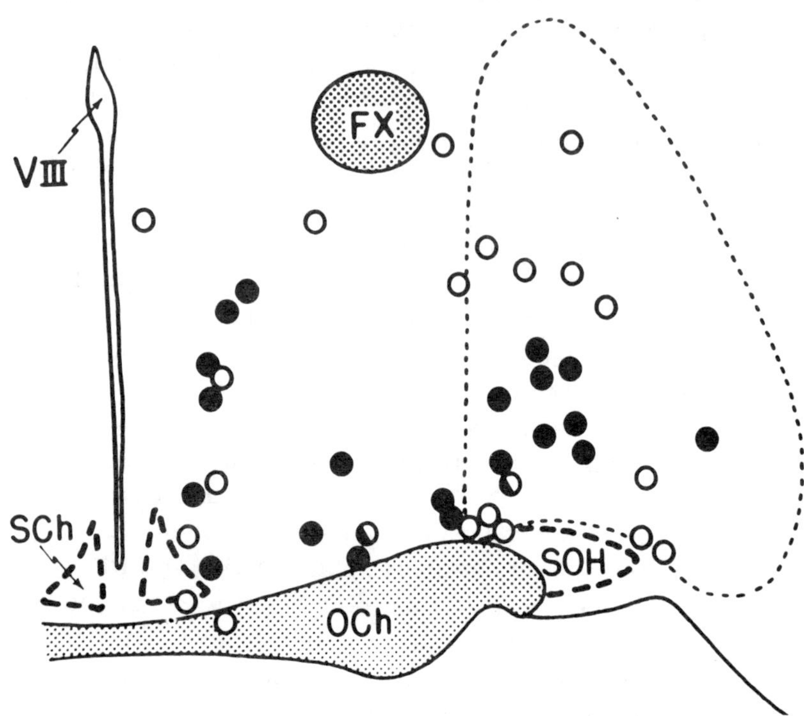


Fig. 1. Diagrams of a frontal section of the rat brain through the suprachiasmatic region of the hypothalamus showing positions of electrode tips in attempts at electrochemical stimulation of ovulation. Key: FX, fornix; OCh, optic chiasma; SCh, suprachiasmatic nucleus; SOH, supraoptic nucleus; $V_{III}$, third ventricle. Broken line circumscribes lateral hypothalamus. Black circles: positive. White circles: negative. Black and white circles: partial effect.

antero-lateral segment which were probably cut in the first operation. At the end of the experiments there was no histologic evidence of scarring which if present might have obstructed vascular recovery. We tentatively conclude that the neuronal system in question is both crossed and uncrossed, with decussation in the retrochiasmatic area. Furthermore, connections ipsilaterally in the rostral segment of the median eminence appear to be inadequate by themselves to cause release of the full ovulation quote of LH. Thus, some ipsilateral connections probably extend caudally beyond the mid-VMH plane.

A surprising development in the course of Tajasen's work was the finding that although none of the unilateral cuts in any of the three planes by themselves brought about LH release that could be detected by our methods, bilateral transections did so in numerous control experiments in which the preoptic stimulus was omitted. The effect was most pronounced in the case of transections through the VMH. Furthermore, the midsagittal cut, while not producing by itself any sign of LH release, did cause ovulation when combined with unilateral mid-VMH transection. McCann, Ramirez and Abrams (1964) reported that the mere insertion of a needle into the hypothalamus released an amount of LH detectable by the ovarian ascorbic acid depletion test. Such amounts of LH, if released by the unilateral cuts in Tejasen's experiments, were clearly too small to induce detectable histologic changes in the ovaries. It does seem strange, however, that merely doubling the stimulus by means of the bilateral cut, can produce a full ovulation quota of LH. Perhaps the answer to this puzzle lies in the considerable variation in ovulation quotas for LH noted earlier, coupled with the fact that only 5 proestrous rats were given unilateral VMH cuts. Were the number of such trials considerably increased, an occasional animal might give an ovulatory response.

If our notions are correct, that the septal-preoptic-tuberal pathway is in control of spontaneous ovulation it follows that such normal activity is selective and that some other central mechanism governs prolactin secretion, since rats normally ovulate without subsequently becoming pseudopregnant. When cyclic rats are subjected to preoptic electrochemical stimulation in the manner described earlier, they do not ordinarily become pseudopregnant (Everett, et al., 1964; Everett and Quinn, 1966). This was true not only when small unilateral stimuli were applied, as by passing a 10 μamp direct current for 60 seconds, but also when the stimulus was greatly increased by passage of 100 μamp D.C. for 30 seconds. The great majority of animals thus treated continued to have regular estrous cycles. Pseudopregnancy occurred in only 8/38 rats (21%). We were challenged by this result to search for other stimulation sites and/or parameters of stimulation which would lead predictably to the pseudopregnancy response.

The basic procedure first used in this search was to block spontaneous ovulation in the usual way with pentobarbital on the afternoon of proestrus and to place an ovulation-inducing lesion in the medial POA. Immediately thereafter a concentric bipolar electrode of either stainless steel or platinum was introduced in another site to deliver a stimulus of the following characteristics: matched biophasic pairs of rectangular 1 msec pulses, 100 pairs/sec, 30 sec/min x 10, 200 μamp peak-to-peak. Pseudopregnancy regularly followed whenever this second stimulus was applied unilaterally to any of a variety of sites in the medial hypothalamus, including the anterior hypothalamic area, the paraventricular, dorsomedial and ventromedial nuclei, and the premamillary complex. Electrode insertion without passage of current was essentially without effect.

The next step was to omit the preoptic stimulus and only to stimulate for pseudopreganancy in the manner just described on the afternoon of proestrus during the pentobarbital anesthesia. While not inducing ovulation, except for one case, this stimulus applied to the medial tuberal region always led to pseudopregnancy. But now, with that one exception, its onset was delayed a day until after the spontaneous ovulation occurring on the second night.

"Delayed pseudopregnancy" has been known for many years, since first described by Greep and Hisaw (1938). Electrical stimulation of the uterine cervix in rats during late diestrus is commonly followed by pseudopregnancy beginning after the ensuing estrus. I encountered delays much longer than this in mating experiments with pentobarbital-blocked rats (Evertt, 1952, 1967). Approximately 50% of the animals thus blocked during proestrus accepted coitus during the succeeding night. A few ovulated "reflexly" in response to the copulatory stimulus, but the usual result, if additional barbiturate was given on the second afternoon at the critical time, was that corpus luteum formation failed entirely during the current cycle. A new, brief diestrus followed and then a new estrus, at which time corpora lutea formed and became functional. Pseudopregnancy of normal duration dated from that estrous period--consistently. By a different method, Zeilmaker (1965) has demonstrated equally long delayed responses to copulatory stimulation. Female rats bearing a grafted ovary on the kidney but otherwise intact were mated, and on the day after copulation the normal ovaries were removed. The grafts developed rapidly, a new estrus occurred a few days later, corpora lutea formed in the grafts, and pseudopregnancy ensued. Zeilmaker concluded that the effect of the copulatory stimulus is retained for 7 or 8 days, including the several days required for the grafts to mature and luteinize plus at least two days for positive feedback action of progesterone from the corpora lutea to establish a self-sustaining pseudopregnancy. He and I agree that the simplest interpretation of our results is that prolactin secretion is immediately elevated by the copulatory stimulus and that it cannot express itself until competent corpora lutea are present. But whether or not this is true, one cannot escape the conclusion that some change takes place in the nervous system in immediate response to the stimulus and that this change in state persists for over a week, provided that the stimulus was large enough. (It should be mentioned that brief electrical stimulation of the cervix, on the morning of estrus following pentobarbital blockade on the previous day, was not adequate to give the long-delayed response although consistently effective with short delays—Everett, 1967).

Quinn extended our studies with successful attempts to induce long-delayed responses to stimulation of the hypothalamus (Quinn and Everett, 1967). Not only could he produce delays like those obtained by cervical stimulation during diestrus, but by increasing the length of stimulation from 10 minutes to 30 minutes or longer, he reproduced the week-long delays that I had obtained with copulatory stimuli in pentobarbital-blocked rats. In fact, his experiments were modelled closely on that earlier work. Four-day cyclic rats were blocked with pentobarbital on the day of proestrus and again on the following day. During the proestrus anesthesia the concentric platinum electrode was inserted into the dorsomedial-ventromedial (DMH-VMH) region of the hypothalamus to deliver the usual stimulus of matched biphasic pulse pairs (Fig. 2). Electrical parameters were exactly as described earlier. Over-all duration of the stimulus was varied, however, from 10 to 60 minutes. The 10-minute stimulus was not followed by pseudopregnancy, but we did note one curious feature. Animals thus stimulated failed to ovulate or luteinize on the third night as they would have done had they merely been blocked with the barbiturate for the two days. That effect I had seen regularly in similarly blocked rats that copulated during the first night. Increase of the brain stimulation to 30 or 60 minutes not only had this action of preventing ovulation of the current set of follicles, but also led to pseudopregnancy that began with the next estrus, when new follicles ripened and luteinized. Thus, in three respects the effects of the selective type of brain stimulation employed closely simulated the effects of genital stimulation: (1) There was an apparent temporary depression of gonadotropin secretion, exemplified in the atresia of the current set of follicles. (2) The greater the stimulus, the longer was its effect "remembered". (3) When the stimulus was large enough, the onset of pseudopregnancy was delayed until the next cycle.

A propos of the proposition that there is no one "sex center" in the brain, we have noted: (A) in control of the acute release of LH for ovulation, a diffuse neuronal system extending from the septal complex to the medial basal tuber, and (B) in control of prolactin

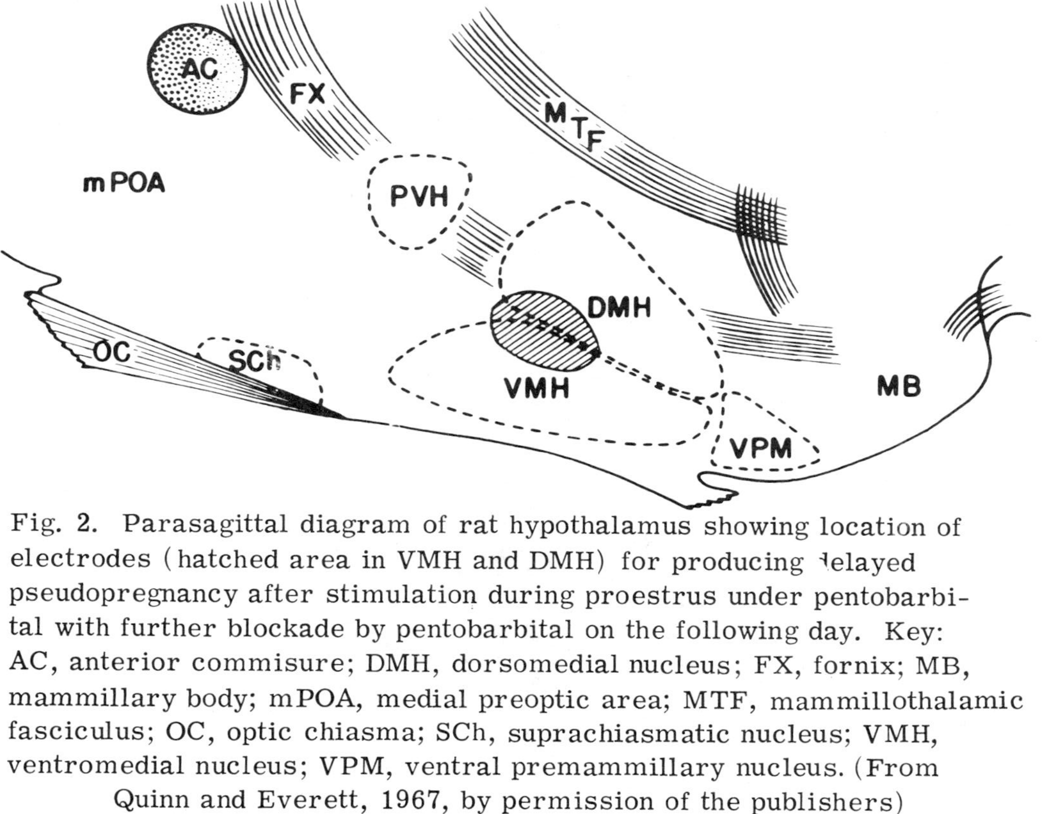


Fig. 2. Parasagittal diagram of rat hypothalamus showing location of electrodes (hatched area in VMH and DMH) for producing delayed pseudopregnancy after stimulation during proestrus under pentobarbital with further blockade by pentobarbital on the following day. Key: AC, anterior commisure; DMH, dorsomedial nucleus; FX, fornix; MB, mammillary body; mPOA, medial preoptic area; MTF, mammillothalamic fasciculus; OC, optic chiasma; SCh, suprachiasmatic nucleus; VMH, ventromedial nucleus; VPM, ventral premammillary nucleus. (From Quinn and Everett, 1967, by permission of the publishers)

secretion as expressed in pseudopregnancy, another system, perhaps equally diffuse in the dorsal-posterior hypothalamus. Clearly much remains to be learned about both of these systems, how each acts enroute to and at the median eminence selectively to exert control of the appropriate pars distalis secretions. Interaction of the two systems is apparent in the suppression of ovulation during periods of corpus luteum secretion, yet there is little knowledge at hand about how this comes about. Although secretion of the folliculotropins and secretion of prolactin characteristically bear a reciprocal relationship, it is increasingly evident that both processes proceed together under some conditions (see Everett, 1964c). Thus, prolactin secretion has been evident in rats that were persistent-estrous as a result of old age or continuous illumination (Aschheim, 1962). In the delayed-pseudopregnancy phenomenon, it is likely that prolactin secretion is at once activated by the appropriate stimulus and yet, in spite of its continuation, at some later time the processes leading to ovulation come into play. The estrogen surge on pregnancy day 3 presents an analogous circumstance (Shelesnyak, 1960, Shelesnyak & Kraicer, 1963). It is tempting to speculate that the septal-preoptic-tuberal system is responsible for this surge as for ovulation. It so, the analogy comes closer: the presence of competent corpora lutea soon after the copulatory stimulus leads to a continuing high level of progesterone secretion; that in turn suppresses ovulation at the time of the next expected cycle. Yet LH release and the subsequent estrogen surge may very well take place on schedule, the amount of LH being inadequate for ovulation and the vaginal effects of estrogen being obscured by the progestogen.

## ACKNOWLEDGMENT

Investigations in the author's laboratory as reported above were largely supported by grants from the National Science Foundation (G 4431, G 9841, GB 1737).

## REFERENCES

Aschheim, P. (1962). Oestrus permanent et prolactine. C. R. Acad. Sci. (Paris) 255, 3053-3056.

Critchlow, V. (1958). Ovulation induced by hypothalamic stimulation in the anesthetized rat. Am. J. Physiol. 195, 171-174.

Daniel, P. M. (1966). The anatomy of the hypothalamus and pituitary gland. In: Neuroendocrinology, Eds. L. Martini and W. F. Ganong. Academic Press, New York. Vol. 1.

Everett, J. W. (1952). Presumptive hypothalamic control of spontaneous ovulation. Ciba Found. Colloq. Endocrinol. 4, 167-177.

Everett, J. W. (1956). The time of release of ovulating hormone from the rat hypophysis. Endocrinology 59, 580-585.

Everett, J. W. (1964a). Preoptic stimulative lesions and ovulation in the rat: 'Thresholds' and LH-release time in late diestrus and proestrus. In: Major Problems in Neuroendocrinology, Eds. E. Bajusz and G. Jasmin, S. Karger, Basel.

Everett, J. W. (1964b). LH-quotas, apparent preoptic thresholds and LH-release times for ovulation in proestrous vs. late-diestrous rats. Fed. Proc. 23, 302 (abstract).

Everett, J. W. (1964c). Central neural control of reproductive functions of the adenohypophysis. Physiol. Rev. 44, 373-431.

Everett, J. W. (1965). Ovulation in rats from preoptic stimulation through platinum electrodes. Importance of duration and spread of stimulus. Endocrinology 76, 1195-1201.

Everett, J. W. (1967). Provoked ovulation or long-delayed pseudopregnancy from coital stimuli in barbiturate-blocked rats. Endocrinology 80, 145-154.

Everett, J. W., and Quinn, D. L. (1966). Differential hypothalamic mechanisms inciting ovulation and pseudopregnancy in the rat. Endocrinology 78, 141-150.

Everett, J. W. and Radford, H. M. (1961). Irritative deposits from stainless steel electrodes in the preoptic rat brain causing release of pituitary gonadotropin. Proc. Soc. Exptl. Biol. Med. 108, 604-609.

Everett, J. W., Radford, H. M., and Holsinger, J. (1964). Electrolytic irritative lesions in the hypothalamus and other forebrain areas: Effects on luteinizing hormone release and the ovarian cycle. In: Hormonal Steroids, Eds. L. Martini and A. Pecile. Academic Press, New York.

Everett, J. W., and Sawyer, C. H. (1950). A 24-hour periodicity in the "LH-release apparatus" of female rats, disclosed by barbiturate sedation. Endocrinology 47, 198-218.

Greep, R. O., and Hisaw, F. L. (1938). Pseudopregnancy from electrical stimulation of the cervix in the diestrum. Proc. Soc. Exptl. Biol. Med. 39, 359-360.

Halasz, B., and Gorski, R. A. (1967). Gonadotrophic hormone secretion in female rats after partial or total interruption of neural afferents to the basal hypothalamus. Endocrinology 80, 608-622.

Halasz, B., Pupp, L., and Uhlarik, S. (1962). Hypophysiotrophic area in the hypothalamus. J. Endocrinol. 25, 147-154.

Hillarp, N.-A. (1949). Studies on the localization of hypothalamic centres controlling the gonadotrophic function of the hypophysis. Acta Endocrinol. 2, 11-23.

Hohlweg, W., and Junkmann, K. (1932). Die hormonale-nervose Regulierung der Funktion des Hypophysenvorderlappens. Klin. Wochschr. 11, 321-333.

McCann, S. M., Ramirez, V. D., and Abrams, R. (1964). Regulation of luetinizing hormone (LH) secretion by a hypothalamic LH-releasing factor. In: Hormonal Steroids, Eds. L. Martini and A. Pecile. Academic Press, New York, Vol. 1, p. 253.

Pasteels, J. L. (1960). Étude expérimentale des différentes catégories d'eléments chromophiles de l'hypophyse adulte de Pleurodeles waltlii, de leur fonction et de leur controle par l'hypothalamus. Arch. Biol. 71, 409-471.

Quinn, D. L., and Everett, J. W. (1967). Delayed pseudopregnancy induced by selective hypothalamic stimulation. Endocrinology 80, 155-162.

Reichlin, S. (1966). Control of thyrotropic hormone secretion. In: Neuroendocrinology, Eds. L. Martini and W. F. Ganong, Academic Press, New York, Vol. 1.

Shelesnyak, M. C. (1960) Nidation of the fertilized ovum. Endeavour, 19, 81-86

Shelesnyak, M. C. and Kraicer, P. F. (1963) Role of Estrogen in Nidation in Delayed Nidation, Ed. E. C. Enders, Univ. Chicago Press pg 265-280.

Szentagothai, J. (1964). The parvicellular neurosecretory system. Progr. Brain. Res. 5, 135-145.

Tejasen, T., and Everett, J. W. (1967). Surgical analysis of the preopticotuberal pathway controlling ovulatory release of gonadotropins in the rat. Endocrinology 81, 1387-1396.

Zeilmaker, G. H. (1965). Normal and delayed pseudopregnancy in the rat. Acta Endocrinol. 49, 558-566.

## DISCUSSION

M. C. Shelesnyak: I will take the privilege of making a few remarks, to initiate the discussion on this particular subject, since it concerns pseudopregnancy, which, for a long time has been of interest to me. My first publication, a number of years ago, was on the induction of pseudopregnancy by electrical stimulation, [Shelesnyak, M. C., Anat. Rec. 49, 179. 1931]

I'd like to invite attention to two things about induction of pseudopregnancy. It has certain characteristics in common with the induction of decidualization in that, it can happen with tremendous ease when not desired, but when desired sometimes succeeds only with difficulty. Certainly, in the original laboratory method of Long and Evans, mechanical stimulation, and then the electrical stimulation technique I originally described, was applied at what we considered to be the optimal time, the time of the female's receptivity to the male, under the impression that this would give us the best results. We did find, as a matter of fact, that in proestrus and estrus, electrical stimulation gave us a maximum response. In our laboratory, stimulation on diestrus was not nearly as effective as in the work of Greep and Hisaw in 1938 [R. O. Greep and F. L. Hisaw, Proc. Soc. Exp. Biol. Med. 39, 359, 1938]. However, recently, Mr. Shalom Joseph, my associate and senior technician, carried out a study in which fifty females at each stage of the estrous cycle were electrically stimulated. These were rats with regular, four-day cycles. The results were as follows: when animals were stimulated on proestrus or estrus or metestrus, in each case, 49 out of fifty animals became pseudopregnant, on the basis of vaginal smear patterns.

J. W. Everett: You are talking about immediate pseudopregnancy, I assume.

M. C. Shelesnyak: Yes, but in the last case, when animals were stimulated on diestrus, 49 out of fifty went into delayed pseudopregnancy, that is, stimulation was followed by a proestrus, estrus and then the pseudopregnancy. Another bit of information I'd like to draw attention to is that Psychoyos [A. Psychoyos, Mem. Soc. Endocrin. 6, 13, 1959], reported that the subcutaneous injection of very large amounts of saline, 5 ml, induced pseudopregnancy. And this, of course, reminds one of the work of Swingle and co-workers in which they managed to induce pseudopregnancy in rats by an infinite minus one number of techniques including irritants, stresses and even injections of substances which seemed rather innocuous [W. W. Swingle, P. Seay, J. Perlmutt, E. J. Collins, G. Barlow, Jr., and E. J. Fedor, Am. J. Physiol. 167, 586, 1951].

E. S. Kisch: I would like to discuss some of the points raised by Prof. Everett and I am motivated in this, partly by my personal taste and partly by work done in our department which is directly related. These points come under the headings of: "Control of stimulus for ovulation, associated with LH release"; "Initiation and control of luteal function, associated with LtH release, as expressed in pseudopregnancy".

J. W. Everett: Can you call it prolactin?

E. S. Kisch: I interchange the two. For future reference, I'll use the two terms indiscriminately.

My third topic is: "Termination of luteal function". And I am very happy that Dr. Everett mentioned something about the estrogen surge, as that will give me a chance to talk also on that subject. These are my four points.

The first point, central control of ovulation. As Dr. Everett has done, we have studied this primarily by pharmacological means. I won't say much about this. We have blocked ovulation with nembutal and roughly find the same critical time and time limits for the effectiveness of the nembutal block as Dr. Everett.

In this connection, I would like to bring up the subject of the very exciting drug ergocornine, which has been one of our principal tools in investigating diencephalic regulation of ovarian function. Ergocornine is an ergot alkaloid introduced by Prof. Shelesnyak as a tool in the study of reproductive processes [Shelesnyak, M.C. Am.J.Physiol. 179 301. 1954]. He found that the drug causes interruption of progestation or pseudopregnancy, followed by a genuine (ovulatory) estrus within two or three days. Prof. Shelesnyak interpreted this response to mean that the ho: monal balance of progestation is disturbed by this and, a was later shown, by other closely related ergot alkaloids. Later investigation by Prof. Shelesnyak, Dr. Kraicer and, more recently by Zeilmaker, Varavudhi and most recently, by myself, has shown that the drug depresses the availability of prolactin or luteotrophin, either by direct action on the pituitary, or indirectly, via the hypothalamus, by initiating the release of PIF, prolactin inhibiting factor, or by both actions together. But this is not all: ergocornine not only affects luteotrophic function, it also affects other central mechanisms such as diencephalic regulation of ovulation. But Dr. Kraicer will tell you something of this.

It is clear that ergocornine is responsible for termination of luteal function by its termination of luteotrophic secretion by the pituitary. About 24 hours after ergocornine has been administered subcutaneously to progestational rats, 1 milligram is the usual dose, luteal failure is apparent. I mean, functionally as evidenced by decreased progesterone production. This has been demonstrated by Dr. Linder and his collaborators.

Regarding initiation of luteal function, Dr. Shelesnyak mentioned that many diverse stimuli will induce pseudopregnancy and it is practically certain that the common denominator of all these stimuli is a pathway through the brain. I myself have used the mechanical methods for induction of pseudopregnancy, electrical stimulation of the cervix as introduced by Dr. Shelesnyak in 1931, and I have used one other method--painting the cervix with xylol. All these methods effectively induce luteotrophic activity as indicated by the pseudopregnancy which follows treatment. But I was really interested in that borderline area between induction of pseudogregnancy and failure of induction or in incomplete induction of pseudopregnancy. My question was, is the triggering of centrally-dominated lutoetrophin secretion an all or none phenomenon? Is there something in between or is some "switch" in the brain "flipped."

We tested this by studying the effect of stimulating anesthetized rats, where the effectiveness of

TABLE I: The Influence of Cervical Stimulation on the Duration of Diestrus.

| Cervical Treatment | Anesthesia* | Number of rats treated | Duration of Diestrus 4 days. | 5 days. | 6 days | Psp. |
|---|---|---|---|---|---|---|
| Xylol | - | 11 | 0 | 2 | 1 | 8 |
| Xylol | + | 6 | 1 | 2 | 3 | 0 |
| Electrical stimulation | - | 10 | 0 | 0 | 0 | 10 |
| Electrical stimulation | + | 10 | 0 | 7 | 0 | 3 |
| None | + | 6 | 2 | 3 | 0 | 1 |

Rats were selected for regularity of 4-day cycles (2 days of diestrus). Treatments were administered at 11.00 hrs on the day of estrus of a normal cycle. The rats were anesthetized. (*Avertin, 1 ml of a 2% solution/100 g body weight, i.p.) at the time of cervical stimulation as indicated.

stimulation would be reduced or by giving a minimal stimulus which would not cause a real pseudopregnancy.

M. C. Shelesnyak: May I ask whether you would consider the persistence of leucocytes for four or five days as meaning an incomplete or minimal effect?

E. S. Kisch: I would be very happy if my results were as clear-cut or simple as that.

All treatments were given on the day of vaginal cornification at 11.00 hrs. Painting of xylol on the cervix is a fairly effective stimulus for inducing pseudopregnancy (Table 1). Unfortunately, there aren't many animals in the groups, but when an anesthetic, in this case Avertin, was given just before the xylol painting, instead of the pseudopregnancy pattern, we got prolongation of the leucocytic phase of the subsequent cycle. However, Avertin did not suppress the effectiveness of electrical stimulation completely; some animals became pseudopregnant and others had a prolonged cycle. I should emphasize that all the animals used in these experiments had been selected for regularity of four-day cycles and whatever their response, they all later returned to the normal four-day pattern. Avertin itself caused irregularity in the cycle and effectively diminished the response to mechanical stimulation. It also induced pseudopregnancy in one case.

J. W. Everett: Do you ever find spontaneous pseudopregnancy in rats with four-day cycles?

E. S. Kisch: Never as far as I know.

J. W. Everett: It's very rare in my colony.

E. S. Kisch: As I have said the animals selected for regularity of cycle, responded to an "incomplete" stimulus with prolongation of the luteal phase of the cycle in 15 out of 16 cases. Maybe it's not prolongation of the luteal phase of the cycle, but just is deferring the next central stimulus for ovulation. I couldn't tell the difference between the two.

J. W. Everett: May I comment here and refer back to the effect we found on the current set of follicles, blocking with nembutal for only two days. Ordinarily, this would be followed by ovulation on the third night. But, if there was in addition a minimal stimulation of the posterior hypothalamus for only ten minutes, the current set of follicles was suppressed. There was apparently some effect on gonadotrophic secretion.

E. S. Kisch: As far as I am aware from your work, you never got this prolongation of the cycle. You got delayed pseudopregnancy.

J. W. Everett: That is more or less correct, but we did get some prolongation, to five day cycles. Also, in one series [D. L. Quinn and J. W. Everett, Endocrinology, 80, 155, 1967] we obtained long pseudopregnancy-like periods of diestrus in which deciduomal reactions could not be obtained.

E. S. Kisch: Is the five-day cycle, that is, in which there are three days of leucocytes due to greater activation of the corpora lutea than in the four-day cycle? Would this be due to any influence of LtH? We are fortunate to have Prof. Everett with us because in 1944 he had evidence that LtH may play a role even in the four-day cycle and I would be very interested to learn what he thinks about this 23 years later.

J. W. Everett: My evidence [Endocrinology, 35, 507, 1944] was based on the fact that one strain of rats, the so-called DA strain, had no detectable cholesterol in the corpora lutea of cycling animals, unless I gave a small amount of prolactin. This was Schering prolactin, which I had tested to be essentially free of LH by the interstitial cell histology in hypophysectomized subjects.

On the day after ovulation, the corpora lutea from the preceding cycle contained, in normal rats, a rich store of cholesterol. The DA strain of rats, however, failed to show this unless a small amount of prolactin, not enough to produce a pseudopregnancy, was given during diestrus.

E. S. Kisch: I have never been able up to now by my "incomplete" stimulus to induce a cycle lasting longer than six days, that is 4 days of leucocytes. I'm not sure whether I'll be able to fill up this area between the frank diestrus period of 13 to 14 days and the prolongation of the cycle that I've managed to get. So far, I haven't been able to get anything in between.

Prof. Everett has spoken about quantitation of the stimulus for both induction of ovulation and of delayed pseudopregnancy. But it appears that, just as I did for pseudopregnancy, you get only an all-or none-response. Either you flip the switch and get delayed pseudopregnancy or you get no response. There is no intermediate response.

J. W. Everett: No stimulus between 10 minutes and 30 minutes was investigated.

E. S. Kisch: Zeilmaker [G. H. Zeilmaker, Acta Endocr. (Kbh.) 49, 558, 1965] recently proposed that copulation triggers a period of LtH secretion lasting about 8 days. His experimental design was quite different from that of Prof. Everett in which delayed pseudopregnancy was induced. Zeilmaker used normal cycling rats bearing homografts of immature ovaries under the kidney capsule. The grafted ovaries were quiescent during the period of cycling. He mated his rats and removed their own ovaries the following day. After this intervention, the grafted ovaries developed, ovulated and an estrus was expressed in the vaginal smear. The corpora lutea arising from this ovulation could now support a period of pseudopregnancy. By varying the time of removal of the orginal, the animal's own ovaries he could bring the time of the ovulation by the grafted ovaries to beyond the period of luteotrophin dominance centrally induced by copulation and defined as lasting 8 days. During this period LtH is available. If the ovulation from the grafted ovaries occurred within the 8-day period, a new pseudopregnancy followed. If it occurred after the 8-day period, there was no pseudopregnancy. In other words, it's all or none. Either the switch is flipped or not.

Now we are all agreed that this must be determined at the level of the central nervous system and the mechanism is maintained independently of the presence of functional corpora lutea or, as in Zeilmaker's work, of corpora lutea at all. Zeilmaker's hypothesis of an eight-day "memory" could be treated readily with our wonder drug ergocornine.

If ergocornine is given on day $L_2$ of pseudopregnancy induced by electrostimulation, it will cause an estrus two or three days later on $L_4$ or $L_5$. This is well within the range of 8 days. We should see a new pseudopregnancy following that pseudopregnancy, a delayed pseudopregnancy. If ergocornine is given on day $L_7$ of pseudopregnancy, estrus is induced on $L_9$ or $L_{10}$. It should be outside the range and no pseudopregnancy should be seen. And this was more or less the case. In the group treated on $L_2$, 18 out ot 20 animals showed a real pseudopregnancy following their ergocornine-induced estrus. In the group treated on $L_7$, only 4 out of 20 animals showed a pseudopregnancy, which agrees with eight day period; maybe it lasts nine and maybe it lasts ten days, but my data roughly agree with Zeilmaker's findings. It also shows that the pseudopregnancy so often seen after ergocornine [P. F. Kraicer and M. C. Shelesnyak, J. Reprod. Fertil. 8, 225, 1964; G. H. Zeilmaker, Acta Endocr. (Kbh.) 49, 558, 1965] is not due to an intrinsic capacity or quality of the drug, but it is only associated with when the drug is injected.

S. Katsh: So it's a non-specific effect, is that what you're saying?

E. S. Kisch: It's not associated with the ergocornine itself. Other methods, such as those of Zeilmaker, will give similar effects.

J. W. Everett: Can we not say that it's as if you were to take out the first set of corpora lutea. New corpora lutea forming several days later (but within the 8-day period), then become activated.

E. S. Kisch: Indeed, luteëctomy, about which Dr. Kraicer will have something to say, in the progestational rat, produces sequelae which are quite similar to what I have just described for ergocornine.

H. R. Lindner: By the way, in this instance where you give ergocornine on $L_2$, you have again one of those situations that Dr. Everett mentioned; where you have coincident secretion of prolactin and of luteinizing hormone.

J. W. Everett: So it appears.

E. S. Kisch: Now to come to my last point. Dr. Everett has mentioned that there is a possible analogy between the central happenings inducing the estrogen surge by the ovary on day $L_3$ and what happens on proestrus. It's tempting to postulate that something happens on day $L_3$ of gestation which is similar to what would have happened at the time of the esrtwhile next proestrus, had copulation not taken place. Pursuing this analogy and working with Dr. Everett's own weapons, I tried to block nidation, just as is so beautifully possible for ovulation if you pick the right time. We administered nembutal,

30 mg per kg., intraperitoneally on the morning of day $L_3$ of pregnancy. I'm not the first to think of this approach. Zeilmaker [Doctoral Thesis, University of Amsterdam, 1964] has done something similar, giving nembutal about the critical time. He noted that the implants in these animals were smaller on day $L_7$ than normal for this day but concluded that they were not as small as they would be had there been a delay in implantation of one day, and therefore, he dismissed the theory that nembutal might block central control of implantation. De Feo also tried to block the stimulus initiating the estrogen surge using the time of sensitivity to decidual induction as his parameter [V. J. De Feo, Endocrinology, 72, 305, 1963]. He started daily injections of nembutal on day $L_1$ of pseudopregnancy, but, as Dr. Everett has pointed out, if you want to block ovulation for more than one day, you have to give two injections of nembutal, or increase the dose, which De Feo did not do. Also, De Feo used scratching to induce decidualization and the period of sensitivity to traumatic stimuli is rather broad so that a shift of only 24 hours or less wouldn't be apparent.

In our experiments, we gave nembutal on day $L_3$, at 12.00 hrs, and performed a laparotomy on day $L_5$. Usually, in the pregnant animal at this time we find the implants as discrete swellings spaced neatly along the uterus, and this was the case in this experimental group. However, when nembutal was given at 14.00 hrs on day $L_3$, which seems to be the critical time, four animals out of twelve had no visible implants on $L_5$, and, even more significantly, we were able to flush blastocysts out of the uterus. Now I cite a personal communication from Dr. Kraicer that never, in his experience, can blastocysts be washed out of the uterus after about 18.00 hrs on day $L_4$ at the very latest. I don't want to stick my neck out too far, but whatever has happened, there has been delay of implantation. Not in very many animals, but it's there.

I have also attempted to block implantation with ergocornine just as Dr. Kraicer has done for ovulation. The results are not very convincing yet, but I think ergocornine as well as nembutal can delay the central stimulation for the ovarian estrogen surge--not by resetting the biological clock 24 hours, but for about eight hours or so.

P. F. Kraicer: If you will excuse the historical digression, I would like to discuss some relevant work that nevertheless seems rather curious and out of place here unless one understands where it came from. I'm referring to work done in our laboratory with ergocornine. Ergocornine knocks out corpora lutea. And I think this is quite obvious from the response to ergocornine which, in a pregnant animal, is almost instantaneous termination of pregnancy. The vagina is usually full of blood, if the pregnancy is sufficiently advanced, by the next day. The animal reverts to an estrous state, and we have demonstrated that this is a true ovulatory estrus, and the number of ova present is the number of ova we have in an average size ovulation in our colony, 11.7 ova per clutch.

M. C. Shelesnyak: May I make one interruption. Ergocornine works invariable in pregnancy, provided that it is given prior to day $L_7$ of pregnancy. The reason I make this point is that there is a historical confusion about the ergot alkaloids being abortifacients. Such a property is not the basis of our investigations.

P. F. Kraicer: Thank you for your correction. The action of ergocornine then would indeed be a block of luteal function, a stoppage of luteal progesterone whatever way one cares to look at it, but in a sense it is analogous to the stoppage of thyroid secretion when one removes the hypophysis; it is not a true thyroidectomy. In this sense, ergocornine treatment is not a true luteëctomy. The corpora can be stimulated by prolactin [M. C. Shelesnyak Rec. Progr. Hormone Res., 13, 269. 1957] and by luteotrophic factors of placental origin, [E. S. Kisch Doctoral Thesis,Rehovolt 1968]. At any rate, we tried to establish what it was that ergocornine was doing to turn off, ultimately, corpora lutea. As a working hypothesis, we postulated that ergocornine went directly to somewhere, and once there, it turned off luteotrophic activity. It is also possible that (and this was the hypothesis we chose to test because the first is rather difficult) as Rothchild had orginally proposed [I. Rothchild, Endocrinology, 67, 9, 1960], luteotrophic influences are a direct response to the presence of progesterone in a self stimulating system of positive feedback. Assuming that progesterone, acting on the hypothalamus and/or hypophysis, stimulates secretion of the luteotrophic principles, we postulated that ergocornine competes with progesterone at this level. Once ergocornine displaces or inhibits the progesterone, the animals cease to be under the stimulus of luteotrophic activity.

In order to test this, we looked for an action of exogenous or endogenous progesterone on the hypothalamic-hypophyseal axis that wasn't concerned with pregnancy. We were very pleased when reports began appearing that if you gave the animal progesterone during proestrus, she subsequently would become pseudopregnant. Here was precisely the system we looked for, here is a direct action of progesterone presumably at the center. Would ergocornine block it? Unfortunately, in our colony progesterone, in doses ranging from 2 to 50 milligrams, does not induce pseudopregnancy.

J. W. Everett: There are three reports of induction of pseudopregnancy by progesterone: by Alloiteau, Rothchild and myself [J. J. Alloiteau, C. R. Acad. Sci., 246, 2804, 1958; I. Rothchild and R. Schubert, Endocrinology, 72, 969, 1963; J. W. Everett, Nature, 198, 695, 1963].

H. R. Lindner: What is your experimental procedure?

J. W. Everett: I gave a single injection of 10 mg of progesterone at 9 to 10 am. on the day of estrus, that is, on the day after ovulation. This was usually followed by pseudopregnancy, provided that several females remained together. If they were isolated, it didn't go.

E. S. Kisch: Does it make a difference whether they are animals with four-or-five-day cycles?

J. W. Everett: Yes, the animals with five-day cycles were much more responsive.

E. S. Kisch: Perhaps that was our problem.

P. F. Kraicer: So, we weren't able to test our hypothesis on this phenomenon. However, it had been known for some time that progesterone is involved in ovulation and this prompted us to attempt to block ovulation with ergocornine, and demonstrate that the block is due to antagonism to progesterone. We used rats with regular 4-day cycles. In our colony, about 92 per cent of animals who show more than two consecutive four-day cycles will continue to show consecutive four-day cycles. In general, the animals used in our study had at least four cycles checked before we used them. Ovulation occurs in our colony at 4 o'clock plus or minus about half an hour, on the morning of the day of estrus (the day of the cornified vaginal smear). Now, we tried the effect of nembutal in our colony to find out if the biological clock regulating ovulation is the same as in Dr. Everett's colony. At 12 o'clock noon, on the day of proestrus, we gave nembutal and checked for ovulation the next day. Two out of ten had ovulated. If we gave it at 2 o'clock in the afternoon or 4 o'clock in the afternoon, none out of five in either case had ovulated. If we gave it at 6 o'clock in the evening, we still got blockage in five out of ten animals. Even as late as 8 o'clock in the evening, we got some blockage, 7 out of 10 did ovulate, 3 didn't. But since the controls showed only 90 per cent ovulation, perhaps there was no significant inhibition. At any rate, the critical period of our colony appears to be somewhat longer.

J. W. Everett: That is true of Charles River CD rats [Endocrinology, 80, 790, 1967].

P. F. Kraicer: Good, then our colony is not unique in this regard.

U. S. von Euler: Would you clarify one point? Is the effect of ergocornine specific or are other alkaloids effective?

P. F. Kraicer: There is a very distinct relationship between the structure of the polypeptide moiety of the ergot alkaloid and its efficiency against pregnancy. The only alkaloid we have tested in the effect I am about to describe is ergocornine.

M. C. Shelesnyak: I could add another bit of information. In some collaborative work with Dr. Ian Silver at Cambridge doing unit cell activity recordings of hypothalamic cells, we found that ergocornine is highly specific in flipping the progestational pattern to the estrous pattern. Ergokryptin, which is also effective in inhibiting pregnancy and decidualization is, however, less effective, but, nevertheless, effective in reversing the hypothalamic firing pattern, and nothing else is. None of the other ergot alkaloids tested were effective.

U. S. von Euler: Hydergin (dihydroergotamine) for instance?

M. C. Shelesnyak: No, not at all.

P. F. Kraicer: We injected the ergocornine at various times and found that beginning about 48 hours before the expected ovulation until about 15 hours before the expected ovulation, one milligram of ergocornine will block ovulation in two thirds of the animals. By 15 or 16 hours before the time of ovulation, that is at about 13.00 hours on proestrus, the same dose blocks ovulation in 90 per cent of the animals. This period of maximal effectiveness lasts for about two hours and after that administration of ergocornine becomes ineffective.

In summary: one, ergocornine does block ovulation; two, the blockade does exhibit a distinct critical period effect; but, three, there is also an extended period of reduced effectiveness occurring before the critical period.

When we investigated the dose-response relation for the critical period we found that the 1 mg dose of ergocornine was a little low; to obtain maximal blockage, one needs a higher dose. The median effective dose or $ED_{50}$ works out to about the same as that for interfering with pregnancy, about 340 micrograms.

J. W. Everett: Is follicle development affected?

P. F. Kraicer: If the animals hadn't ovulated by the time of autopsy, we aspirated ova out of the follicles, examined them under the microscope, and classified them as either normal-preovulatory or post-ovulatory type. In 80 per cent of the ovaries the ova were preovulatory and the follicles were large Graafian follicles. The uterus retained its proestrous appearance and was still distended with fluid in 82 per cent of the animals. So there was every evidence of there having been adequate estrogen and follicular development seemed to be normal, but arrested at the Graafian follicle stage.

It appears that the ergocornine turns off the preovulatory surge of gonadotrophin secretion, even, in a certain percentage of cases, when given 40 hours before the surge is due, but it is difficult to fit all these data into the Procrustean theory of progesterone-hypothalamus interactions, since there is no evidence of stimulation of ovulation by progesterone 48 hours before follicular rupture.

J. W. Everett: Radford and I have tried to block ovulation by giving nembutal a day earlier in the cycle, without success--if that has any bearing.

P. F. Kraicer: Yes, that's also discouraging, thank you.

H. R. Lindner: We have some observations that may be relevant to this discussion. They concern the effects of ergocornine treatment on ovarian content of progestins, as determined by gas chromatography. We have noted that during diestrus, the ovary produces small, but definite amounts of progesterone [H. R. Lindner and A. Zmigrod, Acta Endocr. (Kbh.) 56, 16, 1967]. I think this has also been shown by others, recently, though it has not yet penetrated the textbooks. Another point that is now well established is that at diestrus and proestrus, there is a predominance of 20α-hydroxypregnenone (20α OHP) over progesterone. By contrast, during pseudopregnancy, the ratio is reversed, progesterone predominates over 20α OHP. During the cycle, ovarian content of progesterone is minimal on the morning of proestrus; there is a rise in the afternoon and evening of proestrus, presumably the preovulatory rise postulated by others on physiological grounds. From our data, we cannot say, of course, whether this rise in progesterone formation is a cause of ovulatory hormone release by the pituitary, or rather, the result of increased gonadotrophic stimulation.

Figure 1 shows the effect of ergocornine administered on day $L_4$ of pseudopregnancy. During the first 12 hours, at least, there was no significant difference between the ergocornine-treated rats and the controls. However, 24 hours after giving the drug, there was a significant drop in ovarian progesterone content, to about 40 per cent of the control level, and this was further depressed to one-third or one-quarter the normal content after 30-72 hours. At the same time, there was a dramatic rise in the ovarian content of $20\alpha$ OHP, which is not an effective progestational hormone. This could explain the effects of the drug in blocking pregnancy when given before the placenta is established.

E. S. Kisch: This again fits the picture you have found for proestrus. Here again the animal is about to ovulate.

H. R. Lindner: Yes, the picture entirely resembles that in a proestrous ovary. Wiest [W. G. Wiest, J. Biol. Chem. 234, 3115, 1959] has shown that $20\alpha$-hydroxysteroid dehydrogenase activity in rat ovaries is higher during proestrus than during pregnancy. We have recently measured this enzyme activity after ergocornine treatment [S. Lamprecht, J. F. Strauss III and H. R. Lindner--unpublished observations] and found that this enzyme activity increased markedly between the

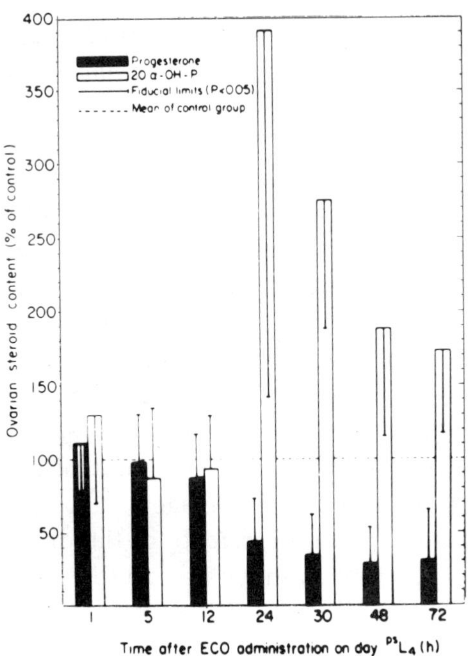


Fig. 1. Ovarian content of progesterone and 20α-hydroxyprogesterone in rats following ergocornine (1 mg s.c.) administration on day $L_4$ of pseudopregnancy, expressed as percent of the level in control pseudopregnant rats. (From Lindner and Shelesnyak, 1967. Reprinted with permission.)

24th and 72nd hour administration of the drug to pseudopregnant rats (Fig. 2); in pregnant rats a similar picture was obtained, though in this series of assays no significant increase in enzyme activity was demonstrable at 24 hours. The time-lag suggests that the effect of the drug is not a direct one on the ovary, and is consistent with the idea that the response is mediated by the hypothalamus and the pituitary gland.

J. Gorski: Are you actually getting an increase in steroid synthesis?

H. R. Lindner: No, the total content was roughly the same except at 48 hours after treatment when it was significantly reduced. But there is a marked shift from progesterone to 20$\alpha$-OHP.

J. W. Everett: You are getting more LH aren't you?

H. R. Lindner: Probably, yes, since the animal will ovulate on the third day. We have not measured this directly.

G. J. Marcus: There have been some reports, recently, concerning "over-ripe" eggs, that is ova which have been ovulated following delay and have reportedly produced abnormal foetuses [N. W. Fugo and R. L. Butcher, Fertil. Steril. 17, 804, 1966; R. L. Butcher and N. W. Fugo, Fertil. Steril. 18, 297, 1967]. Since both Prof. Everett and Dr. Kraicer have discussed inhibition or postponement of ovulation, would they comment on this "overripeness"?

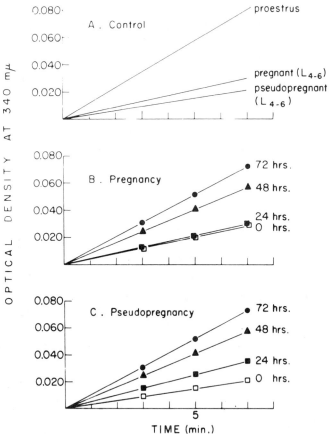

Fig. 2. Ovarian 20 α-hydroxysteroid dehydrogenase activity in rats treated with ergocornine (1 mg s.c.) at 10.00 a.m. on day $L_4$ of pregnancy (B) or pseudopregnancy (C). Controls (A) were injected with vehicle only. Assays were performed at 24-hour intervals as indicated. Each vessel contained the 20,000 g supernantant from a homogenate of 1.25 mg of ovarian tissue, 2.8 μmoles of EDTA, 2.8 μmoles of cysteine, 28 μmoles of nicotinamide, 1 μmole of NADP and 0.316 μmoles of 20 α-hydroxypregn-4-ene-3-one (added in 0.1 ml EtOH) in a final volume of 3.0 ml of 0.1 M potassium phosphate buffer, pH 8.0. Incubation was carried out at 37° and the absorption at 340 mμ was recorded continuously as a measure of NADP reduction.

J. W. Everett: I will say this, that a five-day cycle, as I interpret it, is one in which there is a spontaneous delay. Follicles grow an extra day and are larger at proestrus than at proestrus in the 4-day cycling rats. They are like follicles in the four-day cycle in which blockade has been produced by drug action. One can readily obtain normal pregnancies from five-day cyclic animals. On the other hand, we have a number of assorted experiments in which animals have been mated on the day after one blockade by nembutal or phenobarbital and some of these pregnancies were rather abnormal. I'd like to drop it right there, for want of sufficient data.

M. C. Shelesnyak: What do you mean by the pregnancies, the offspring?

J. W. Everett: No, the number of eggs implanting.

G. J. Marcus: But, of those that did implant, were there malformations? One paper reported chromosomal abnormalities.

J. W. Everett: I don't know. I have one case in which only one egg was implanted and the animal continued cycling. I picked her up only by accident later on. The foetus was oversize, incidentally.

U. S. von Euler: I was going to ask Dr. Kraicer a question. Can you exclude here an action of a more general type, I mean adrenolytic? You mentioned that there is a very specific effect of ergocornine. But, on the other hand, one must ask whether that can have something to do with the, say, penetration into the brain and the time of destruction, and such things. Do you have any evidence for any action of a similar kind by some other adrenolytic agent? One must not forget that the hypothalamus is just criss-crossed by adrenergic neurons, and it is not unlikely that they have something to do with this induction of changes which you measure here as inhibition of implantation and of ovulation.

P. F. Kraicer: I would prefer that Dr. Everett, who has worked with Dibenamine, answer this.

J. W. Everett: That was in collaboration with Drs. Sawyer and Markee [Endocrinology, 44, 234, 1949]. We used Dibenamine as a blocking agent and, at the time, we were reasonably confident that the transmitter substance going down the portal vessels was adrenergic. We have changed our viewpoint as to the site of action of Dibenamine and its congeners since then, though I am, of course, much interested in the recent evidence for a high concentration of adrenergic agents in the median eminence [K. Fuxe, Zeitschr. Zellforsch., 61, 710, 1964].

U. S. von Euler: But this may be at a higher level of the brain and come in before the actual release of the releasing substances. I think it would be of interest to try a large number of adrenolytic blocking agents, because they differ so much in their penetration, time of action and so on. There are many of them and one may be successful. Has reserpine been tried?

J. W. Everett: Reserpine does block in the rat [C.A. Barraclough and C. H. Sawyer, Endocrinology, 61, 341, 1957].

P. F. Kraicer: But only during the critical period, and not before. It does not produce an extended block. Many drugs have been found to confirm the critical period (which ergocornine does also, although only at the end of its period of effectiveness).

U. S. von Euler: And chlorpromazine?

P. F. Kraicer: It also matches the critical time.

U. S. von Euler: And that is also effective?

J. W. Everett: Yes. And incidentally - Psychoyos, I remember used chlorpromazine in the pregnant rat to get delayed nidation [J. Endocrinol. 27, 337, 1963].

E. S. Kisch: Mayer's group used reserpine for this purpose [G. Mayer and J. M. Meunier, C. R. Acad. Sci., 248, 3355, 1959].

P. F. Kraicer: And Chambon [Y. Chambon, Bull. Acad. Nat. Med., No. 9-10, 243, 1958]. This is very well documented, not only for reserpine and chlorpromazine, but a whole group of so-called tranquillizers will delay implantation.

U. S. von Euler: Chlorpromazine is a good adrenolytic agent, too. There is quite a number of them which might be tried systematically, I think.

J. W. Everett: I think it's a good point to mention here that Sawyer and associates working with the rabbit in which Dibenamine is an effective blocker of the rabbit reflex ovulation, found that in spite of Dibenamine, or treatment with one of the analogues of Dibenamine, stimulation of the basal tuber would, nevertheless, induce ovulation [C. H. Sawyer, in Endocrinology of Reproduction, C. W. Lloyd, ed., Academic Press, 1959, p. 1]. Partly on that basis, it seemed that Dibenamine and similar agents must be acting at a considerable distance away from the basal hypothalamus.

M. C. Shelesnyak: We have really been concerned with the effectiveness of ergocornine as an agent producing progesterone deprivation. With respect to the reversal of its action by the administration of reserpine and with regard to its influences on decidualization and implantation, we have studied the alkaloids of the ergotoxine series and the ergotamine series including the hydrogenerated derivatives. Ergocornine, ergosine and ergokryptine are effective; ergokryptine has about one tenth or one twentieth the activity and ergosine about one half the activity of ergocornine. But ergosine doesn't affect the hypothalamic cell discharge pattern nor does ergotamine or any of the hydrogenated alkaloids. I'm referring to influences on the phenomenon reported by Cross and Silver [B. A. Cross and I. A. Silver, J. Endocrin., 31, 251, 1965; Brit. Med. Bull. 22, 254, 1966]. The hypothalamic cells produce a characteristic spiking or firing frequency in their discharge pattern when the rats are under progesterone dominance and a different pattern when they are under estrogen dominance. If you give a progestating animal ergocornine by any route, the discharge pattern flips over to that characteristic of the estrous pattern and persists in this pattern for a long time. It can be reversed to the progestational pattern by intravenous progesterone administration, but the reversal only lasts about 40 minutes and then the pattern reverts to the estrous pattern. So it seems that the ergocornine acts right up there, and very quickly.

A. Barnea: Referring back to Dr. Everett's paper, with reference to the degree of stimulation of the preoptic nucleus or the surrounding area in relation to the amount of LH release, it seems to me that when you need a longer or shorter stimulus, at different times of the cycle, it might be related to the physiological condition of the neurons within this region which somehow regulate or control the secretion of the releasing-factors from the median eminance.

There is some evidence for conditioning of neurons in the work of Meyerson in Uppsala [B. J. Meyerson, Psychopharmacol. 6, 210, 1964]. He induced estrous behavior in ovariectomized animals by the well-known procedure of injecting estrogen, and after a certain period of time, injecting progesterone. Meyerson found that he could replace the injection of progesterone by biogenic amine-releasing substances like reserpine or tetrabenazine which act on the central nervous system, and when he did the whole study of these things more carefully, he found that the effect of reserpine or the other drugs he used probably was due to a depletion of a serotonin in the hypothalamus: he could reverse the effect only with injections of serotonin; injections of noradrenaline or dopamine which were also depleted by these drugs were ineffective. And a very interesting observation that he reported, was that when he gave the single dose of estrogen and two days later the reserpine, the effect of the reserpine lasted for about three weeks, that is he could wait two or three days, give another shot of estrogen, and again get estrous behavior without any progesterone, reserpine, or any other treatment. He waited again two or three days and again, another dose of estrogen produced estrous behavior. This effect of reserpine, lasted about two or three weeks, and during the whole period, the content of serotonin in the hypothalamus remained low. Progesterone didn't reduce the amount of serotonin in the hypothalamus, so the reserpine action cannot be compared directly to what progesterone is doing, but at least it concerns a type of memory. Perhaps it's not so much memory as it is a physiological conditioning of certain neurons.

J. W. Everett: Yes, I would use "memory" very loosely in quotes. I am well aware of Meyerson's observations and I find them very interesting.

U. S. von Euler: How were the amines administered? Intraventricularly?

A. Barnea: No, he administered the precursor. In certain cases, where he wanted to overcome the effects of reserpine by increasing the amount of serotonin in the hypothalamus, he gave 5-hydroxytryptophan or DOPA.

P. F. Kraicer: I thought there was no blood-brain barrier in the hypothalamus. Isn't that true?

J. W. Everett: That's true in the basal hypothalamus, that is, the tuber. But, at the higher levels there is a barrier.

P. F. Kraicer: The number of drugs which have been used to block ovulation, ranging from the barbiturates to atropine, are so diverse in their known pharmacological actions that it is difficult to extract from their actions any common feature which allows you to say that this must be a feature of the neurons affected. As a matter of fact, there doesn't seem to be any really common feature in the whole collection. What is the characteristic, do you think, of the hypothalamic neurons that makes them sensitive to this tremendous spectrum of pharmacological agents?

J. W. Everett: On the contrary, portions of the hypothalamus remain sensitive in spite of these agents, e.g., the medial preoptic region, and the anterior hypothalamic area.

P. F. Kraicer: Sensitive to direct electrical stimulation?

J. W. Everett: Yes.

P. F. Kraicer: Therefore, the nerves presumably are not firing and you have to make them fire.

J. W. Everett: However, the drugs cut off something else at a higher level.

P. F. Kraicer. I correct the question. What is the common characteristic of the something else?

J. W. Everett: That's one of the great questions that we hope to get at sometime. So far, I cannot give you an adequate answer.

M. Tausk: I think it has been made quite clear, particularly when Dr. Barnea quoted Halasz and the other Gorski (R. Gorski), that there are many influences from everywhere in the brain which somehow can influence the hypothalamus, so that a drug which ultimately shows up by some influence on ovulation or pseudopregnancy may have its point of attack, almost any where in the brain. This is exaggerated, but perhaps not too much exaggerated. And, therefore, I could imagine all sorts of pharmacological mechanisms coming into play. Would you say that is nonsense?

J. W. Everett: No, indeed.

M. Tausk: May I add to this another question? You showed, I think that there are changes in the sensitivity of the ovary, depending on the day of the cycle, and this you showed in two ways. One was that on certain days of the cycle you need more electric current or a longer period of stimulation of certain hypothalamic centers. You assume that, therefore, the pituitary will be forced to release more of its LH. On the other hand, you approach the problem by showing that on various days of the cycle the ovaries need different quantities of exogenous LH to ovulate. Now, the tacit assumption in this argument of yours, if I have reproduced it correctly, is that the sensitivity of the pituitary does not change. I just wonder whether, notwithstanding the proven changes in the sensitivity of the ovary, which, I think you have demonstrated by having to give varying quantities of exogenous LH, the sensitivity of the pituitary to hypothalamic stimuli or to, let's call it, LHRF, may not also vary. I would have thought that the only way of proving that would be by determining the level of LH in the blood, and, I believe, that this can be done. Have you any comment on that?

J. W. Everett: I think we have to look very closely at the amounts of LHRF required to stimulate the pituitary under different conditions as well as the possible variations in threshhold within the median eminence itself. I think all the way down the line, it may be desirable to test threshhold and amounts very critically.

M. Tausk: That may be perhaps too complicated. What I am suggesting is a somewhat simpler approach. If, on one day of the cycle, you have to stimulate the animal for 30 minutes and another day for 60 minutes to make it ovulate, it would be interesting to see whether there are differences in the secretion of LH into the blood by the pituitary.

J. W. Everett: By direct measurement?

M. Tausk: Of LH. Not of the releasing factor or anything, but simply of LH. I think it is being done, first, by radioimmuno assays, and it has been done particularly in Holland by Swelheim [Acta Endocr. 49, 231, 1964] in his analysis of the so-called Hohlweg effect. You know that Hohlweg showed 30 years ago that if you give a large dose of estrogen, the rat will ovulate. It has been assumed that this is due to an extra release of LH from the pituitary. Swelheim has actually shown that the castrated rat, maintained on a low maintenance dose of about 0.5 micrograms of estradiol benzoate, when you give a 100-fold larger amount will release LH within 24 hours, but in the female only, not in the male.

J. W. Everett: Has he shown this with the radioimmune assay?

M. Tausk: He did it by bioassay, but I think the radioimmuno assay would really be the royal route. Midgley and his group have determined LH in human plasma by a radioimmuno-assay [A. R. Midgley, Jr., Endocrinology, 79, 10, 1966].

J. W. Everett: One complication that occurs to me, is that we might be testing by radioimmuno-assay something which is totally inactive biologically.

So, a number of different kinds of assay need to be compared.

J. Gorski: I'd like to add a comment to that. It seems to be running through the course of this discussion so far, that it would be nice if there were more quantitative assays for these things. It seems to me it would be worth thinking, at least at this stage of the game, of trying to really mobilize energies in this direction. In so much of this, it seems to me you can go so far, as you have, but you are always talking sort of around the point that could be settled only by direct measurements.

H. R. Lindner: This also applies I think to the question of prolactin secretion during the latent period of delayed pseudopregnancy. Methods are now becoming available for measuring this in blood and I think, following the first principle of scientific research, it should be measured. The first principle, as you know, is that nothing is too much trouble as long as somebody else does it.

M. C. Shelesnyak: I wouldn't disagree with Jack (Gorski). It would be nice to have some of these things tied up and really measured. In many instances, though, we have a tremendous problem in knowing what to measure.

B. L. Lobel: I wonder whether quantitative differences in stimulation necessary on different days of the cycle might not have something to do with the sensitivity of the ovary at that time. In an animal with a short cycle, such as the rat, you would have great differences in the degree of maturation and development of the follicles on proestrus, estrus, $L_1$ and $L_2$. Therefore, if you stimulate an animal at a later time, it might need less, and if you stimulate an animal at an earlier time, it might need more. Also, I believe it has been shown that estrogen is stimulatory to the growth of the follicles itself.

J. W. Everett: With respect to the second point, it was shown a long time ago, that estrogen does have a growth effect on follicles [P. C. Williams, Proc. Roy. Soc., London, Ser. B, 132, 189, 1944].

On the first question, I think we indicated by LH injection that there are differences in requirements for LH between follicles in proestrus in a 4-day cycle on the one hand, and those in late diestrus in a 5-day cycle on the other hand, in which the follicles are of equivalent size and age since the last ovulation. The diestrous follicles require more LH.

B. L. Lobel: Don't you think this might be related to the degree of development of the follicles?

J. W. Everett: The follicles look alike. Maybe there is a difference in some subtle detail. Clearly, they differ in their responsiveness to LH.

B. L. Lobel: In view of Dr. Schayer's discussion of the intimate involvement of microcirculation in the mediation of so many physiological influences, I just would like to mention here that in the bovine ovary we have observed striking changes in the microcirculation preceding corpus luteum formation [B. L. ,Lobel, and E. Levy, Acta Endocr. (Kbh.) in press]. After ovulation there is extensive expansion of the microcirculation and one may see individual luteal cells surrounded by a network of capillaries. Towards the end of the cycle, the drop in the progesterone level in the blood is preceded by a collapse of the microcirculation within the corpora lutea. The capillaries surrounding the luteal cells lose their characteristic enzyme-histochemical staining properties and the endothelial cells become pyknotic.

R. W. Schayer: I like it. I just would make the general remark that every cell is preset genetically to carry out some function, and a very good way to bring this about is to increase its nutrient supply and let it reach its full potential. There is nothing mysterious about it; we all know that if a single celled animal is well nourished it'll develop and divide, if not well nourished, it won't.

G. J. Marcus: I would just add that Szego has shown that there is a fall in ovarian histamine content associated with immediate ovarian hyperemia in response to LH administration [C. M.Szego and E. S. Gitin, Nature, 201, 682, 1964].

# THE ACTIONS OF PROGESTERONE: FACTS AND THOUGHTS

# THE ACTIONS OF PROGESTERONE: FACTS AND THOUGHTS

M. Tausk

When Dr. Shelesnyak invited me to make a contribution to this meeting he suggested that this should reflect on the history of our concepts of progestation. In expressing my gratitude, I might say that my main relationship with the development of these concepts has been that I watched it for a very long time indeed. I thereby gained the impression that the history of progesterone and of its modern substitutes would be particularly suited to illustrate the development of endocrinology as a whole, which it does indeed reflect.

In 1903 Ludwig Fraenkel in Breslau wrote these sentences: *"The late embryologist Gustav Born is the

---

*Original text: "Der verstorbene Breslauer Embryologe Gustav Born ist der alleinige Vater der ursprünglichen nicht publizierten Hypothese, das Corpus luteum verum graviditatis müsse nach seinen Bau und Entwicklungsgang eine Drüse mit innerer Sekretion sein, ausgestattet mit der Function die Ansiedelung und Entwickelung des befruchteten Eies im Uterus zu veranlassen. Schwerkrank ersuchte er mich, die experi-

sole father of the original unpublished hypothesis that the corpus luteum verum graviditatis according to its structure and development should be a gland of internal secretion, having the function of initiating the settlement and development of the ferfilized egg in the uterus. Gravely ill, he asked me to undertake the experimental pursuit of this idea. The plan according to which I performed the experiments was my own independent work. Only some time after Born's death had the experiments matured so far as to prove the correctness of the theory."

Having stated a number of reasons why certain changes at and shortly after the time of ovulation were probably not brought about either by the ovum itself or by the mature follicle, Fraenkel wrote:* "If therefore we are looking for purpose in the institutions of Nature, we must assume a further function to be vested in the corpus luteum". But as a true son of his time he hurried to add in parenthesis, this apology:** "(Points

---

mentelle Verfolgung dieser Idee zu übernehmen. Der plan, nach welchem ich die Experimente anstellte, war mein selbständiges Werk. Erst längere Zeit nach dem Tode Born's waren die Experimente so weit gediehen, dass der Beweis für die Richtigkeit der Theorie erbracht war."

*Original: "Wenn wir also Zweckmassigkeit in den Institutionen der Natur suchen, müssen wir in dem Corpus luteum eine weitere Function vermuthen".

**Original: "(Die Punkte V and VI sind als teleologische Wahrscheinlichkeitsbeweise nicht uneingeschränkt giltig.)"

V and VI, being teleological circumstantial evidence, are of limited validity.)"

While bowing to the rule of the tribe that banishes teleology, Fraenkel was obviously profoundly convinced of the purposeful organization of life. It is this conviction which made and makes biological research possible. Clearly our mind cannot even for the briefest moment function without the concept of purpose and it is this purposeful mind with which we, the living, searchingly approach the way life is operating.

Fraenkel's experimental animal was the rabbit, in which he showed that early removal of the corpora lutea prevents a fertilized egg from becoming an implanted embryo, and at a later stage causes the termination of pregnancy. That the corpus luteum produces a characteristic lace-like structure in the endometrium of the nonpregnant rabbit was, as we know, shown by the French biologists Bouin and Ancel in 1910. In their classic paper, they give ample credit to Fraenkel and his teacher Born, but they also mention that Prenant in France had simultaneously with and independently of Born discovered the fact that the corpus luteum has the structure of a gland of internal secretion. In their own work, Bouin and Ancel tried to avoid some of the objections raised against Fraenkel's work and therefore they did not operate on their experimental animals, female rabbits. They had them mated with vasectomized males and then observed the histological changes in the ovary and the uterus following the ensuing ovulation.

They found a striking parallelism between the evolution and involution of the corpus luteum on the one hand and of the endometrium on the other. It is in regard to the latter's appearance on the fifth day after mating that they use the word lace-like.*

It was the great American anatomist Dr. G. W. Corner (1946) to whose lot it fell, as he said himself, "to conduct the experiments which tied together the discoveries of Fraenkel and Bouin and Ancel by showing exactly what happens, and when, to embryos deprived of the support normally afforded them by the corpus luteum."

While we all are convinced of the fundamental importance of Willard Allen and George Corner's work leading for the first time in history to the preparation of "progestin" (Allen, 1930) we may wonder at the relative and temporary validity of terms like "showing exactly what happens"; when we have been shown, we know, but to know something is only meaningful in relation to the state of affairs prior to such knowledge; in science this generally means: in relation to what we wanted to know or what we set out to learn. And since the human desire for knowledge is by definition insatiable, knowledge can only for brief moments quench our thirst.

As soon as progesterone became available from natural extracts or from synthesis, pharmacologists, biochemists, and endocrinologists set out to discover everything concerning the biological effects of the compound. Would such effects help us to understand those functions of the hormone, which had originally guided the biochemists in their attempts at isolating it? This we might call one highway of research: elucidation of the mechanism of physiological effects.

*"L'épithélium a envoyé dans la profondeur des invaginations glanduliformes très nombreuses, très allongées, parallèles les unes aux autres, qui decoupent le chorion en une véritable dentelle (l.c., page 11).

A second avenue was and is directed towards destinations of greater practical utility: the preparation of drugs having prolonged or otherwise improved activity (particularly by the oral route). In the laboratories of pharmaceutical companies, this research was nourished and sustained by the fruit of other efforts: large numbers of steroids, synthesized for sometimes entirely different purposes were screened for effects analogous to those of progesterone, a fact which automatically led to enquiries into the nature of structure-activity relationships and the like. In as much as the effects of such drugs are still regarded as analogous to those of the corpus luteum and could be used to substitute for it, we may still speak of a form of natural development from the basic discovery of progesterone.

The third highway on our map, starting from the same point of departure, leads us in a direction which is very much different from those of the first and second one. It is the road that Pincus surveyed and that was built largely according to his plans: the road towards ovulation-inhibition which led to oral contraception, using one of the activities of progesterone but apparently not for the purpose intended by nature.

This symposium is centred around nidation, defined as the period beginning with coition and terminating with placentation. This would mean, that I should concentrate on the mechanisms of effects exerted by progesterone in that period. However, knowledge gained along other lines might prove useful, since the screening of artificial steroids may tell us which activities of the progesterone molecule can be dissociated from others and which of these may or may not be required for nidation. Finally to look now and then on the scenery along the third road--let us call it the Pincus Road--might inspire us to think of methods of contraception based on interference with processes taking place at the critical period defined above.

Now in the classic paper in which Allen (1930) introduced the name "progestin" for the hormone of the corpus luteum, he expressed the view that "its chief action lies in its ability, by alterations of the endometrium to aid gestation in the castrated rabbit." This was a very logical conclusion--as far as the rabbit goes--since the extracts obviously acted on the endometrium, and equally obviously made gestation possible.

Today we have to ask ourselves whether this holds good for other species, whether the action on the endometrium is the one and only activity that makes pregnancy possible and whether the action that helps pregnancy to be established (action on nidation) is identical with the one needed to maintain pregnancy.

We know that the histological effects of progesterone on the endometrium are quite different in various species, which by no means excludes the possibility--indeed the probability that the functional effects may be the same. This would only illustrate another principle of hormone actions as we see them: a hormone, such as testosterone for example, may act on entirely different tissues in various species producing widely different morphological effects, but these seem to be of analogous functional significance.

One of the most remarkable aspects of the effects of progesterone on the endometrium is timing. The effects take a few days to develop, during which the egg is retained in the oviduct. C. G. Hartman (1961) epitomized this in these words: "from mouse to cow, monkey and man, the ovum reaches the uterus in about three and a half days . . . . . ," What does progesterone do to the egg during that stay or how does it influence the structures that harbour it?

I find it difficult to express in a few sentences, what a number of investigators have found by means of different techniques and in various species. The ovum in the Fallopian tube is apparently exposed to rotating, peristaltic and antiperistaltic movements, it is bathed in secretions of the epithelial lining and covered with mucus. It runs quickly through the first part of the tubal ampulla but lingers in the second, before being admitted to the isthmus. Oestrogens and progesterone have been shown to influence muscular activity, rate of transport, synthesis of mucin and discharge of mucus in the tube, (Greenwald, 1958; Koester, 1967), and it seems to be proven that the survival of the ovum in the tube depends on a subtle balance of these hormones. Tubal lock under the influence of oestrogens is one of the first dangers threatening the fertilized ovum and progesterone may be its protector at this early phase. It is to Dr. Pincus, who was to have been the moderator of this symposium, that we owe a good deal of our basic knowledge on this stage (see: Pincus, 1963). The ovum must enter the uterus not too early, not too late. What has progesterone done to prepare its settling there?

Once more it acts in concert with the oestrogenic hormone, in a quantitative relationship, precisely studied by Courrier and Kehl (see Courrier, 1945). Psychoyos' work led him to conclude: "A secretion of progesterone for at least 48 hours and the presence of oestrogen at the end of this period is the basic hormonal sequence necessary for implantation." We know of the great importance Prof. Shelesnyak attaches to the "estrogen surge" (Shelesnyak and Kraicer, 1963) and its biochemical implications. But returning to progesterone, it will be remembered that at a time when the uterus is conditioned to permit a blastocyst to implant itself, it will also respond to little traumas by the formation of nodules of decidualized cells, of which G. Mayer (1960) says: Progesterone sets them up, trauma makes them manifest.* It is here that we may for the first time resort to synthetic analogues of progesterone to show that the ability of a compound to produce the progestational lace-like structure of the rabbit's endometrium, does not mean that it will enable a mouse to produce a deciduoma. This was studied by Madjerek, de Visser, van der Vies and Overbeck (1960) in the Organon Laboratories in Holland.

So at least these two effects of progesterone can be separated and can appear independently in other, synthetic molecules. It stands to reason that they require different biochemical receptors. The same group of investigators have also shown that the ability of a substance to maintain pregnancy in a rat, castrated on the 10th day after fertile mating, is not reflected by its activity in the endometrial-lace-test, but as Madjerek (1967) recently expressed it: "an agent with a poor activity in the deciduoma test in mice usually does not maintain pregnancy in rats." (It should not be forgotten that in the maintenance of pregnancy the effect of progesterone on the uterine muscle may be of great importance, as shown by the fundamental work of Csapo (1961)). So it becomes clear that we must not look for one mech-

*"La progestérone les installe, le traumatisme les actualise" (l.c. page 4).

ism of action of progesterone but we may have to look for many.

The same impression is gained when we look at carbonic anhydrase activity which, according to Lutwak-Mann (1955, 1956) and to Pincus, Miyake, Merrill and Longo, is increased in the rabbit's endometrium (but not in the pig, the rat or the mouse) during pregnancy, and under the influence of exogenous progesterone, in parallel with the progressive histological transformation of the mucosa. The correlation may get lost, when other, synthetic substances are substituted for progesterone (Madjerek, unpublished data).

Data like these should warn us not to rush into accepting any biochemical effect of progesterone as primary. Many things may happen once a hormone like progesterone has started to influence any of its natural substrates. This was beautifully demonstrated in a paper by Erika Bontke (1960) who found increases in 10 different enzymes and other substances in the premenstrual, progesterone dominated endometrium in women.

We are again confronted with the dissociation of activities vested in the progesterone molecule when we look for compounds imitating its effects on the hypothalamus. There progesterone can facilitate ovulation but also inhibit it, the latter action being more popular nowadays. But as Kincl and Dorfman (1963) have shown (and we know from our own studies), the antiovulatory activity of a synthetic compound is not related necessarily to its progestational activity, the latter term referring, of course, to the rabbit's endometrium.

By inhibiting ovulation progesterone would appear to exert another protecting function for the benefit of ova already fertilized, but again this is not the only one of its actions which serves this particular purpose. After ovulation (and fertilization), when progesterone becomes dominant, the female organism seems to become hostile to spermatozoa. Thus we know that the cervical mucus in women changes conspicuously and becomes unfavourable to the penetration of sperm. But it has also been demonstrated by Chang (1958) that under the influence of progesterone (endogenous or exogenous) rabbit endometrium loses its ability to capacitate spermatozoa. Capacitation probably consists of the destruction of a decapacitation factor which occurs in seminal plasma (Weinman and Williams, 1964; see also Austin, 1967).

I am afraid, I have wandered a little too far afield, away from the main subject of this symposium. However, any feeling of guilt I might be expected to show, is relieved by the simple fact that every single member of this audience knows ten times more about the preimplantation stages of pregnancy that I do. I was told I should speak about the historical roots of our current understanding of progestation. Understanding sounds like an ambitious word when applied to the phenomena of life, but perhaps it expresses longing rather than ambition. Looking at hormones we are impressed, time and again by the remarkable fact that there are these relatively simple substances in the living body, which obviously fit into a great number of systems—as in our case the ovary, the tube, the uterus, the hypothlaamus--and may find a great variety of receptors there to react with. Most or perhaps all of the effects so produced leave us with the inescapable conclusion that they are converging towards purposes inherent in the preservation of life. While we may be hopeful of elucidating the physical and chemical mechanisms of every one of these reactions I doubt whether science is equipped with tools to reduce to physics and chemistry the overwhelming organisation of life as a whole.

## LITERATURE

Allen, W. M. (1930). Physiology of the corpus luteum V. The preparation and some clinical properties of progestin, a hormone of the corpus luteum which produces progestational proliferation. Amer. J. Physiol. 92, 174-188.

Austin, C. R. (1967). Capacitation of Spermatozoa. Internat. J. Fertil. 12, 25-31.

Bontke, E. (1960). Histochimie de l'endomètre prémenstruel et gravide. In: Les fonctions de nidation utérine et leurs troubles. Colloque de la Société Nationale pour l'étude de la stérilité et de la fécondité. Masson et Cie., Paris.

Bouin, P. and P. Ancel (1910). Recherches sur les fonctions du corps jaune gestatif. J. de Physiologie et de pathologie générale 12, 1-16.

Chang, M. C. (1958). Capacitation of rabbit spermatozoa in the uterus with special reference to the reproductive phases of the female. Endocrinology, 63, 619-628.

Courrier, R. (1945). Endocrinologie de la gestation. Masson et Cie., Paris.

Csapo, A. (1961). The role of progesterone in the maintenance and termination of pregnancy. In: Progesterone. Brook Lodge Symposium. A.C. Barns, Ed.

Fraenkel, L. (1903). Die Function des Corpus Luteum. Arch. Gynaek. 68, 438-545.

Greenwald, G. S. (1958). Endocrine regulation of the secretion of mucin in the tubal epithelium of the rabbit. Anat. Record. 130, 477-495.

Hartman, C. G. (1961). A half century of research in reproductive physiology. Fertil. and Steril. 12, 1-19.

Kincl, F. A. and R. I. Dorfman (1963). Anti-ovulatory activity of steroids in the adult oestrous rabbit. Acta Endocr. Suppl. 73.

Koester, H. (1967). Zur Physiologie der Eileitersekretion während der Eipassage durch die Tube. Lecture held at the 69th meeting of the Nordwestdeutsche Gesellschaft für Gynakologie, Göttingen, May 5-7. To be published.

Lutwak-Mann, C. (1955). Carbonic anhydrase in the female reproductive tract; occurrence, distribution and hormonal dependence. J. Endocrinol. 13, 23-28.

Lutwak-Mann, C. (1956). La carbonico-anidrasil nell'utero di mammiferi. Boll. Soc. Ital. Biol. sper. 31, 511-514.

Madjerek, Z., J. de Visser, J. van der Vies and G. A. Overbeek (1960). Allylestrenol, a pregnancy maintaining oral gestagen. Acta Endocr. (Kbh.) 35, 8-19.

Madjerek, Z. (1967). Bioassays. In: Progestational drugs and antiferility agents. Section Ed.: M. Tausk; The International Encyclopedia of Pharmacology and Therapeutics. Pergamon Press. London. To be published.

Mayer, G. (1960). Morphologie et physiologie comparées de l'ovoimplantation. Résultats et problèmes. In: Les fonctions de nidation utérine et leurs troubles. Colloque de la Société Nationale pour l'étude de la stérilité et de la fécondité. Masson & Cie. Paris.

Pincus, G. (1936). The eggs of mammals. MacMillan Co., New York.

Pincus, G., T. Miyake, A. P. Merrill and P. Longo (1957). The bioassay of progesterone. Endocrinology 61, 528-533.

Psychoyos, A. (1966). Recent researches on egg implantation. In: Egg Implantation. Ciba Foundation Study Group No. 23. Ed.: G. E. W. Wolstenholme and Maeve O'Connor. J. & A. Churchill Ltd. London.

Shelesnyak, M. C. & Kraicer, P. F. (1966) Role of estrogen in nidation. p. 265-280. In: Delayed Implantation. A. C. Enders, Ed. Univ. of Chicago Press.

Weinman, D. E. and Williams, W. L. (1964). Mechanism of capacitation of rabbit spermatozoa. Nature 203, 423-424.

## DISCUSSION

M. Tausk: I forgot to show one slide, the latest on in the historical picture gallery. As everyone probably knows, this was Gregory Pincus, the man who invented the Gregorian calendar which begins on the fifth and ends on the twenty-fifth day of the cycle.

P. F. Kraicer: I have taken the liberty of arranging some of the discussants in what I consider to be a reasonable order, especially since the things that Dr. Tausk spoke about are so pertinent to the work we have been doing.

We have utilized one of the earliest techniques, that of Fraenkel, which Dr. Tausk has described, that is, the extirpation of the corpora lutea in order to study not only the effects of the extirpation of of the corpora lutea, but also the endocrine activities of the non-luteal tissues as they relate to progestation and pregnancy. The animals in our experiments are treated with trypan blue at a time before the corpora lutea are formed. As a result the animals become completely blue, but the new corpora lutea, when they are formed, are not blue. This makes the latest generation of corpora stand out beautifully. Now, with an electrocautery needle, we can burn out the corpora. The electrocautery we used was particularly convenient for this purpose, because there is no contact between the electrode and the tissue, but rather, if one brings the electrode close to the tissue, a spark jumps the gap and combusts the tissue. This seals off blood vessels so that one doesn't get all blood all over everything and it allows one to follow the course of the destruction of the corpus luteum because the cauterization leaves nothing but a hole. We even managed to get the ovarian bursa back on so that if the animal ovulates we can collect the ova in the oviduct.

The tissue which remains we refer to as nonluteal ovarian tissue. It's quite a mixed bag though, not uniform composition by any means. It consists of small and large follicles, interstitial tissue and older corpora lutea which are in various stages of involution.

The day after the surgery, the interstitial tissue is red in color. The remaining ovarian tissue is inflamed. Nevertheless, it seems to be capable of endocrine function at a fairly normal level.

We have burned out corpora lutea on day 4 of pregnancy and then watched the vaginal smears. The number of corpora left intact was verified subsequently, at autopsy. When we left no corpora, the animals reverted to estrus two or three days later and none of eleven rats so treated had nidation sites. Of 18 rats left with one corpus luteum, only one had nidation sites on day 7; she also had an estrous vaginal smear. Fifteen of the remaining 17 showed frank vaginal cornification and the two that didn't had ovaries full of corpora lutea at autospy so I suspect that they did have a wave of luteinization, probably accompanying ovulation which was not reflected in the vaginal smear. With 2 corpora lutea, 11 animals had nidation sites, but nine of the eleven showed vaginal estrous configurations. Three of the four animals without nidation sites had estrous smears. And finally, with three corpora lutea left intact, all of the animals had nidation sites and six out of the eleven had original cornification. Pregnancy continued normally. Of 4 rats allowed to go to term, 3 delivered living, term foetuses.

Conclusions: Extra-luteal tissue is capable of functioning after luteëctomy. Among other things, it is capable of secreting estrogen. This is absolutely certain. And what is curious, it is capable of secreting estrogen even in the presence of enough corpora lutea to maintain some of the foetuses to term. This is a curious association. Estrogen in the presence of physiologically adequate quantities of progesterone does not cause vaginal cornification; it causes vaginal mucification. What we saw here, however, was frank cornification, a finding which I am not able to interpret.

What does this extra-luteal tissue do? It is known that if rats are spayed sometime between one and three days after copulation, and treated with progesterone, nidation will be delayed. Until when will it be delayed? It will be delayed until estrogen is added to the previous treatment. With estrogen plus progesterone, there is nidation at the normal time. When we removed the corpora lutea, and treated the luteëctomized rats with progesterone giving no exogenous estrogen, ova implanted at the normal time and developed into perfectly normal foetuses. This indicates that the non-luteal tissues of the ovary can secrete estrogen in pregnant animals.

Since it is widely believed that estrogen synergizes with progesterone in the maintenance of gestation, we examined the ability of progesterone to maintain foetal development to term in the presence and absence of the non-luteal ovarian tissues.

In our control series, which were injected with 4 mg of progesterone every day from 4 to day 20 of pregnancy, we found 75 percent of normal foetuses as well as a few resorbed foetuses (resorbed foetuses are represented by myometrial glands in the mesometrium).

M. C. Shelesnyak: Were these normal pregnancies?

P. F. Kraicer: Yes, these were normal pregnancies, but the rats got daily progesterone injections. These results are not different from those obtained with another group which was not treated with progesterone.

M. C. Shelesnyak: In other words, there was 25 per cent pregnancy wastage.

P. F. Kraicer: Yes, 25 per cent of the ova originally present, as estimated from counts of corpora lutea. All of the animals were vitally stained to give accurate counts of corpora lutea.

Now, when we ovariectomized animals on day $L_4$ and maintained them on progesterone to term, only 6 live foetuses were obtained from 12 rats. The number of resorbing foetuses was 14; there were only macerated placentae in most cases. The number of metrial glands only, was 43; these presumably represent embryos which were resorbed soon after implantation. The total number of implantations was a little under half of the number of corpora lutea counted.

If we luteëctomized the rats instead of ovariectomizing them (these animals were also maintained with exogenous progesterone) the ova count again turned out to be half the corpus luteum count, but, in contradistinction to the ovariectomized, progesterone-treated group, most of the implanted ova were maintained to term and the number of resorbing or resorbed embryos was very small. That is, the extra-luteal tissues allowed exogenous progesterone to bring the foetuses to term as live, normal pups, which progesterone without the extra-luteal tissue was unable to do.

If, instead of removing the corpora lutea by surgery, we removed them pharmacologically, with ergocornine, we got much the same picture. We were able to maintain 72 per cent of the ova to term with progesterone and had only 10 per cent resorbing and resorbed embryos. We must conclude from the discrepancy between the numbers of implants in the various groups, that just exposing the ovary and handling it surgically causes a certain amount of pregnancy wastage--a loss of 25 to 30 per cent of the ova, which, never implant. Had they implanted and then been lost there would have been bleeding into the vagina two or three days afterwards, but we never found this.

M. C. Shelesnyak: There is a tendency for referees to ask for sham operations for everything nowadays, and a tendency for certain authors to say sham operations were done. What would you consider sham operations for this type of approach?

P. F. Kraicer: Our original technique for luteectomy was to open the animal up and check both ovaries. One ovary usually has more corpora lutea than the other. The one with most of the corpora was removed and the corpora from the second ovary were cauterized. This ensured that the extra-luteal tissue which remained had suffered minimal damage. Our sham operation was to take out the ovary which had the minimum number of corpora and then burn out half a dozen follicles in the other ovary leaving in as many corpora lutea as possible untouched. This operation had no effect except on $L_1$, the day after insemination, when a certain amount of pregnancy wastage was caused. At this time, however, the corpora lutea are not very well formed. The ruptured follicles are still undergoing luteinization. For this reason, it is difficult to speculate on what the effect of sham luteëctomy, that is, ovarian trauma, may be.

M. C. Shelesnyak: It seems that the ideal of sham operation is something which is close to, but assures you of not getting any results.

M. Tausk: May I say a few words with respect to this phenomenon that puzzles you, that is, the cornification in the vagina of the animals which have a reduced number of corpora lutea. I wondered whether this isn't just a matter of a ratio between the quantities of estrogen and progesterone. Apparently the thresholds, or more precisely perhaps, the required ratio between progesterone and estrogen is not the same for a) vaginal cornfication, b) nidation, and c) maintenance of pregnancy. I can well imagine that you only have an estrogen: progesterone ratio which gives you enough progesterone for nidation and still gives you cornification of the vagina. I think these things, to be extent that you haven't done it yourself, can probably be worked out quantitatively. I am sure Courrier has done a lot of this work already.

The other thing is about the maintenance of pregnancy. Our experience, that is to say, of Madjerek and his group, is that we always castrated rats on the tenth day of pregnancy for the purpose of testing new compounds for their ability to maintain pregnancy. If you do that, then with progesterone alone you maintain about 70 to 80 per cent of the foetuses. On day ten of pregnancy, the rat is spayed, the number of implants counted and thereafter you inject progesterone daily and count the number of viable foetuses extracted by caesarean section at term. I don't know what your experience is, but these castrated animals don't spontaneously deliver, which is another queer and interesting phenomenon.

P. F. Kraicer: But the luteëctomized do.

M. Tausk: They do? Castrated rats do not normally deliver.

H. R. Lindner: The sheep does.

M. Tausk: The only point I wanted to make is that in these rats, castrated on day ten of pregnancy, you don't have to add estrogen to the progesterone in order to get about 70 per cent of live foetuses, but in general, it helps.

P. F. Kraicer: The largest pregnancy wastage in the rats receiving only progesterone in our experiments was represented by small metrial glands with nothing in the uterine lumen beside them. I assume that this pregnancy wastage occurred at approximately the time of ovariectomy or, in other words, soon after implantation. If you take out the ovaries later, you found foetuses already well on their way to placentation. These are at a far more advanced stage of development, than were the embryos which died in our experiments, and have probably passed the sensitive stage.

M. Tausk: Quite possible.

P. F. Kraicer: If there is no further discussion on this point, perhaps Dr. Lobel would discuss some of the morphological manifestations of progesterone action on the rat endometrium.

B. L. Lobel: Unfortunately, we have little information on the independent effects of progesterone acting on the uterus in ovariectomized rats. I would just mention that in pseudopregnant rats, progesterone withdrawal 48 hours after induction of decidualization, either due to ovariectomy or to ergocornine administration, leads to disintegration of the deciduomata and extensive hemorrhage into the endometrial stroma and into the lumen.

M. Tausk: I can only say that it's highly interesting. Hemorrhage on withdrawal of hormones is, of course, a very familiar phenomenon in the primate. I didn't know that is occurs in rodents, and apparently under very specific conditions. It might be interesting to see whether these conditions in any way resemble those prevailing in the primate on withdrawal of steroids.

M. C. Shelesnyak: The parallelism with the situation in the primate is very good here because the hemorrhage in the rat is not simply the result of estrogen and progesterone withdrawal, but of withdrawal of progesterone after estrogen action during progestation and after decidual tissue has formed, which is precisely the situation in the human endometrium at the end of the secretory or luteal phase. There is decidual tissue from which hormonal support is withdrawn. I'm referring to what pathologists call predecidual cells, because there is no pregnancy, but the cells are essentially decidual cells.

G. J. Marcus: There has been a great deal of attention paid to synergism between estrogen and progesterone in their actions on the uterus. Such synergism has been demonstrated, usually only after extended pretreatment with estrogen or in response to extended treatment with both hormones [cf, Reviews by R. Courrier, Vitamines Hormones 8, 179, 1950; K. Fotherby, Vitamins Hormones 22, 153, 1964].

Although increases in uterine protein, RNA and weight are readily demonstrated within twenty four hours after administration of estrogen or estrogen plus progesterone, to the best of my knowledge no increase in the uterine content of DNA within 24 hours in reponse to hormone administration has been demonstrated.

Nevertheless, during progestation in the rat, a brief period of estrogen action, that is, when estrogen is secreted by the ovary within an interval of less than 12 hours [M. C. Shelesnyak, P. F. Kraicer and G. H. Zeilmaker, Acta Endocr. (Kbh) 42, 225, 1963] results in an increase in total uterine DNA within 24 hours [M. C. Shelesnyak and L. Tic, Acta Endocr. (Kbh) 41, 465, 1963; V. J. De Feo, Endocrinology, 72, 305, 1963]. We recently attempted to duplicate this growth effect using exogenous hormones in various ratios. We have used a constant amount of progesterone, viz. 4 mg which we have found to be the minimal daily dose which would maintain a decidual growth in our colony. We were able to demonstrate a highly significant increase in total uterine DNA as well as of protein, RNA and uterine weight at 24 hours after administration of estrogen plus progesterone, but under specific conditions only: we ovariectomized rats at 08.00 hrs on day $L_3$ of pseudopregnancy, that is, before the estrogen surge has begun, and administered 4 mg of progesterone and 0.02 micrograms of estradiol benzoate at 12 noon [L. Tic, P. Levinson and G. J. Marcus, unpublished observations]. At 24 hours, we found a significant increase in uterine weight, protein, RNA and DNA. With larger doses of estrogen, as the benzoate or as free estradiol, no increases in DNA nor in protein were observed, although increases in RNA and uterine weight were obtained. Progesterone alone or estrogen alone were unable to produce these increases, although progesterone prevented decreases and a high dose of estradiol produced an increase in RNA only.

No synergistic effects could be demonstrated in rats which had been spayed 3 weeks before the hormonal treatment. Now this failure to obtain synergism between estrogen and progesterone illustrates a point which I believe is frequently overlooked, and that is that when one investigates the action of hormones on the uterus one must not forget the previous status of the uterus influences the response obtainable on subsequent treatment. I only want to emphasize that the standard assay animal, that is the immature or long-time castrate rat may not respond to experimental treatment in the same way as the normal mature animal and misleading or conflicting data may result from observations in such experimental animals.

H. R. Lindner: The induction of implantation is one of the more sensitive responses to estrogen. You can induce implantation with 50 to 60 nanograms of estrogen in the rat that is under progesterone domination. You obviously couldn't do it without the progesterone. This dose, incidentally, is of the same order as that which appears to be synergistic with progesterone in your experiments.

M. Tausk: This whole problem of estrogen and progesterone antagonism and synergism I think is rather perplexing. I think we should not forget that progesterone practically never acts except together with estrogen. If you take an infantile or castrated rabbit, without estrogen priming, progesterone does nothing, or certainly does not give any typical response. It must be preceded by estrogen, and certainly under physiological circumstances there is always estrogen present whenever progesterone acts. The corpus luteum itself produces estrogen.

G. J. Marcus: But in the rat, at least, there doesn't appear to be any estrogen present during progestation except for that brief period which is necessary for implantation, that is, the estrogen surge. Also decidual growth, once initiated, can be supported by progesterone alone. As a matter of fact, although glycogen deposition in the uterus seems to be controlled by estrogen, this only applies to the myometrium, at least in the rat. The endometrium normally contains very little glycogen, if at all. We found that endometrial tissue scrapped out of the uteri of pseudopregnant rats with a trocar (and, therefore, possibly contaminated with some myometrial tissue) contained only about 25 mg per cent glycogen but decidual tissue from spayed rats maintained on progesterone only contained several hundred milligrams per cent glycogen. This was dependent on the dose of progesterone in the sense that if you reduce the dose very much, you can't get decidualization and therefore no glycogen. So, at least, in the decidual tissue of the rat progesterone acting alone does something.

However, would the reverse not be true, that is, that whenever estrogen acts, progesterone is present?

M. Tausk: No, no.

A. Barnea: In immature rats there is estrogen secretion which very likely precedes any progesterone secretion.

G. J. Marcus: I was referring to the mature animal. Can one assume that the mechanism or nature of the action of estrogen is the same in an immature animal, where estrogen may always act in the absence of progesterone, as in the mature animal where there may always be some progesterone present.

H. R. Lindner: You can get responses in castrated rats and mice to estrogen alone. There in doubt about that.

P. F. Kraicer: But that's not the question. Does one find estrogen in an animal when there is no progesterone present, since progesterone is a precursor, and they both are coming out of the same place, I seriously doubt it.

M. Tausk: Do you mean there will be a little bit of progesterone from the adrenal?

P. F. Kraicer: I have been tremendously impressed by the high concentrations of progesterone which have been identified in follicular fluid and follicular tissue generally. I seriously doubt that none of this leaks out into the blood system.

The question is, when one gets away from the assay animal, and deals with the animal which is running a normal life; does she ever exist in a purely estrogenic status, devoid of progesterone? Surely it's possible; surely it also isn't known.

H. R. Lindner: Probably not.

M. Tausk: Now, with respect to the question of glycogen, may I just briefly say that in the human, estrogen is known to produce glycogen in the vagina, the famous nutrient medium for the Döderlein bacilli. In the endometrium, a small dose of progesterone will produce a very thin layer of glycogen in the basal part of the cells, underneath the nucleus, and large doses of progesterone will produce a large quantity of glycogen in the apical or top layer of the cells which will overflow into the secretion. But I think all these observations in women are practically always done in women who have some estrogen production, because if you do it in ovariectomized women, as for instance, Ferin is doing in the University of Louvain in Belgium, then I don't think that with progesterone alone anyone has ever produced the full maturation of the endometrium with the full overflow of glycogen as occurs under physiological conditions.

G. J. Marcus: Are the cells in which glycogen can be seen in the human endometrium those which are referred to by some as predecidual cells?

M. Tausk: No, these are epithelial cells, glandular cells.

H. R. Lindner: I just wanted to make a few comments on Dr. Tausk's presentation. I had some sympathy with you in your wistful remarks about the usefulness of the concepts of teleology, and the purposefulness of nature which seems to be an essential guiding principle to any biological investigator. And sometimes it happens that a concept which we are really still attached to falls into disrepute or becomes odious, and the way out is often to invent a different name for the same thing: Dr. Pittendrigh in 1958 [C. S. Pittendrigh in Behaviour and Evolution, ed. A. Roe and G. G. Simpson, Yale University Press, New Haven, 1958 p. 391] proposed the use of the term teleonomy for teleology in the sense in which the latter is used by modern biologists, implying that natural selection rather than divine foresight is the responsible agent. The distinction is analogous, perhaps, to that between astrology and astronomy. Someone has proposed recently that maybe we should substitute bionomy for biology in the same way. I feel, just as Prof. Tausk, that this concept, the seeming purposefulness, usefulness and elegance in the design of nature is helpful to us; I would, nevertheless, insist that the belief that all biological phenoma can eventually be reduced to the principles of physics and chemistry is equally essential to the biological investigator, although we may not as yet be able to explain many problems in these terms.

M. C. Shelesnyak: I would like to take issue. One must realize that the biophysical and biochemical terms and the methods that we use to approach the examination of certain biological processes, are valid for the examination but not necessarily for the complete understanding. There is a difference in the final analysis—I always like to come back to this rather naive generalization—that with all due respect to Jack and to Jensen and everybody else who works out the precise mechanism of action receptors of estrogen, it is a long, far cry from providing a basis for explaining why a spayed rat, if given estrogen will suddenly change her personality. It's true one can say it's working on the brain and does all sorts of things but there is still a totality of biological behavior that must be accepted.

J. Gorski: You can't explain a computer by just looking at a piece of copper wire, but you would surely be in trouble trying to explain it if you didn't know about the copper wire. I think I really agree with Hans. I don't think you really disagree, either, but you are saying that it's complex and that it may be sometime before we can explain the whole process.

M. Tausk: May I say something, since you are provoking me. I like this discussion, and first of all, I'd like to state again exactly what I have said so as to avoid any misunderstanding. What I said literally at the end of my lecture was: "while we may be hopeful to elucidate the physical and chemical mechanisms of everyone of these reactions (the reactions which are elicited by hormones), I doubt whether science is equipped with tools to reduce to physics and chemistry the overwhelming organization of life as a whole."

Let me elaborate on this for just a moment, and then I will try to reply more specifically to what you have said. I do not for one moment suggest that there are any reactions taking place in living organisms which are not subject to the laws of physics and chemistry. That would be preposterous, it would be foolish, and I haven't said anything of the sort. But, I am equally convinced that all these reactions take place within the framework of an organization. That organization is provided by the structure, the immensely complicated structure, and even at the electromicroscopical level, there is always this requirement of an organized structure. Only within that structure do these reactions occur so that they have a biological function.

Now, gentlemen, during these past days, knowing that something like this would happen after I said my last sentence, I was tempted—I didn't do it—to jot a little mark on my paper whenever any speaker spoke about the function of a thing in an organism. Function is nothing else but the definition of the purpose of a thing within the organization. If you try to take out purpose or function, you are no longer practicing biology. I once heard a very fine lecture by the Viennese ethologist, Konrad Lorenz, who is studying animal behavior so profoundly. In a lecture at the New York Academy of Sciences, Lorenz said that if you were to find a man from some other planet and give him all the parts of which a Cadillac is made and ask him to put them together, he would not succeed unless he knew what the thing was made for, what the function of the whole is.

Now you said one thing, Dr. Lindner, which provokes me very much. You said that we should introduce the word teleonomy instead of teleology, just as we use astronomy instead of astrology, the difference, of course, being that astrology is some charlatanism and astronomy is a science. We would then treat the subject by means of the principles of natural selection. The point I am trying to make now is this. Your aversion to the introduction of the word "purpose" or teleology, rests upon a belief of yours, a basic conviction, and that itself is a prescientific. Before you even start any scientific work, you are starting from a belief, from a faith, which says that all we are dealing with in science are matters of cause and effect, and that there is no place for anything like purpose or an overall plan or something like that. Introducing that would, in your mind, and in the minds of many people who argue the same way, somehow introduce the principle of the governing spirit, and that you don't want. You don't want it for the same reason for which the people who believe in God want God. You have a negative religion and a negative belief. Now, I say that any attempt to explain life as a whole should take into account the fact that part of this life is our spirt, our thinking, the thing with which we approach this science. We approach the corpus luteum with our thinking. How would you explain that by the process of natural selection such a thing as my, for or that matter, your very much greater intelligence has come into being, and that you can now with this intelligence, which is part of our life, approach the phenomena of life, if you want to eliminate from it the only one and characteristic element of this intelligence, and that is the element of purpose? I said in passing in my lecture that "not even for the briefest moment can our mind function without the concept of purpose."

H. R. Lindner: You are thinking now of the purpose of a creator or a divine force?

M. Tausk: No. I am not saying anything about the creator. I respectfully leave that alone. I said just now that people who are so much afraid of using the argument of teleology are those who are afraid that by using it they are somehow introducing God into science and there God should not be. This is a religion, a negative religion, but it is a religious belief. If you observe life, you must be prepared to include within the phenomena which you observe what your mind does. It seems to me, that purely for statistical reasons, it is exceedingly improbable that life could have developed by pure chance and by natural elimination of lethal mutations, although I do not for one moment dispute the importance of mutations and lethal mutations. It is the famous story of the monkey and the typewriter which you certainly know. If you put enough monkeys in front of enough typewriters, then you might say that statistically it is possible that one day a sonnet of Shakespeare will come out. But you would never make such an improbable assumption in any of your laboratory experiments. You are making this highly improbable assumption because you are driven by basic beliefs that something should not be. This basic belief is in contradiction with your own behavior and with the behavior of your own mind, and it is an attempt to explain away the obvious.

H. R. Lindner: I would just say two sentences. I would not dispute anything Prof. Tausk has said. I only think that in my scientific endeavors I confine myself to hypotheses that can be disproved. Dr. Schayer's hypothesis, for example, is one which I at the moment regard as marginal in this respect. It has not been formulated in such a form as to be readily amenable to experimental test. But I think we both agree that the existence of God or the operation of divine foresight or purpose in nature is a proposition which cannot be disproved by any scientific hypothesis that I take into account in any of my experimentations.

M. Tausk: Perfectly right.

H. R. Lindner: I don't say it doesn't exist, but in my mind it doesn't belong to the realm of scientific experimentation as such.

M. Tausk: May I just say in conclusion that, like you, I would be violently opposed, to any attempt to explain any biological reaction by what Dr. Shelesnyak called this morning "an act of God." We do not introduce God into any biological reaction, and I am not proposing to do so. I am perfectly convinced that the whole raison d'etre of the scientist is that he should explain everything that happens by means of pure chemistry and physics, and nothing is more fascinating for me than to see other people do that because I don't do it. But I very modestly remarked and I repeat, that while we may hope to explain chemically and physically every single reaction in the living organism, I doubt whether science is equipped with the tools to reduce to chemistry and physics the overwhelming organization of life.

H. R. Lindner: I don't think we are terribly far apart.

J. Gorski: Maybe with purpose we can get the tools.

M. C. Shelesnyak: I'd just like to point out that the phrase "act of God" is a legal phrase--

M. Tausk: I know, I was joking.

M. C. Shelesnyak: And also I don't think I should get credit for originating that statement. I mean it's only fair that reference be made to the earliest, not to the most recent publication.

# IMMUNOLOGICAL ASPECTS OF REPRODUCTION

# IMMUNOLOGICAL ASPECTS OF REPRODUCTION

Seymour Katsh, Ph.D.
Department of Pharmacology
University of Colorado Medical Center
Denver, Colorado

## INTRODUCTION

It is a comfort to scientists generally to be able to point to a juncture in time or literature when realization of a phenomenon was first made evident. In respect to immunological interference with fertility, we have no definitive reference point. We could speculate that here in the cradle of civilization the first recorded instance of such an event had occurred. In the Bible it is related that Sarah was sterile for much of her married life but conceived in her later years. This could be interpreted to mean that following her initial coital exposures to male antigens, she had become immunized to her mate's spermatozoal and seminal plasmal antigens. Then, during the long period of continence while Abraham had Hagar as a second wife, her antibody response declined and conception was possible. A stronger inference can be drawn from the stipulations in the ancient Assyrian Laws: "If a woman has crushed a man's testicle in an affray, one of her fingers shall be cut off: And if although a physician has bound it up, the second testicle is affected with it and becomes inflamed, both her nipples shall be torn off" (Driver and Miles, 1935; Sigerist, 1955). Using today's knowledge, this stipulation could be interpreted as an observation that trauma to one testicle caused the release of antigen and the resulting auto-antibody induced damage in the contralateral gonad. In this context the ancient observation is noteworthy because legal restriction of human behavior is invariably _ex post facto_ and, consequently, the laws recognized the event had occurred.

Even Darwin's writings suggest a relationship between immunology and fertility. In the Descent of Man (Darwin, 1898), there are a number of statements relating the profligacy of women to reduced fertility. The inference could be drawn that repeated exposure to antigenic material in the male ejaculate caused antibody response that resulted in sterility. Clearly, the speculations, inferences and interpretations entertained here could only be made meaningful with experimental evidence. The experimental literature has been summarized earlier in a historical review (Katsh, 1959) and has since been reviewed extensively (Tyler, 1961; Katsh, 1965; Katsh, 1967). It will not, therefore, be the objective here to report the depth of the literature in view of constraint of time. It can be said that subsequent to the initial reports of Landsteiner (1899), Metchnikoff (1900) and Metalnikoff (1900) on the antigenicity of spermatozoa and testis, a considerable literature has been accumulated relative to the abilities of testicular, spermatozoal and seminal plasmal preparations to induce antibody formation. Our discussion will focus on the following five points relating primarily to experimental observations that are of fundamental interest and can be presumed to bear on problems of fertility and sterility in humans. In so doing it is readily admitted that certain topics (e.g. blood group substances, trophoblastic and placental antigens, etc.) will be slighted: full treatment would require lengthy sessions.

In this discussion, one will find questions, points for further development, allusions to incompleteness of information interwoven with the warp and woof of anointed evidence. Hopefully, these rights and privileges appertaining to the philosopher will be acceptable.

The main topics to be considered here are as follows:

I. Antigenicity of Testis, Sperm, and Seminal Plasma.

II. Antigencity of Female Genital Materials.

III. Experimental Induction of Infertility in Male Laboratory Animals.

IV. Experimental Induction of Infertility in Female Laboratory Animals.

V. Evidence for Immunological Reactions in Certain Human Cases of Infertility.

VI. Why do not Males and Females Normally React to Reproductive Antigens to the Extent that Sterility Ensues.

VII. Lines of Investigation regarding Correction of Existing Immunologically-Based Infertility and Control of Fertility.

## I. Antigenicity of Testis, Sperm and Seminal Plasma.

The topic of male reproductive antigens deserves priority consideration not only because more is known of male antigens than those of the female but also for the obvious reason that infusion of the female with foreign antigens would logically occupy a dominant role if fertility could be influenced by immune reactions to coitally deposited antigens.

As mentioned in the Introduction considerable evidence is available demonstrating that spermatzoal and testicular antigens from a variety of species can induce complement-fixing, sperm-immobilizing, sperm-agglutinating, sperm-cytolyzing (fish) and anaphylactic-type antibodies. Antibodies to specific seminal plasmal constituents have also been found.

Evidence for the localization and nature of these antigens has also been obtained. Thus, for example, Henle, Henle and Chambers (1938) found bull sperm contained heat-labile, head-specific and tail-specific antigens and a heat-stable antigen common to both heads and tails. One of the head antigens was detectable only after rupture of the sperm. The specificity of antigenic materials contained in the heads or tails of spermatozon could account for the head-to-head or tail-to-tail types of agglutination of spermatozoa in the presence of antisera as witnessed by many workers including Smith (1949 a,b). Although it is recognized that non-specific sperm-agglutination must also be reckoned with, the careful observations of the Henle group, Smith, Pernot (1956) —who immunized with guinea pig sperm head and tail fractions—, Dallam and Thomas (1953) —who immunized with a lipoprotein extracted from sperm heads of ram, dog, bull, boar and human—, and many others present compelling evidence that sperm-agglutination can be effected by specific antibodies. Inasmuch as agglutination of spermatozoa is correlatable in humans with infertility, this phenomenon deserves investigation which it is not receiving.

Additional information on localization of spermatozoal antigens was made available when the acrosomal antigenic material was traced to its origin in the primary spermatocytes through the secondary spermatocyte, spermatid and sperm stages of metamorphosis (Katsh, 1960). Subsequently the fluorescent-labelling of antibody revealed further information (Willson and Katsh, 1965): spermatozoa from the distal epididymis of guinea pigs have antigens not only in the acrosome, but also in the mid-piece and principal piece: testicular spermatozoa have similar antigenic constituents; the protoplasmic droplet (the function of which has not been elucidated) contains antigenic material; cross-reactivity occurs between human and guinea pig sperm, but not between human and rat sperm (confirming previous observations obtained in a different manner, Katsh, 1962); treatment of motile guinea pig sperm with fluorescent-labelled globulins from sera of immunized guinea pigs results in agglutination and immobilization of the sperm.

In addition to the variety of antibodies to sperm mentioned above, a number of precipitin bands can be detected upon reacting washed guinea pig epididymal sperm with the respective antiserum (Fig. 1) in the

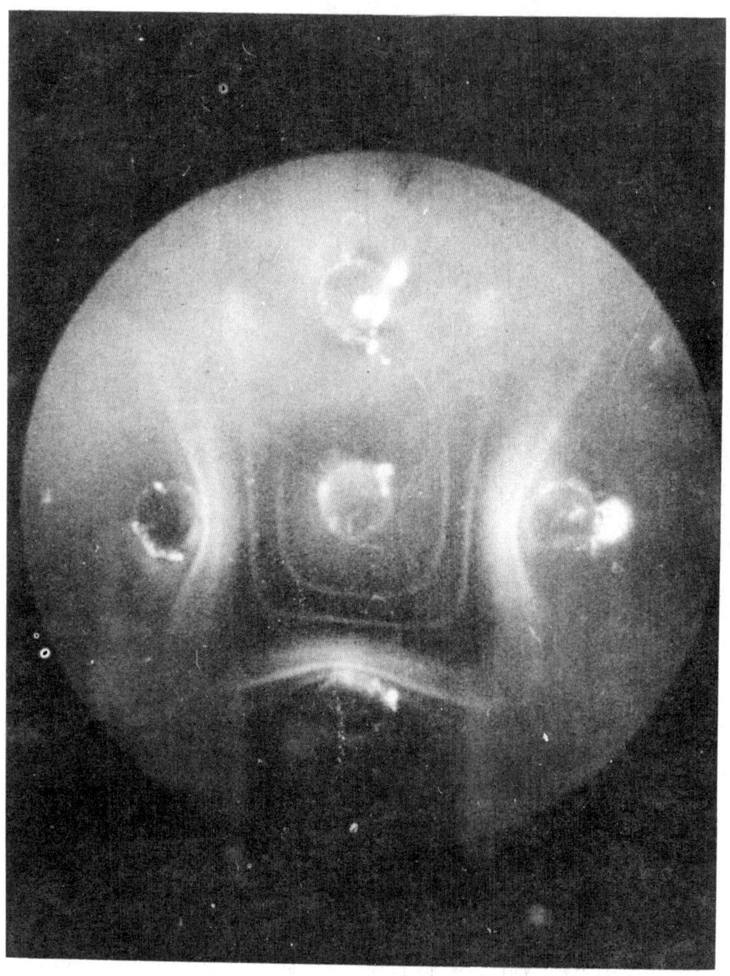

Fig. 1 Photograph of an agar gel double diffusion slide in which rabbit antiguinea pig sperm (center well) was reacted with guinea pig sperm (3-, 6-, and 9-o'clock wells). The precipitin bands indicating antigen-antibody complexes are easily discerned.

immuno-double-diffusion test. One such antigen that reacts in this test is the aspermatogenic antigen (A. S. A.) which will be discussed in section III.

A survey of the prospective antigens associated with testis or sperm would be incomplete without mention of certain enzymatic constituents. Hyaluronidase occupies a prominent position in this regard because it has been suggested that this family of enzymes permits penetration of the spermatozoan to the ovum. The presence of this enzyme (regardless of function) makes it a candidate for an antigenic moiety to be considered in relation to immune response. Using the isolated organ technique, it was shown (Katsh, 1960) that hyaluronidase is antigenic and that a species difference exists in hyaluronidase obtained from guinea pig and bull testicles and sperm and both of these could be distinguished from staphylococcal hyaluronidase. In fact, cross-reactions were absent, indicating a high degree of species-specificity. While there is as yet no evidence that antibodies to hyaluronidase can be responsible for an infertile state, the topic cannot be terminated without further investigation. If, for example, neutralization of the enzyme by antibody occurs, the suggested function of the enzyme (penetration of the cumulus cells) could be inhibited or abolished, preventing fusion of the gametes.

Other enzymatic systems of sperm and testis (e. g. the dehydrogenases, lysozymes, acetylcholinesterase) have not been sufficiently explored in this context. It is worth noting the importance such studies may hold. An acetylcholinesterase system may have a motility function in sperm. Antibodies to this enzyme could be responsible for sperm-immobilization. Our unpublished findings in guinea pig sperm with acetylcholinesterase assays revealed little, if any, superficially available enzyme. However, it was possible to induce antibodies to true (specific) acetylcholinesterase. Work in this area should be continued.

The Y-chromosomal antigen also deserves further attention. In inbred strains of mice, skin transplantation can be successfully achieved between females, between males and from females to males. Skin transplants from males to females are rejected (Eichwald, Silmser and Wheeler, 1956; Billingham and Silvers, 1958; Katsh, Talmage and Katsh, 1964). The presumed cause of rejection of male skin by the female is the presence of Y-chromosomal antigenicity in the male skin. When females of such inbred strains of mice are immunized with isologous sperm and male skin is transplanted to the immunized females, such grafts undergo accelerated rejection (Katsh, et al., 1964). The questions whether transplantations or blood transfusions may affect fertility are still receiving attention.

As mentioned previously, seminal plasma also contains antigenic materials. Indeed, many of the early workers in the field of immunogenicity of spermatozoa who used whole ejaculate as an antigenic source were undoubtedly detecting seminal plasmal antigens as well. Since then, others have recognized that seminal plasma contains antigens distinct from blood constituents (Larson, Gray and Salisbury, 1954; Hermann, 1959). Weil and colleagues (Weil, Kotsevalov and Wilson, 1956; Weil and Rodenburg, 1962) have provided evidence that human seminal plasma contains an antigen that is unrelated to sperm. The antigen can be traced by immuno-fluorescent methods to the seminal vesicle and can be detected on sperm to which it adheres strongly.

Other agents present in ejaculate, notably the prostaglandins, require brief mention. Eliasson and Posse (1960) suggest a function of the prostaglandins in the facilitation of sperm migration from the vagina to the uterus. These agents, amongst others, are of interest in the pharmacology of fertility (a field ripe for exploration, Katsh, 1961) but future investigation may reveal an immunological potential. If antibodies to prostaglandins can be induced, an immunological contribution of these substances would need elaboration.

It must also be remembered that seminal plasma also contains antibodies (Katsh, 1964; Katsh and Katsh, 1965) that could be implicated in immune mechanisms affecting fertility.

## II. Antigencity of Female Genital Materials.

By comparison with knowledge of the male antigens, the volume of literature relating to female reproductive antigens is sparse, indeed and that which is available in the early literature is tenuous at best. For example, the report of Bruck (1907) indicating induction of complement-fixing antibodies in rabbits injected with monkey ova and that of Ricketts (1911) mentioning the production of antisperm toxins after injection of the "plasma of ova" provide inadequate data for evaluation.

Lewis' (1941) work, however, did reveal that the corpus luteum has antigenic qualities: cross-reactivity between this organ and testicle as well as brain was observed.

Insofar as antigens specific to the ovary are concerned, we have been unable to detect any (unpublished). This is also the conclusion to be drawn from the work of Isojima and Stepus (1959). It must be said, however, that efforts to extract specific antigens from ovarian material have not been revealed in the literature.

Placental tissue seems to possess antigenic materials (Dobrowolski, 1903; Cohen and Nedzel, 1940; Siegal and Loeb, 1940) but the uniqueness of these antigens remains to be determined.

Trophoblastic cells have been reported to contain antigenic material. Hulka and Brinton (1963) and Hulka, Brinton, Schaaf and Baney (1963) noted antibodies to trophoblastic tissue were increasingly apparent in the maternal serum beginning on the fourth post-partum day in normal pregnancies. In toxemic pregnancies such antibodies could influence the course of gestation significantly.

Awareness of the antigenicity of placenta as well as its competence to form antibodies (Douglas, Samuels and Dancis, 1962) reinforced analogies of the fetus and its membranes to that of a homograft and led to the speculation that parturition is a normal homograft rejection phenomenon. Many serious reservations could be entertained about this speculation (such as parturition in inbred strains of mice with female fetuses; the contribution of the delicately poised endocrine system evolved through eons, etc.). The theory seems more remote now that the claim has been made that the trophoblast acts as an immunological buffer, normally preventing maternal sensitization to fetal antigens and rejection of the fetus by the mother (Simmons and Russell, 1962) but could explain abnormal expulsion of the fetus.

III. Experimental Induction of Infertility in Male Laboratory Animals.

A monograph would be required to discuss this topic adequately. The summary which follows emphasizes the major points derived from recent experimentation.

It has already been mentioned that sperm-agglutinating and sperm-immobilizing antigens offer promise for fertility control. These approaches would prevent fusion of the gametes. Considerable work remains to be done in these areas to isolate and identify these antigens. Meanwhile, another approach which involves the induction of aspermatogenesis has received much attention.

Aspermatogenesis can be induced in the guinea pig consistently and reproducibly in the following manner. Homogenates of homologous or autologous testis, suspensions of sperm or extracts of these materials are incorporated into Freund adjuvant (paraffin oil, emulsifier and M. butyricum or tubercle bacilli) and injected into recipient guinea pigs. Within 2 to 3 weeks after this single injection, exfoliation of the seminiferous epithelium can be observed. Within 2 months, the testes are essentially devoid of spermatogenic tissue except for spermatogonia. Meanwhile, the androgen production of the interstitial cells continues and the accessory organs of reproduction are maintained as in the normal animal. The aspermatogenic response is reversible within 6 to 8 months. Periodic immunization prevents repopulation of the seminiferous epithelium and maintains the animal in as sterile state. (Detailed information regarding aspermatogenesis can be found in references Nos. 18, 25,

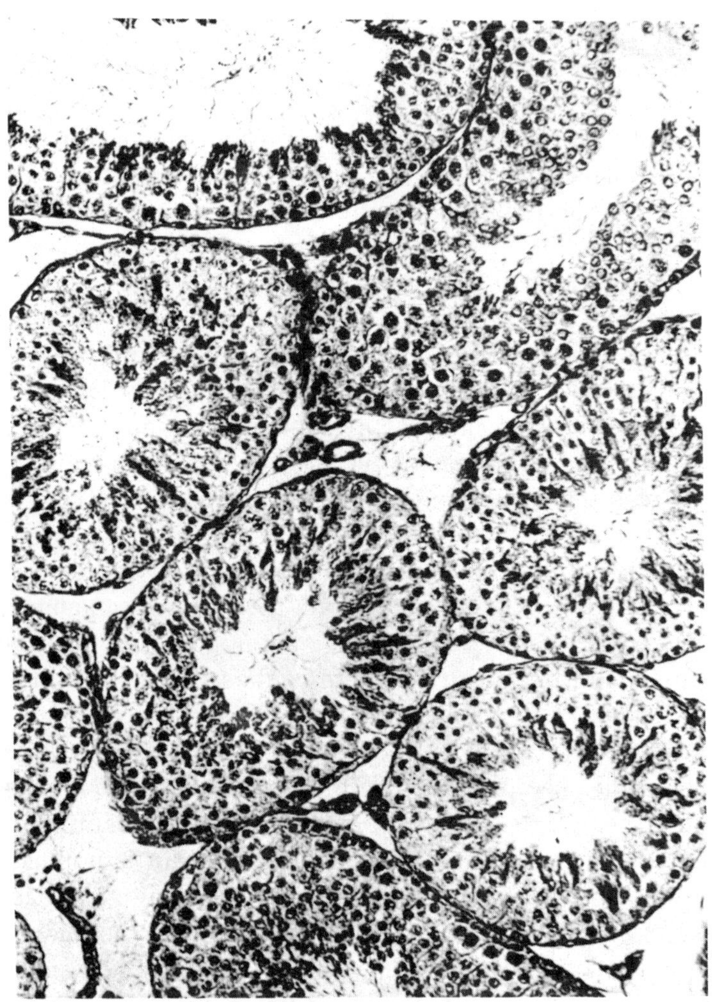

Fig. 2 Section of a testis of a guinea pig injected 60 days previously with complete adjuvant plus saline. This figure illustrates the histology of the normal testis (Reproduced at x150).

28, 30, 33, 34, 36, 40). Figures 2 and 3 provide illustration of the aspermatogenic response.

Considerable interest pertains to the aspermatogenic response quite apart from the implications regarding fertility: The specific cell deletion achieved in this manner holds import for the cell biologist. It is worth, therefore, mentioning current experimentation in this model of an auto-immune phenomenon accompanied by cell depletion.

One phase of interest centers about the role of adjuvant in the induction of aspermatogenesis. Since incomplete adjuvant (paraffin oil plus emulsifier but lacking Mycobacteria) is ineffective in inducing the disorder, the deduction that Mycobacteria participate is a simple one and can be verified by extracting the bacilli for active agents which will mediate aspermatogenesis (Katsh, 1958, 1959, 1960). Acid-fast organisms are not the sole possessors of this factor (termed a lipo-polysaccharide or glycolipid) since other bacterial forms including C. rubrum can replace the Mycobacteria (Katsh, 1964; Katsh, Crowle and Katsh, 1966). Similarly, the paraffin oil and emulsifiers can be replaced (although not so effectively) with materials of plant origin (Katsh, 1964). The oil is presumed to act as a depot at the site of injection to which macrophages and other inflammatory cells are attracted. In this depot, the antigen is incubated at skin temperature with the bacterial factor and may couple to form an antigen-hapten complex.

The antigen has been the subject of intensive investigation: the amino acid composition has been reported (Kirkpatrick and Katsh, 1964) but the saccharidic and lipid moieties remain to be completely elucidated. A single injection of the purified antigen is effective in

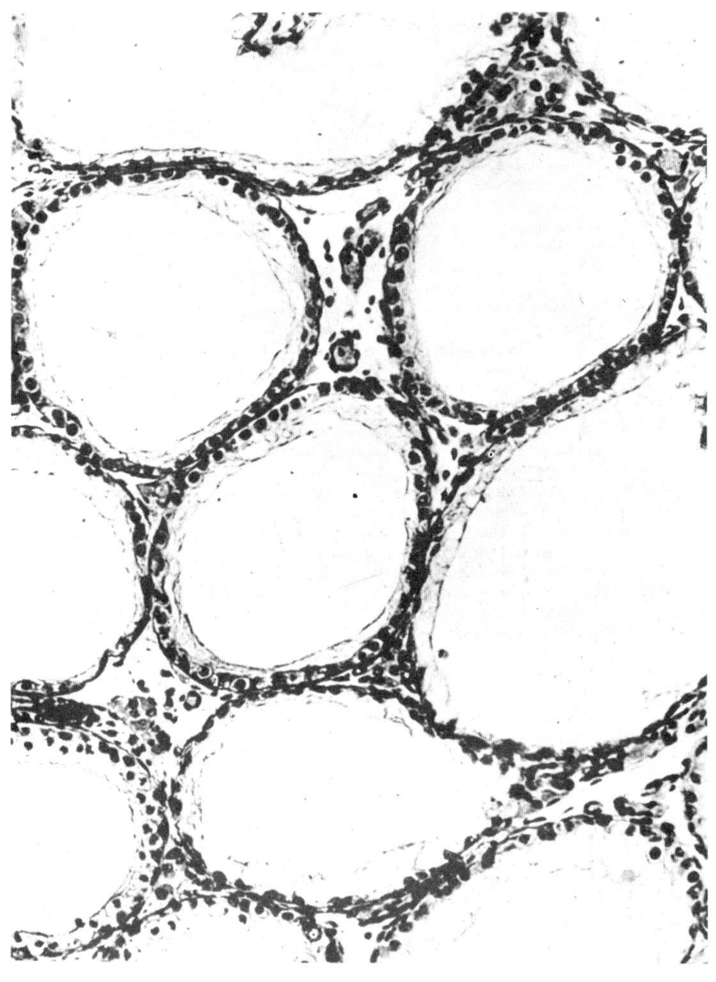

Fig. 3 Section of a testis of a guinea pig injected 60 days previously with aspermatogenic antigen (A. S. A.) extracted from guinea pig epididymal sperm. This figure illustrates the aspermatogenic response (rated as +4 damage). (Reproduced at x150).

TABLE I: Enzymatic Inactivation of Aspermatogenic Antigen: I "Proteases"

| I.U.B.C. | Enzyme | No. of Aspermatogenic Guinea Pigs per Experimental Group |
|---|---|---|
| 1.4.3.2 | L-Amino acid oxidase | 0/6 |
| 3.4.1.1 | Leucine amino peptidase | 1/6 |
| 3.4.4.10 | Papain | 0/4 |
| 3.4.4.12 | Ficin | 0/4 |
| - | Pronase | 0/4 |
| 3.4.4.4 | Trypsin | 4/8 |
| 3.4.4.5 | Chymotrypsin | 4/8 |
| 3.4.4.1 | Pepsin | 6/6 |
| 1.4.3.3 | D-Amino acid oxidase | 4/4 |
| 1.10.3- | Polyphenol oxidase | 4/4 |
| 3.4.2.1 | Carboxypeptidase A | 5/6 |
| 3.4.2.2 | Carboxypeptidase B | 5/6 |
| 3.4.3.7 | Prolidase | 4/4 |

TABLE II: Enzymatic Inactivation of Aspermatogenic Antigen: II Non-Proteases

| I.U.B.C. | Enzyme | No. of Aspermatogenic Guinea Pigs per Experimental Group |
|---|---|---|
| 3.2.1.4 | Cellulase | 0/6 |
| 3.1.3.1 | Alkaline phosphatase | 0/4 |
| 3.1.4.1 | Venom phosphodiesterase | 0/4 |
| 3.2.1.1 | $\alpha$-Amylase | 1/5 |
| 3.2.1.21 | $\beta$-Glucosidase | 1/5 |
| 3.1.4.3 | Phospholipase | 1/5 |
| 3.1.1.1 | Lipase | 2/5 |
| 3.1.3.2 | Acid phosphatase | 2/4 |
| 3.1.4- | Micrococcal nuclease | 3/4 |
| 3.2.1.2 | $\beta$-Amylase | 5/5 |
| 2.4.1.1 | Phosphorylase | 4/4 |

inducing aspermatogenesis in amounts as small as 4 μg. Enzymatic inactivation of aspermatogenic antigen has been accomplished (Tables I and II), providing additional information regarding its composition (Katsh, 1966; Katsh and Katsh, 1966). In work still progressing, enzymatic levels in immunized animals are being measured. Sorbitol dehydrogenase (SDH) levels of the epididymides and testes decline precipitously through the 8 weeks postimmunization whereas in control animals (adjuvant plus saline), SDH levels are returning to normal at 6 weeks. Leucine amino peptidase (LAP) levels rise significantly in the antigen-treated animals but in the controls, LAP levels have returned to normal by the fourth week. Alkaline phosphatase levels are still rising 8 weeks postimmunization whereas in the controls, the levels of this enzyme are close to normal at the 8th week. The objective of these studies is not only to determine the metabolic responses of immunized animals (information sadly lacking in immunology) but also to evaluate the possible mechanisms involved in the aspermatogenic response. One would think immediately of the activation of lysosomal systems. Work is continuing in this area.

In this brief discussion we simply want to emphasize the various methods whereby fertilization may be thwarted. Interest in aspermatogenesis centers not only around the phenomenon *per se* but involves also attempts to separate aspermatogenic antigen from those inducing sperm-immobilization and agglutination.

## IV. Experimental Induction of Infertility in Female Laboratory Animals.

Attempts to induce infertility in females using immunization procedures have been made for over half a century. Space does not permit enumeration of these attempts here but the topic has been reviewed (Katsh and Katsh, 1965; Katsh, 1967). Pertinent here are the following points. One can detect specific antibodies in the uteri of female guinea pigs after copulation using the isolated organ technique (Katsh 1957, 1958). Immunization of females with homologous testicular homogenate or sperm can confer sterility upon females (see reviews). The mechanisms involved in the induced sterility have not been adequately explored. Whether agglutination or immobilization of sperm are the main responses, whether inhibition of hyaluronidase, etc. are cofactors, remain to be determined. It would appear, in any case, that fusion of the gametes has been prevented.

## V. Evidence for Immunologic Reactions in Certain Human Cases of Infertility.

Antibodies can be found in the fluids of patients who have been classified as infertile. For example, Wilson (1954, 1956) recorded case histories of 3 patients with auto-agglutinated sperm and observed that the seminal plasma and blood serum of these patients could cause agglutination of normal human sperm. The wives of 2 of the men conceived promptly after A. I. D. (artificial insemination by donor other than the mate which, latter, should be called A. I. M., artificial insemination by mate. The identifying initials, A. I. M., may never gain popularity because of the implied humor.) Rümke and Hellinga (1959) also observed auto-agglutination of sperm in a small percentage of infertile males and suggested a correlation of the agglutination with infertility. We have made similar observations (Katsh, 1961, 1964). Cruickshank and Stuart-Smith (1959) examined the sera of patients with granulomatous orchitis or epididymitis and found 2 cases of auto-agglutination but both sired offspring. Phadke and Padukone (1964) concluded that the presence of sperm-agglutinating antibodies in the serum of the male does not interfere with fertility.

These few citations are sufficient to illustrate the lack of concert of opinion regarding the influence of auto-agglutinating antibodies in male fertility but that certain cases seem to indicate a strong correlation. In our experience, many ejaculates have been observed in which agglutination occurs in varying degrees from sparse clumps with many freely motile sperm to complete agglutination with no free sperm. The latter instances, it has been our impression, are most likely to continue to be infertile and follow-up studies support this impression. Attempts to disrupt the clumps mechanically have been unrewarding for the usual result is immobilization (an interesting observation meriting further attention). On the other hand, semen specimens with small clumps of agglutinated sperm do not presage sterility even if antibody is detectable. In the latter cases where, nevertheless, infertile status exists, the suggestion of pooling 2 to 3 ejaculates and conducting A. I. M. has met with success. The degree of agglutination, in summary, needs to be qualified in such observations and the antibody titers in serum may not be as directly pertinent as some may conclude: after all, the antibody in ejaculate may not be truly reflected in the serum.

Auto-sensitization of the female to her own reproductive antigens as a cause of infertility has not been accorded the efforts applied to the male. Nonetheless, it would be folly to dismiss the topic. It is not impossible that antibodies to ovarian constituents (e. g. corpora lutea), placental or secretory products of the reproductive tract could prevent fertilization or result in abortion. When added to antibody responses incited by pituitary and steroidal hormones, the list becomes imposing enough to impel activity in this unattended area. We have, for example, noted precipitin band formation when serum and cervical mucus of certain infertile females are reacted in immunodiffusion tests. Similarly, precipitin bands have been observed when serum is reacted with placenta in certain habitual aborters.

Regarding immune response of the female to male antigens delivered during coitus, a considerable literature is being accumulated. Indeed, Franklin and Dukes (1964) have claimed that 75% or more of infertile females are sterile for this reason. Unfortunately, the methodology and resulting evidence upon which such conclusions have been drawn are open to serious reservation. At this time, it is only possible to state that in certain idiopathic cases of sterility, antibodies in serum and cervical mucus can be found and the antibody levels persist for years. Blood types appear not to be involved; rather, the reactivity is related to seminal components (sperm and seminal plasma). Attempts we have made to relate antibody response with exposure to coital antigens have not been satisfactory. We have, for example, explored the responses of prostitutes in a local county jail and, while antibodies to ejaculates can be found in the serum and cervical mucus of these females, the reactions are not notably different from the general population of fertile women we have investigated. The evidence does show that antibodies to ejaculate can be found in the secretions of fertile women and that the antibody responses in these individuals wax and wane, seeming never to be a strong response in contrast to the relatively small percentage of infertile patients in whom antibody response is strong and is maintained. Nevertheless, there can be little doubt that the female does, on occasion, respond to coital antigens by forming antibody. The question, why do not all females become immunized in this way, is the topic of the next section.

## VI. Why Do Not Males and Females Normally React to Reproductive Antigens to the Extent That Sterility Ensues.

If, as we have said, it is possible for certain males to experience auto-immunization and for certain females to respond to male antigens delivered during coitus, by forming antibodies, the question posed above must be answered satisfactorily: otherwise, the observations are mysterious and the experimental evidence philosophically meaningless.

Referring to the male first, there can be little doubt that auto-immune response can result in seminiferous epithelial degeneration as well as agglutination and immobilization of sperm. The genesis of the auto-immune response in the male has been elaborated upon previously (Katsh, 1958, 1961, 1964). Briefly, trauma to the testes or the associated ducts can cause release of antigen. The released antigen incites antibody production. Because sperm can induce granuloma formation as Friedman and Garske (1949) have shown, cells of the macrophage and antibody-forming series are called to the locus. Since sperm are acid-fast (Katsh, 1959), no doubt the inflammatory response is exacerbated. In the presence, furthermore, of infectious agents, antibody response may be pronounced, akin to an adjuvantal effect. Antibody response could be directed towards any or all of the spermatozoal antigens (immobilization, agglutination, aspermatogenic). Quite apart from release of antigen by trauma, such immune reponse could occur naturally or during infections(measles, etc.). The problem, really, is to explain how the body prevents reaction to its own antigenic constituents. Without dwelling upon the recognition of self vs. non-self theories, I would confine my remarks to other built-in safeguards because in spite of the self-recognition (or foreign-recognition) systems, autoimmune responses do occur. We searched for enzymatic systems in the testes and epididymides of guinea pigs that could inactivate the antigenic materials since we conceived of enzymatic inactivation as the most effective method of contravening auto-immunization due to released antigens. Having demonstrated that authentic enzymes are capable of destroying aspermatogenic antigen (Table I), it remained to perform similar studies with testicular homogenate, epididymides and serum. The results demonstrated clearly that inactivation of the antigen was accomplished (part of the results are included in Table III). Further, such enzymes as leucine amino peptidase, $\alpha$-amylase, lipase, alkaline phosphatase, etc. have been found in the reproductive organs and sera. It is reasonable, therefore, to make the following account as a response to the question heading this section. Normally, released antigen is inactivated promptly at the site

TABLE III: Inactivation of Sperm Antigens by Male and Female Organs and Female Serum

| Organ or Serum | No. of Trials: Inactivation/Total |
|---|---|
| Normal Guinea Pig Testes | 5/7 |
| Normal Female Guinea Pig Serum | 4/5 |
| Normal Guinea Pig Uterus | 6/6 |
| Normal Guinea Pig Endometrium | 4/4 |
| Normal Guinea Pig Myometrium | 3/4 |

so that incitement to antibody production is absent. When, however, deficiency of enzymatic inactivation systems is present, excaped antigen can result in antibody production. One or all enzymatic systems for antigenic degradation may be deficient and, thus, the response could include immobilizing, agglutinating or aspermatogenic antibodies, singly or together. Further, if the escaped antigen complexes with endogenous substances (including infectious agents such as lipopolysaccharide of bacteria), enzymatic destruction could be impeded if not prevented and a similar spectrum of antibodies could result.

The female, presented with coital antigens, is faced with the challenge to dispose of these materials. Soluble substances could be expected to be absorbed through the mucosa of the genital tract. Particulate matter requires a more specialized method of disposal. Kohlbrugge had long ago (1912) reported that after copulation in rats, mice, bats, rabbits and fowl, sperm penetrated the epithelial lining of the female reproductive tract. More recently, Austin (1957, 1959) demonstrated that sperm are phagocytized in the Fallopian tubes and uteri and our observations in the guinea pig also reveal phagocytosis of sperm occurs in the genital tract. Absorption and/or phagocytosis of antigens represent the first step in incorporation of foreign material into body comparments. Unless these antigenic materials are inactivated, they would be suspect as incitors of antibody production. Again, therefore, we examined the ability of female serum and uteri of guinea pigs to inactivate male antigens, selecting aspermatogenic antigen because it is the only one concerning which our present knowledge permits definitive assay. The results indicated in Table III demonstrate clearly

| Inactivator Source | Antigen (mg./animal) | No. of Trials Inactivation/Total |
|---|---|---|
| Incubated Female Guinea Pig Serum | 10 | 6/7 |
| Non-Incubated Female Guinea Pig Serum | 10 | 6/12 |
| Electrophoretic Fractions of Female Guinea Pig Serum | | |
| $\gamma$, $\beta$ and $\alpha$ Fractions | 10 | 5/5 |
| albumin Fraction | 10 | 0/2 |
| Ammonium Sulfate Fractions of Female Guinea Pig Serum | | |
| Guinea Pig Serum | 10 | 7/7 |
| Precipitates of 40-70% fractions | 10 | 1/4 |
| Incubated Female Guinea Pig Uterine Homogenate | 10 | 10/10 |
| Non-incubated Female Guinea Pig Uterine Homogenate | 10 | 2/8 |
| Incubated Guinea Pig Myometrial Homogenate | 10 | 8/8 |
| Incubated Guinea Pig Endometrial Homogenate | 10 | 5/6 |
| Non-incubated Guinea Pig Endometrial Homogenate | 10 | 0/5 |
| Human Serum | | |
| Male | 10 | 12/12 |
| Female | 10 | 8/9 |

TABLE V: Enzymes Present in Guinea Pig Sera and Uteri That Hydrolyze Sperm Antigen

| Source | Enzyme | Avg. No. of Units of Enzyme per mg. Protein (range) |
|---|---|---|
| Serum | Leucine Amino Peptidase | 50 (30-100) |
| Endometrium | Leucine Amino Peptidase | 36 (24-46) |
| Myometrium | Leucine Amino Peptidase | 22 (16-31) |
| Serum | $\alpha$-amylase | .099 (.068-.138) |
| Endometrium | $\alpha$-amylase | .169 (.021-.332) |
| Myometrium | $\alpha$-amylase | .091 (.050-.161) |
| Serum | Lipase | .111 (.07-.189) |
| Endometrium | Lipase | .169 (.053-.460) |
| Myometrium | Lipase | .11 (.021-.167) |
| Serum | Alkaline Phosphatase | $4.7 \times 10^{-6}$ ($1.8$-$7.9 \times 10^{-6}$) |
| Endometrium | Alkaline Phosphatase | $1.06 \times 10^{-3}$ ($.027$-$3.0 \times 10^{-3}$) |
| Myometrium | Alkaline Phosphatase | $6.6 \times 10^{-3}$ ($.2$-$20 \times 10^{-3}$) |

that female uteri and sera are capable of inactivating this antigen. Further, we are learning what fractions of uteri and sera contain these inactivators in guinea pig and human material (Table IV). These studies are continuing. Meanwhile, it can be demonstrated that certain enzymes as leucine amino peptidase, $\alpha$-amylase, lipase and alkaline phosphatase as were found to be effective in hydrolyzing A. S. A. are present in uteri and sera of female guinea pigs (Table V).

On the basis of evidence accumulated, it seems clear that evolutionary processes providing for continued fertility of the female despite repeated exposure to antigen have incorporated safeguards against immune responses which would prevent reproduction of the species.

If such safeguards are present, how can one explain instances of infertility attributable to immune response ? A hypersensitivity of the female's antibody-forming tissue to reproductive antigens (as may also be true in the male) is one possibility. Another possibility is as follows. A deficiency or absence of the normal complement of enzymatic systems in the uterus could permit the escape of antigens from being degraded. The undegraded antigen is now available as an incitor for antibody production. On this basis, the immunologically infertile female might be viewed as a model of molecular deficiency. The deficiency might not be apparent from assay of serological or other (than reproductive) tissue enzymes. These may be entirely normal. Because of the periodic desquamation of the uterine epithelial lining, this organ presents a unique situation. Indeed, perusal of Table V reveals that the endomentrial enzymatic content is significantly different from that of serum. For example, the content of alkaline phosphatase (although it fluctuates throughout the cycle) is several orders of magnitude higher in the endometrium than in serum, indicating that the endometrium must provide its own enzyme content.

In addition to deficiency of inactivating mechanisms, one must also consider the presence of foreign agents (derived from viral, microbial, fungal infections) that could serve as adjuvants in enhancing antibody response to intromitted antigens.

The degree to which any or all of these possibilities exist would determine the degree of antibody response. It is not surprising, then, to find a spectrum of responses (in a population) from zero to the highest degree of sensitization. Gradations include mild sensitization with no observable effect upon fertility; antibody production to a single antigenic moiety (e. g. sperm agglutination or sperm immobilization).

The inability to correlate circulating antibody with immune response to ejaculate antigens is understandable. Fixed (cellular) antibody may not be reflected in the serological titers. Moreover, local antibody production in the female's genital tract does not presuppose the level of serum antibody would be equivalent. It has been shown that the female reproductive tract can produce antibodies. Batty and Warrack (1955) and Broome and Lamming (1959) have demonstrated that resistance to bacterial infections of the reproductive tract in experimental animals is in part a function of the antibody response of the uterus. Furthermore, Straus (1961) used typhoid vaccine and soluble typhoid bacillus antigen to demonstrate the occurrence of specific antibody in human vaginal mucous following active immunization: Vaginal antibody production occurred also after local application of antigen and was not affected by menstruation or pregnancy.

VII. Lines of Investigation Regarding Correction of Existing Immunologically-Based Infertility and Control of Fertility.

With regard to correction of existing immunologically-based sterility of the female due to ejaculate antigens, it is instructive to recall the case history of Sarah (see Introduction). The suggestion has been made, and followed with some success, that continence or use of a male sheath be practiced to prevent continued contact of female tissues with male antigens. Such practice, continued for several months, permits decline in antibody production and when coitus is practiced close to ovulation, chances for successful fertilization are apparently increased. In an aside, it is of more than passing interest to note that granulomatous lesions in the abdominal cavity of a female were attributed to condom emulsion transmitted through the tubes (Saxen, Kassinen and Saxen, 1963). It is worth asking whether emulsions from diaphragms or condoms could lead to sensitization processes that cause infertility.

In intractable situations, immunosuppressive agents might be used. Experimentally, we are finding that aspermatogenesis in guinea pigs may be prevented with corticosteroids.

In order for full development of the program to relieve infertility and to induce sterility we need to provide adequate experimental models and the sub-human primate must be included in such studies. From our point of view, however, basic mechanisms involved in explaining processes of fertilization and inhibition thereof are vital. These are the approaches toward which our laboratory has been devoted. Understandably, then, this Symposium dedicated to this theme is of profound significance.

## ACKNOWLEDGMENTS

The studies reported herein have been supported by grants from the following sources: The Ford Foundation, The National Science Foundation (GB-603 and GB-6309) and The University of Colorado Medical Center (GRS-10).

## REFERENCES

1. Austin, C. R. (1957) Fate of spermatozoa in the uterus of the mouse and rat. J. Endocrinol. 14, 335-342.
2. Austin, C. R. (1959) Entry of spermatozoa into the Fallopian tube mucosa. Nature 183, 908-909.
3. Batty, I. and Warrack, G. H. (1955) Local antibody production in the mammary gland, spleen, uterus, vagina and appendix of the rabbit. J. Path. Bact. 70, 355-363.
4. Billingham, R. E. and Silvers, W. K. (1958) Induction of tolerance of skin isografts from male donors in female mice. Science 128, 780-781.
5. Broome, A. W. I. and Lamming, G. E. (1959) Studies on the relationship between ovarian hormones and uterine infection. III The role of the antibody system in uterine defense. J. Endocrinol. 18, 229-235.

6. Bruck, D. (1907) Zur forensischen Verwertbarkeit und Kenntnis des Wesens der Komplementbindung. Berl. klin. Wchnschr. 44, 1510-1513.
7. Cohen, H. R. and Nedzel, A. J. (1940) Specific action of an anti-serum for placental proteins on placenta and normal progress of pregnancy. Proc. Soc. Exp. Biol. Med. 43, 249-250.
8. Cruickshank, B. and Stuart-Smith, D. A. (1959) Orchitis associated with sperm-agglutinating antibodies. Lancet I, 708.
9. Dallam, R. D. and Thomas. L. E. (1953) Chemical studies on mammalian sperm. Biochim. Biophys. Acta 11: 79-89.
10. Darwin, D. (1898) The Descent of Man and Selection in Relation to Sex. Appleton, Co., New York.
11. Dobrowolski, M. S. (1903) Uber Cytotoxine der Plazenta. Bull. Int. Acad. Sci. Cracovie 5, 256-260.
12. Douglas, G. W., Samuels, B. D. and Dancis, J. (1962) Immunologic competence of mouse placental cells. Am. J. Obstet. and Gynec. 84, 1126-1133.
13. Driver, G. R. and Miles, J. C. (1935) The Assyrian Laws. Oxford Univ. Press, New York.
14. Eichwald, E. J., Silmser, D. R. and Wheeler, N. (1956) The genetics of skin grafting. Ann. N. Y. Acad. Sci. 64, 737-740.
15. Eliasson, R. and Posse, N. (1960) The effect of prostaglandin on the non-pregnant human uterus in vivo. Acta Obstet. et Gynec. Scandinav. 39; 112-126.
16. Franklin, R. R. and Dukes, C. D. (1964) Antispermatozoal antibody and unexplained infertility. Am. J. Obstet. and Gynec. 89, 6-9.

17. Friedman, N. B. and Garske, G. L. (1949) Inflammatory reactions involving sperm and the seminiferous tubules: Extravasation, spermatic granulomas and granulomatous orchitis. J. Urol. 62, 363-374.

18. Freund, J., Thompson, G. E. and Lipton, M. M. (1955) Aspermatogenesis, anaphylaxis and cutaneous sensitization induced in the guinea pig by homologous testicular extract. J. Exp. Med. 101, 591-604.

19. Henle, W., Henle, G. and Chambers, L. A. (1938) Studies on the antigenic structure of some mammalian spermatozoa. J. Exp. Med. 68, 335-352.

20. Hermann, G. (1959) Immunoelektrophoretische Untersuchungen am menschlichen Spermaplasma. Clin. Chim. Acta 4, 116-123.

21. Hulka, J. F. and Brinton, V. (1963) Antibody to trophoblast during early postpartum period in toxemic pregnancies. Am. J. Obstet. and Gynec 86, 130-134.

22. Hulka, J. F., Brinton, V., Schaaf, J. and Baney, C. (1963) Appearance of antibodies to trophoblast during the postpartum period in normal human pregnancies. Nature 198, 501-502.

23. Isojima, S. and Stepus. S. (1959) Antigenicity of guinea pig testis and ovary. Int. Arch. Allergy 15, 350-359.

24. Katsh, S. (1957) *In vitro* demonstration of uterine anaphylaxis in guinea pigs sensitized with homologous testis or sperm. Nature 180, 1047-1048.

25. Katsh, S. (1958) Host-graft interrelationship and the effects of injection of organ homogenates and of cells upon the testes of experimental animals. Ann. N. Y. Acad. Sci. 73, 698-706.

26. Katsh, S. (1958) Demonstration in vitro of anaphylactoid response of the uterus and ileum of guinea pigs injected with testis or sperm. J. Exp. Med. 107, 95-103.
27. Katsh, S. (1959) Immunology, fertility and infertility: A historical survey. Am. J. Obstet. Gynec. 77, 946-956.
28. Katsh, S. (1959) The contribution of the bacterial components of adjuvant in the induction of aspermatogenesis and in the sensitization of the ilea of guinea pigs. Int. Arch. Allergy 15, 172-188.
29. Katsh, S. (1959) Acidfastness of sperm. Anat. Rec. 133, 397.
30. Katsh, S. (1960a) Localization and identification of antispermatogenic factor in guinea pig testicles. Int. Arch. Allergy 16, 241-275.
31. Katsh, S. (1960b) The anaphylactogenicity of testicular hyaluronidase demonstrated by isolated organ anaphylaxis. Int. Arch. Allergy 17, 70-79.
31. Katsh, S. (1961) The pharmacology and immunology of human ejaculate relating to problems of fertility and infertility. Int. J. Fertil. 6: 53-66.
32. Katsh, S. (1962) Antigenicity of human testis. J. Urol. 87, 896-902.
33. Katsh, S. (1964) Adjuvants and aspermatogenesis in the guinea pig. Int. Arch. Allergy 24, 319-331.
34. Katsh, S. (1964) Studies on immunological aspects of reproduction in laboratory animals and man. Excerpta Medica. 72, 513-526.
35. Katsh, G. F., Talmage, D. W. and Katsh, S. (1964) Acceptance or rejection of male skin grafts by isologous mice: Effect of injection of sperm. Science 143, 41-42

36. Katsh, S. and Katsh, G. F. (1965) Perspectives in immunological control of reproduction. Pacific Med. and Surg. 73, IA 28-43.

37. Katsh, S. (1966) Immunological control of reproduction in experimental animals: Implications regarding human fertility and infertility. Ann. Allergy 24, 615-620

38. Katsh, S. and Katsh, G. F. (1966) Enzymatic inactivation of aspermatogenic antigen. Nature 212: 1486.

39. Katsh, S., Crowle, A. J. and Katsh, G. F. (1966) A non-mycobacterial adjuvant mediating aspermatogenesis. Nature 212, 1486-1487.

40. Katsh, S. (1967) Immunological Aspects of Infertility and Conception Control In Advances in Obstetrics and Gynecology, Vol. I, Chap. 34, 467-485. Ed. Marcus and Marcus, Williams and Wilkins Co., Baltimore, Md.

41. Kirkpatrick, C. H. and Katsh, S. (1964) Amino acid content of antispermatogenic antigen. Nature 201, 197-198.

42. Kohlbrugge, J. H. F. (1912) Die Verbreitung der Spermatozoiden im weiblichen Körper und im befruchteten Ei. Arch. Entwicklungsmechanik, 35, 165-188.

43. Landsteiner, K. (1899) Zur Kenntnis der spezifisch auf Blutkörperchen wirkenden Sera. Zbl. Bakt. 25, 546-549.

44. Larson, B. L., Gray, R. S. and Salisbury, G. W. (1954) The proteins of bovine seminal plasma. II. Ultracentrifugal and immunological studies and comparison with blood and milk serum. J. Biol. Chem. 211, 43-52.

45. Lewis, J. H. (1941) The antigenic relationship of alcohol-soluble substances of corpus luteum to those of testis and brain. Am. J. Path. 17, 725-730.
46. Metalnikoff, S. (1900) Études sur la spermatoxine. Ann. Inst. Pasteur 14, 577-589.
47. Metchnikoff, E. (1900) Recherches sur l'influence de l'organisme sur les toxines. Sur la spermatoxine et l'antispermatoxine. Ann. Inst. Pasteur 14, 1-12.
48. Pernot, E. (1956) Recherches sur les constituents antigéniques des spermatozoides de cobayes. Bull. Soc. Chim. Biol. (Paris) 38, 1041-1054.
49. Phadke, A. M. and Padukone, K. (1964) Presence and significance of autoantibodies against spermatozoa in the blood of men with obstructed vas deferens. J. Reprod. Fertil. 7, 163-170.
50. Ricketts, H. T. (1911) Infection, Immunity and Serum Therapy. Amer. Med. Assn. Press, Chicago, Ill., 165-166; 2nd ed. pp. 295-296, 1911.
51. Rumke, P. and Hellinga, G. (1959) Autoantibodies against spermatozoa in sterile men. Amer. J. Clin. Path. 32, 357-363.
52. Saxen, L., Kassinen, A. and Saxen, E. (1963) Peritoneal foreign-body reaction caused by condom emulsion. Lancet I, 1295.
53. Seegal, B. C. and Loeb. E. N. (1940) Effect of anti-placenta serum on development of the foetus in the pregnant rat. Proc. Soc. Exp. Biol. Med. 45, 248-252.
54. Sigerist, H. E. (1955) A History of Medicine. Vol. I. Primitive and Archaic Medicine. Oxford Univ. Press, New York.

55. Simmons, R. L. and Russell, P. S. (1962) The antigenicity of mo· e trophoblast. Ann. N. Y. Acad. Sci. 99, 717-732.

56. Smith, A. U. (1949a) Some antigenic properties of mammalian spermatozoa. Proc. Roy. Soc. London (B) 136, 46-66.

57. Smith, A. U. (1949b) The antigenic relationship of some mammalian spermatozoa. Proc. Roy. Soc. London (B) 136, 472-479.

58. Straus, E. K. (1961) Occurrence of antibody in human vaginal mucus. Proc. Soc. Exp. Biol. Med. 106, 617-621.

59. Tyler, A. (1961) Approaches to the control of fertility based on immunological phenomena. J. Reprod. Fertil. 2, 473-506.

60. Weil, A. J., Kotsevalov, O. and Wilson, L. (1956) Antigens of human seminal plasma. Proc. Soc. Exper. Biol. Med. 92, 606-610.

61. Weil, A.J. and Rodenburg, J.M. (1962) The seminal vesicle as the source of the spermatoza-coating antigen of seminal plasma. Proc. Soc. Exp. Biol. Med. 109, 567-570.

62. Willson, J. T. and Katsh, S. (1964) Cyto-immunological studies of guinea pig sperm antigens. I. Testicular versus epididymal spermatozoa. Zeit. Zellforsch. 65, 16-26.

63. Wilson, L. (1954) Sperm agglutinins in human semen and blood. Proc. Soc. Exp. Biol. Med. 85, 652-655.

64. Wilson, L. (1956) Sperm agglutination due to autoanticodies. A new case of sterility. Fertil. Steril. 7, 262-267.

## DISCUSSION

G. J. Marcus: First of all, I would like to thank Prof. Katsh, not only for a most engrossing lecture but for shoring up our egos and reminding us that the male has something to do, after all, in reproduction. You referred to the presence of immunologically competent cells in the uterus. Could you be more specific; what is the evidence that these particular cells are immunologically competent?

S. Katsh: A variety of other workers of course have performed such experiments. I mentioned the works of Batty and Warrack in England and others in which the local introduction, topical application, of various antigens, cellular antigens as well as discrete antigens that have been isolated, resulted in detectable antibody. The work of Straus is rather important too. Incidentally, she did this work on a population of students at a woman's college. She introduced a variety of typhus organisms and spermatozoa. The data provided unequivocal evidence that local antibody production had occurred. I think the more recent information, including that obtained by fluorescent labelling techniques, substantiates the conclusion that local antibody production can occur. Lymphocytes and plasma cells appear in the uterus.

G. J. Marcus: This reminds me of a study or survey carried out by Jan Behrman in which he looked for titers of antibodies to spermatozoa in unmarried female college under-graduates, finding a rather surprising incidence [cf. W. B. Schwimmer, K. A. Ustay and S. J. Behrman, Obstet. Gynec. 30, 192, 1967]. He allowed the audience at the lecture in which he reported this to draw its own conclusions.

S. Katsh: We didn't go quite that far. In fact, we approached it from the other angle. I suppose Denver is no different from any of the other metropolitan areas in the United States. It does have its population of prostitutes. Now we can find some serological indications, but we were taking curettage material as well as cervical mucus and quite strangely, we did not find a very high incidence of antisperm antibodies. In the female partner of an infertile couple, however, we often find antisperm antibodies in the precipitin test. This is not the only kind of antibody one should look for, because one should also look for fixed antibodies, which I think are more pertinent and related to the infertile condition. Nevertheless, the idea is that in the infertile female one can detect a fairly high level of antibody which is maintained. In contradistinction to those females, there are many in our group of volunteers, who have as many as four or five children and also show evidence of antibodies. However, the antibody level appears to wax and wane and at any rate is a very low order of response. I think the point should be made that there must be a disposal system—a very effective disposal system—for these antigens that are introduced, and it must be fairly rapid one too, and I don't think one can account for it alone on the basis of phagocytosis which is after all a fairly slow response, but the enzymatic system should be explored intensively.

G. J. Marcus: You asked a question as to why one normally does not obtain an effect of sterility as a response to copulation. Do I understand that correctly? Was it in response to copulation that you would *a priori* assume that there could be reaction resulting in sterility?

S. Katsh: Well, I think this is a key question; I think it's a central question. Please let me amplify. The act of intercourse for the virgin female could be her first exposure to antigens of sperm and/or seminal plasma. Thus, the first exposure might be compared with an initial innoculation to any foreign antigen (even penicillin, for example). As we know, it is not the first exposure to antigen that causes difficulty (again using penicillin as the example) but, rather, this provides the sensitizing dose: following subsequent exposures, the immune response becomes evident. Therefore, to answer your question, the first exposure is essential but, subsequent innoculations will provide evidence as to whether or not sterility will ensue.

G. J. Marcus: What I want to ask in return is whether you would consider the possibility that a mild local reaction of an immunological type is a normal feature of reproductive processes. For example, a response which would invoke production of local antibodies and which is of such a mild degree that this does not result ultimately in infertility but may play a role in the behavior of the uterus in response to the blastocyst. You can see where I am getting.

S. Katsh: Yes, you are ascending the tubes, if I understand you correctly. I quite agree. There's no question but that there could be a local inflammatory response, but I would hesitate to dedicate myself to the philosophy that each time this does occur there could be an immune response. There indeed could be. There are several other factors we haven't covered and I think the pharmacoimmunology, or at least the pharmacology of seminal plasma must be considered here. Now many other people have described certain pharmacologically active agents as being present in the seminal fluid, so I need not describe these to you, but it would not be beyond reason to suggest that upon copulation these pharmacologically active agents could certainly cause what would be a pseudo-inflammatory response, having all of the characteristics that we know. Histamine will induce, for example, an erythema.

H. R. Lindner: Would you then consider it likely or probable that in response to coitus there might normally be an immunological reaction to the introduced spermatozoa or to components of the seminal plasma?

S. Katsh: If the question is asked—does this happen at the first exposure to antigen, my answer would have to be no. I must say, however, that the answer is predicated upon immunological principles, not direct observation.

M. C. Shelesnyak: This is a case reported by Bernard Halperin in Paris [B. N. Halpern, T. Ky and B.

Robert, Immunology, 12, 247, 1967]. I think he has finally published the report, but it's been in the gossip for a long time. A very specific instance in which a woman seemed to be highly allergic to her own husband's ejaculate. What I think really is being attempted, Seymour, is to ask you to make a frank expression of opinion. And I gather you have been willing to say that under certain circumstances this phenomenon may occur.

S. Katsh: Yes, I would have to agree, if the female had previously been sensitized by prior exposure.

M. C. Shelesnyak: I would like to point out that in the human this doesn't necessarily have to be a matter of great concern, because, although in the human, in most instances, the statistical probability of sexual intercourse between the same male and the same female is greater than in other animals, and one would imagine from an immunological point of view therefore that the impact of the same antigen again and again would create a response, a pertinent response, that in the event that we are concerned with a tissue response, endometrial tissue response, that is, the human has a protective mechanism in that, under normal circumstances, every month this whole tissue is shed; menstruation involves the loss of a great deal of the tissue in which one might expect localized antibodies, if you expected localized antibodies in the tissue. I'm not referring to circulating antibodies, we're talking about localized antibodies.

H. R. Linder: Even in the case of local antibody production, can you really assume that the information necessary for recognizing these seminal antigens on reexposure is entirely confined to the decidual part of the endometrium which is shed, and is not transmitted to and stored in other antibody-synthesizing centres? I would hesitate to make such an assumption. Why don't we ask Prof. Billingham to comment on that.

R. E. Billingham: Dr. Katsh's suggestion that sensitization to sperm or seminal fluid antigens may occur locally (or, in an immunological sense, "peripherally") in the uterus is very plausible. However, if a sort of local ad hoc machinery of immunological response is established in the uterus, its effector products, in the form of immunoglobulins and/or "sensitized" lymphocytes, will surely be distributed systemically via the blood stream. Thus, the physiological pathway between the seat of response and the target antigenic material against which the immunity is directed may be a long one. If lymphocytes are the immunologic effectors they may be very long-lived cells, some of them constantly recirculating from the blood to the lymph via the nodes. Hence shedding of the decidual part of the endometrium would not necessarily be expected to erase the immunologic memory.

J. W. Everett: I would like to point out that the oviduct receives a considerable amount of ejaculate and that does not shed tissue regularly.

H. R. Lindner: I might add considering the possibility or plausibility of local production of immune bodies. There is considerable evidence in the bovine that organisms such as *Trichomonas foetus*, which is a non-invasive flaggelate, give rise to local production of antibodies that can be demonstrated in the vaginal and uterine mucus and usually does not give rise to demonstrable circulating antibody [A. E. Pierie, *Veterinary Reviews Annotations* *5*, 17, 1959]; but as Prof. Billingham has pointed out, this does not necessarily mean that what you refer to as informed lymphocytes (or macrophages ?) are not carried to other centers.

S. Katsh: Generally, yes. I am, of course, familiar with the citations mentioned—a human female exhibiting allergy to her husband's sperm—(indeed, we have shown the presence of precipitins in the sera of such females) and the bovine case in which antibodies can be detected in the reproductive tract but not in the circulation. Further, as Dr. Billingham has stated, it seems difficult to perceive how this local "antibody" remains contained without "escaping" to the circulation. Yet the observations made to the effect that antibodies demonstrable in the reproductive tract are not always demonstrable in other body compartments remain. Perhaps the detection systems for such antibodies have not been exhaustively employed.

M. Tausk: Since the main subject is nidation and Dr. Shelesnyak, in his opening lecture, mentioned this local allergic reaction as one of the possible mechanisms, may I ask the simple question: You said you would consider it a possibility that there is such an immune reaction. Would you say that it is possible—I believe that's important—that the uterus could be sensitized during the first contact with sperm and that sufficient immunity would have been built up, so that at the time of implantation, there could be a local reaction which would induce the deciduoma formation? Is this possible, time-wise?

S. Katsh: To induce the deciduoma formation as a result of the release of histamine or some other pharmacological active agent?

M. Tausk: Leaving aside the question of what the mechanism is in deciduoma formation, but assuming that this is, as Dr. Shelesnyak called it in his opening lecture, a delayed sensitization. I believe it is known that even the very first coition can induce fertilization of the female—I believe that is in the literature.

S. Katsh: To the regret of a lot of people, I think this has happened.

M. Tausk: Well, I think we can take this as a fact. Then the sensitization would have to take place during the very first entrance of sperm and the ovum would nidate seven days thereafter and at that time, there would have to be this local reaction of hypersensitivity or an allergy or whatever it is, this would then lead to deciduoma formation. Is it possible time-wise?

S. Katsh: As a result of the second coitus ?

M. Tausk: No, No. As Dr. Shelesnyak suggested in his first lecture and in some of his papers, the ovum would carry some sperm antigen in its zona pellucida or whereever, and it would penetrate the endometrium. Time-wise, is it possible?

S. Katsh: Before responding to that I should say that to my knowledge at least, although tagged antibodies have been shown to pass through the foetal barrier and to coat the surface of ova, to my knowledge, antigens have not been shown to do that, and I really don't know whether or not ova could carry sperm antigens, directly, which would be implied by your question.

M. Tausk: But suppose they do?

M. C. Shelesnyak: Marius, may I try to make your simplification of my complicated statement a little simpler. I think what you are being asked, Seymour, is simply this: that the postulated mechanism, process, that post-coital sperm enter the uterus, sensitize the endometrium—just as you give your first injection in the skin—sensitize the endometrium with some antigen from sperm or seminal plasma or whatever it happens to be, and this reaction begins, and this is the first reaction. Five to six days later, as the blastocyst, which has a male component—it may be only the genetic component but we have already shown that there are other sperm components attached to the blastocyst—carries the original protein which, we speculated on as being antigenic—arrives in the uterus, the uterus, having been sensitized five days previously, is in a position to react. Would you accept this as a theoretical possibility? Was this your question?

M. Tausk: Exactly. Can it be time-wise that this happens seven days later?

S. Katsh: I can't reject it because I don't have the information with which to reject it. But what it demands is that there be present and demonstrable sperm antigens or plasma antigens on the surface of the ovum.

M. Tausk: But assuming they are there.

G. J. Marcus: One thing that Prof. Katsh mentioned, but perhaps didn't emphasize, is that sperm coating antigens would invariably be present in the case of the normal copulation, that is when the sperm are ejaculated together with the usual complement of seminal plasma components, since the sperm coating antigens (SCA) is extremely adherent to the sperm (A. J. Weil, Proceedings of the Conference on Immuno-Reproduction, La Jolla, California, The Population Council, New York, 1962, pg. 43). There is no doubt that some material derived from sperm persists in or on the egg and would be present when the egg enters uterus. Perhaps Dr. Kraicer would expand on this?

P. F. Kraicer: Penetration of the zona pellucida by spermatozoa tends to take place at a very shallow angle in mammals. Because of the shape of the head of the sperm in the rat, the sperm must go through diagonally. However, this is also true of the rabbit in which the sperm head is not hooked. The result is that when the sperm enters the perivitelline space, it comes to lie alongside the ovum [Z. Dickman, in Preimplanatation Stages of Pregnancy, eds. G. Wolstenholme and M. O'Connor; Little, Brown and Co., Boston, 1965, p. 169]. Szollosi and Ris [D. Szollosi and H. Ris, J. Biophys. Biochem. Cytol. 10, 275, 1961] have shown, in a marvelous electron micrograph, that the next stage is a coalescence of the sperm and vitelline membranes. The sperm in incorporated into the egg *in toto*, that is, the plasma membrane of the sperm becomes confluent with that of the egg and the sperm lies within. This implies that a portion of the cell membrane of the fertilized egg is derived from the plasma membrane of the sperm. Now if there is a membrane associated antigen on the sperm, it is reasonable to assume that there is a patch of such antigen on the fertilized egg; it may be the sperm coating antigen.

S. Katch: Even though as I understand it, there is an incorporation of some of the spermatozoa into the blastocyst itself, that does not necessarily imply that this would retain its antigenicity. The demonstration of the presence of a sperm or a part thereof does not necessarily demonstrate the presence of an *antigen*.

P. F. Kraicer: I have always believed that in order to be able to analyse a physiological process, one should know something of the anatomical or mophological basis. An anatomical basis must be established as the first step in supporting the possibility of the occurrence of a phenomenon. This is all that I had intended to do; there is morphological or anatomical evidence that male-derived antigen could survive. I did not, for a moment, mean to imply that I, or to my knowledge anyone else, has demonstrated this.

S. Katsh: I think I have already admitted to the possibility; whether it is probable, I don't know.

P F. Kraicer: To strengthen the hypothesis, let me indicate how the antigenicity may be preserved. In a series of pictures of ova taken both by interferential contrast and by electron microscopy, Mrs. Tachi and I have seen two things: a] there is male-derived material in the perivitelline space about the egg which may be actually attached into the ovum; and b] the perivitelline environment stabilizes the male derived material [S. Tachi and P. F. Kraicer, J. Reprod. Fertil. 14, 401, 1967].

I would like to review our findings because of the implications of immunological response to the egg by the uterus. Supernumerary sperm can and do penetrate the zona pellucida at the time fertilization. Whereas the fertilizing sperm soon loses its identity, the supernumerary sperm remain clearly identifiable for many days. We have isolated blastocysts on the fifth day of pregnancy which have already lost their zonae pellucidae. These blastocysts were isolated by flushing the uterus through the cervix into a polyethylene tube fitted into the vagina. I mention this rinsing procedure to point up the fact that the egg was severely agitated during the isolation procedure. In several cases sperm tails were found adhering to the outside of a naked egg. The explanation of this phenomenon is provided by several elegant electron micrographs, of Mrs. Sumie Tachi. She has found sperm tails "sewing" themselves into a trophoblast cell. She has also found sperm tails between the cells of blastocysts and even in the blastocyst cavity. The remarkable state of preservation of these sperm remnants stands in contradistinction to the breakdown of the tail and middlepiece of the fertilizing sperm. The preservation and stability of these male-derived elements associated with the egg suggests the persistence of male antigen on or in the egg until the time of implantation.

Another interesting aspect of this observation is the interpenetration of sperm tails into the trophoblastic cells. This must indicate something peculiar about these cells since sperm tails probably cannot stick themselves into cells of other organs.

H. R. Lindner: They do it in the Fallopian tubes.

P. F. Kraicer: They are engulfed, they penetrate between cells, and are engulfed by leucocytes, but they don't go sewing themselves in, leaving a free end flapping in space.

J. Gorski: In what percentage of, say, seemingly normal blastocysts do you see this?

P. F. Kraicer: We have seen it in 25 per cent, but if they were inside the trophoblast cells or in an unfavorable plane in the light microscope, we would not see them. The blastocyst is very thick, and it's difficult to resolve something which is a micron in diameter in this 100-micron ovum, unless it happens to fall alongside the egg in a particular orientation or if it overlies a particularly transparent part of the blastocyst.

J. Gorski: Well, what would you estimate it as being?

P. F. Kraicer: I would estimate it as being 30 per cent of free sperm, and I suspect a much higher percentage of sperm cells which may penetrate in and remain inside or between the cells. Apparently, the pieces inside are stable, because peculiary enough if you find supernumerary sperm like this in one egg from an animal, you will probably find them in all.

M. C. Shelesnyak: I would hazard a guess that they are in all blastocysts. Just to allay one qualm of Seymour, of course, the statement that the existence of a structure does not necessarily mean the existence of antigenicity in that structure, is not challenged. The evidence for this would have to be obtained. But the presence of the structure certainly strengthens the possibility of the antigenicity of the structure being retained or that at least antigen has diffused into the blastocyst.

S. Katsh: Yes, I would agree, but I would think that could be readily determined by localization with fluorescent antibody.

M. C. Shelesnyak: Not quite so easily, but theoretically it's true. Again this comes under the category of it being a nice thing to do, but at the moment we'd prefer that someone else do it.

H. R. Lindner: One more question, for those people who have experience in human reproduction. The primates are somewhat unique, particularly the human, in indulging in coitus for its own sake, irrespective of the reproductive receptivity of the female. Do you know whether sperm deposited in the vagina during intercourse outside the period corresponding to estrus in other animals, that is, outside the time of ovulation, penetrate into the womb of the human? Because if this were the case, if they could penetrate the cervix at times other than the time of ovulation, then this exposure could happen at any time during the menstrual cycle, and there would be nothing critical about the time interval between copulation and implantation in relation to the time relationships in inducing a delayed sensitivity.

M. C. Shelesnyak: Quite aside from the question—it's an interesting question—but the critical time remains irrespective, because the interval would be determined solely by the coition associated with fertilization, and the descent of the blastocyst, assuming that the uterus is sensitized before.

H. R. Lindner: Yes, but there may have been three or four more occasions of coitus, in between.

M. C. Shelesnyak: So what? It doesn't really matter.

H. R. Lindner: I was referring to the question of timing raised by Prof. Tausk earlier in this discussion.

G. J. Marcus: But also it is established that the uterine leucocytic response to the deposition of semen is different at different physiological stages, at least in the rabbit, with a maximum response at the time of normal mating [L. E. McDonald, W. G. Black, S. H. McNutt and L. E. Casida, Am. J. Vet. Res., 13, 419, 1952]. There are also cyclic variations in "spontaneous" leucocytic infiltration [R. Yanagimachi and M. C. Chang, J. Reprod. Fertil., 5, 389, 1963; W. M. Allen, Anat. Rec., 45, 65, 1931]. If the leucocytic infiltration can be considered as pertinent to any kind of immunological response, then, by analogy, differences in the stages of the menstrual cycle in humans could account for the lack of a response other than at the time of ovulation. This would emphasize the idea of a critical period. Changes in the viscosity of the cervical mucus might also affect sperm penetration at different times during the cycle thereby limiting possible tissue responses to periods of maximal sperm penetration [cf. G. Gennser, Lancet 7414, 492, 1965].

Is there any variation with the cycle or stage of pregnancy in the activity of antigen-inactivating substances in the uterus?

S. Katsh: We delineate four stages in the guinea pig, and there are certainly significant differences in the enzymatic content, if that is what the question is.

G. J. Marcus: Could this provide a reasonable explanation or answer to Prof. Lindner's question?

S. Katsh: You see the answer to Dr. Lindner's question depends upon the acquisition of evidence that sperm penetration, let's say to the sub mucusa, does occur outside of the ovulation period. I must admit that I do not have that evidence.

H. R. Lindner: Do sperm reach the uterus after coitus outside the time of ovulation?

S. Katsh: Yes.

P. F. Kraicer: If I may just interject another comment, I think the human may not be the best species for this study. If the assumption be made, and I think that it's a logical one, that the function of the antigen-antibody reaction is induction of a reactive state in the endometrium, which, thereafter, leads to decidualization of the area adjacent to the egg, then this is quite superfluous in the human. In the human, cells decidualize in the fundus region of the uterus. This is the <u>deciduum menstrualis</u> and is a concommittant of an ovulatory cycle. The fertilized ovum is engulfed by or invades this already decidualized area.

If one is worried about the process of exogenous induction of decidualization, then nature insists that you restrict your discussion to those animals where decidualization is induced, if at all, exogenously. There is no point discussing decidual induction in the cow. There is no decidual tissue in the cow. In the same way, in the human, you don't have to induce it, except by allowing the proper balance of progesterone and estrogen, and then the cells will carry on by themselves.

H R. Lindner: Granted this, do you still postulate that this immune mechanism has an essential or important function in implantation in the human, or would you like to exclude this a priori?

P. F Kraicer: I would like to investigate the phenomenon to find out if it has a function in the rat. This is conveniently done because we have as our first end point decidualization. If, in the course of such work, it becomes clear that such an interaction has other end points, has other responses, one can then search for these in the human. But I must reiterate simply what I said before. I am not putting the restriction on this. I think nature has done this for us by evolving in the primates an endogenous decidual inducing mechanism.

M. C. Shelesnyak: If Dr. Lindner addresses his question to me, I am perfectly prepared to say that I speculate on an immunological mechanism operating also in the human. I will add that the amount of data available doesn't give me the authority to say any more than that I speculate on the involvement of this mechanism.

H. R. Lindner: If we're talking about rats, there is another problem. If you transplant blastocysts from a pregnant rat tc another rat which has not been inseminated or subjected to coitus, I believe you get fairly good results. You get maybe 70, 80 per cent success of implantation. How can this be explained away?

G. J. Marcus: If I may take a comment on this observation. As you know, we claim that spontaneous decidualization in a non-pregnant rat does not occur [M. C. Shelesnyak and G. J. Marcus, J. Reprod. Fertil. 14, 497, 1967]. When you observe apparently spontaneous decidualization, we feel it can usually be traced to some irritant. Dr. Kraicer has found, for example, that disturbing the oviduct at about the time of ovulation, or just after ovulation, results, later on in the pseudopregnancy, in a decidual response. It is very likely that merely in transferring ova one produces an irritation which is sufficient to produce a degree of decidualization which could then provide a favorable environment for implantation of the ovum.

P. F Kraicer: There is one problem. I would have agreed with what George said, however, unfortunately people do experiments. Dickman has done a series of experiments not directed to this problem, but directed to the question of ovum survival in the uterus after transplantation. He ovariectomized virgin animals at various parts of the cycle, subjected them to various progesterone regimens, transplanted blastocysts into their uteri and then tested whether the ova survive and whether they can implant under the proper hormonal conditions. In this case, the period between trauma and induction of implantation of the ovum was very long. So that it is difficult to imagine that the traumatic stimulus was retained. Certainly, we do know from work here that if you perform almost any treatment which would induce decidualization during the period of blastocyst diapause, wait, then produce implantation, you will not get massive decidual induction, you will just get implantation; the decidualization is restricted to where the egg is. But why postulate only one mechanism for inducing decidualization? I don't think anyone has said that such an immune response is <u>the</u> mechanism; they have said it is <u>a</u> possible mechanism. Legitimate. There is not a mechanism for clotting blood. There are books full of mechanisms.

M. C. Shelesnyak: I think one thing must be remembered. In most reproductive processes, there are primary and secondary and standby mechanisms to take over to assure the continuity of the race. Whether this is an act of wisdom on the part of nature is hard to say, but at any rate, so it is.

There is another point that might be made about the administration of blastocysts into a uterus that has not been sensitized by the antigen. You must remember that you are essentially administering a foreign body. I may sound like a scoundrel or like someone trying to promote a particular thesis, whether it is microcirculation or something else. You can always come around back to something, and that something I am coming around back to is as follows: the admittance of a blastocyst into the uterus as a foreign body may very well provoke enough of a localized reaction, as a foreign body, not as an immunological mechanism at all, to release enough histamine locally, thinking of it as a foreign protein rather than as a part of an immunological response. The idea proposed about the immunological mechanism is a supporting one, in the sense, that this is a way in which it could take place.

H. R. Lindner: I have found the idea in some way attractive that the blastocyst itself, irrespective of the presence of male derived components or spermatozoal remnants may make its presence felt in the uterus by an immunological mechanism; I mean the blastocyst itself is partly male derived and, in a colony which is not closely inbred, and contains immunologically, presumably foreign protein. The uterus may thus, in some way, recognize the presence of some such foreign protein and react to it. Although we know that eventually a barrier is established which prevents such immunological interaction, the possibility of such a transient response to the presence of foreign protein, before this barrier is established, is something which I would find attractive, and would like to have Prof. Billingham's comments. This is independent of the demonstration, which I find convincing, of the presence of remnants of spermatozoa on the blastocyst.

U. S. von Euler: May I ask Prof. Katsh one question? I know very little about immunology, but I wonder very much whether it is possible to influence an immunological reaction by various low molecular substances, and I am thinking particularly of certain constituents of human seminal fluid, namely, prostaglandins. The reason I ask is that these occur, as far as we know, in large quantities only in human seminal plasma, in other primates, in sheep and also in goats. We obtained a number of semen samples collected from infertile marriages. In a certain number of them there was a remarkable lack of prostaglandins. But it was not in any way one hundred per cent. We never published these results. At any rate, in several cases where there was infertility and we couldn't see anything wrong with the spermatozoa, there were low prostaglandin levels in the seminal fluid. I just wonder whether possibly a substance like that could influence nidation, and if one would speculate wildly, one could think of a protective effect of a substance like that under ordinary condition.

S. Katsh: Of course, I have been following the literature on the pharmacologically active and identified materials in seminal plasma, and, of course they are intriguing. Dr. Eliasson has been doing a considerable amount in that area. I cannot answer your question directly with regard to a deficiency here, because we have not examined that. What we have done is to remove the prostate glands from guinea pigs to determine whether there is any effect on the prostaglandins there. But you have already said this is not the best animal to work with. Sheep, yes, but we have very limited animal quarters. What is of interest is the profound effect that prostaglandin does have upon the receptor organ, namely, the uterus; and whether or not it may prepare the uterus for the reception of what is to come is, of course, an interesting question. Apparently, the prostaglandins affect uterine motility *in vivo* or *in vitro*. I think that the pacemaker control of uterine motility should be investigated thoroughly in order to determine the relationship between motility and progesterone or estrogen dominance. The uterine pacemaker actually seems to be very much like the pacemaker in the heart.

M. C. Shelesnyak: There is a technical problem at the moment which prevents us from pursuing such a study. As we conceive the experiment, it should be done in an intact animal that moves around freely, with no wires attached, which means we have to telemeter the information, and all the instrumentation for the telemetry has not been competent. It has to be a small unit. Besides, various things, we recently had a period of tension and a war, you know, diverse things that interfere with the progress of science.

G. J. Marcus: It might have been instructive to know what was the fate, *in utero*, of the spermatozoa in those cases of infertility associated with low prostaglandin levels referred to by Prof. von Euler. Mr. Joshi, in our Department, has been investigating interactions between the ejaculate and the uterus and has made some observations which are apropos of the protective effect of some seminal component as suggested by Prof. von Euler.

M. S. Joshi: We have observed that when epididymal sperm, i. e. sperm without seminal plasma, are incubated, *in vivo*, in the proestrous uterus or *in vitro* in proestrous uterine fluid, the sperm suffer decapitation within five to six hours. We discovered this during our attempts to find out which of the components of the male ejaculate is responsible for the massive infiltration of erythrocytes into the uterus immediately after mating. When we tried epididymal sperm we found they were decapitated and so we checked whether this occurs *in vitro* and found that it does. The decapitation is accomplished by a constituent of uterine fluid which behaves as a phospholipase C; in addition to inhibition of the decapitation by phospholipase C inhibitors such as phosphate, fluoride or sodium lauryl sulfate, seminal plasma or a saline extract of seminal vesicle fluid also prevented the decapitation.

When Dr. Katsh mentioned destruction of sperm antigen in the uterus, he mentioned that the antigens contained a phospholipid portion. I wonder what phospholipase he used in order to destroy the antigens, since we have been concerned with what might be the physiological significance of the phospholipase-like activity in the uterine fluid. Might it not destroy sperm antigen?

S. Katsh: What I said was that we had polypeptide and polysaccharide chains with associated lipid and we don't know quite how to fit that lipid in there. In fact, by Soxhlet extraction, we got just about every bit of free and bound lipid out of there that we can. Yet, there still remains some, so we have a feeling that this may be an integral part of the molecule. But as far as which phospholipase we used, I think we used A and C, but I'm not sure. I'd have to check the records.

Now, with regard to the role of the uterine fluid, you are not saying decapacitation, you are saying decapitation. Yes, now, in general, what one finds is that the entire seminal fluid plus spermatozoa are apparently taken up through the reproductive tract, and it may be what you are demonstrating here when you add back your seminal fluid, that you are actually protecting it as it would be *in vivo*.

M. S. Joshi: We've also tried removing sperm from the uterus, after normal mating, washing them with saline and incubating them then in uterine fluid. We got considerable decapitation so it doesn't seem that the sperm coating antigen is the protective factor because that's supposed to be nearly impossible to remove.

S. Katsh: Well, you have to be careful when you talk about this term coating antigen, because as far as A. Weil has demonstrated, this is true of a rabbit and it's true of man, but I don't think he has progressed to other forms. So I am not sure whether or not this would apply to the rat.

G. J. Marcus: Moyer believes the seminal antigen to be present in the rhesus monkey [D. L. Moyer and H. Maruta, *Fertil. Steril.* **18**, 497, 1967] and in the guinea pig [H. Maruta and D. L. Moyer, *Fertil. Steril.* **18**, 649, 1967]; but, in the case of the rat, there is a technical difficulty in approaching the problem, and that is that the ejaculum or the seminal vesicle fluid clots almost immediately and cannot be redissolved, not even in the way the guinea pig ejaculate can be dissolved with chymotrypsin. This doesn't work with the rat ejaculate.

S. Katsh: It's the best glue or rubber I've ever found. No, that's quite right. It's most difficult to do.

M. C. Shelesnyak: Mr. Joshi: What is your opinion about the possibility that the repression of the decapitation plays a role in capacitation?

M. S. Joshi: I don't think it does, because sperm reach the oviduct within an hour or so after copulation, before ovulation. There is no gradual entry of sperm into the tubes. The sperm that do reach the tubes undergo capacitation while they are waiting for the eggs to come down, the uterine sperm are disposed of either by phagocytosis or by evacuation through the cervix at the end of estrus. Normal capacitation takes place in the oviducts, not in the uterus, in the rat.

E. S. Kisch: As far as I recall, from the observations of Long and Evans [J. A. Long and H. M. Evans, Mem. Univ. Calif. 6, 72, 1922] the copulation plug closes the cervix and extends up into the cervical canal. I wonder how fast the uterine fluid can really disappear and if it does get out through the cervical canal.

M. S. Joshi: The plug remains in the vagina for only 12 to 24 hrs and it has been established that the uterine contents are expelled through the cervix during late estrus [R. J. Blandau and D. L. Odor, Anat. Rec. 103, 331, 1949; C. R. Austin, J. Endocrin. 14, 335, 1957].

B. L. Lobel: Dr. Katsh, earlier you discussed the atrophy of the seminiferous epithelium resulting from the injection of sperm antigens into the testes. Have you any information on exactly where the reaction takes place?

S. Katsh: I'll try to give the smallest answer I can, and that involves, really, the mechanism of destruction of the cells. That's what you are asking for. This is still a puzzle. I will tell you quite frankly that we just don't have this information now. We are looking, as a result of the culling of many alternatives, at the lysosomal responses here, figuring that activation of lysosomes may very well, in the immunized animal, be responsible for the autodestruction. But whether or not it is a direct involvement of cell fixed antibodies with the seminiferous epithelium remains to be determined.

# TRANSPLANTATION IMMUNITY AND THE MAMMALIAN EMBRYO

# TRANSPLANTATION IMMUNITY AND THE MAMMALIAN EMBRYO

R. E. Billingham
Department of Medical Genetics
School of Medicine
University of Pennsylvania, Philadelphia

## INTRODUCTION

Even the layman is now well aware of the remarkable consistency and promptitude with which living cells, tissues or organs are destroyed following their exchange between unrelated individuals of the same species, and of the rather heroic measures necessary to overcome this natural intolerance of vertebrates to homografts transplanted for experimental or therapeutic purposes.

However, the confrontation of adult individuals with genetically alien cells in relatively large dosage is a commonplace natural process in mammals since every pregnancy in an outbred population constitutes an intimate, parabiotic union, and consequent exposure of the mother to fetal tissues that she might have been expected to react against immunologically. This follows since tissue homografts from offspring transplanted to their mothers enjoy no special dispensations. When fertilized eggs resulting from a mating between one pair of unrelated individuals are transferred to the uterus of a third party female host, the immunogenetic relationship between the mother and her adoptive fetuses is exactly similar to that obtaining when homografts are grafted between unrelated individuals. In striking contrast to the fate of artificial tissue or organ homografts is the apparently uniform success of Nature's homografts—fertilized eggs that become implanted in the uterus and the embryos that develop from them. For completeness' sake another, recently discovered example of the natural transplantation of foreign cells may be mentioned—the transmission of lymphomas in hamsters by mosquitos (Banfield et. al., 1966).

The purpose of this review is to present a general account of the relevant principles of transplantation immunology and then to examine critically our knowledge of the peculiar status of the mammalian embryo our homograft.

## GENETIC BASIS OF HOMOGRAFT INCOMPATIBILITY

Appropriate genetic analyses, conducted principally in mice, have revealed the complex nature of the polymorphism responsible for homograft graft incompatibility (see Snell and Stimpfling, 1966). A minimum of 15 so-called histocompatibility loci are widely distributed throughout the chromosomes, including the X and the Y. Multiple allelic co-dominant histocompatibility genes at many of these loci determine antigens that vary considerably in their relative strengths or sensitizing potencies. The genetic requirement for permanant acceptance of a graft is simply that each of the donor's complement of histocompatibility genes must also be represented in the host, so that the latter is not confronted with alien transplantation isoantigens determined by these genes. This requirement is met if donor and recipient are identical twins or if they are members of the same isogenic or inbred strain. Another situation in which it is satisfied is when grafts from either of two unrelated isogenic parental strains are transplanted to their $F_1$ hybrid offspring. There is wide variation in the potency of the isoantigens determined by different histocompatibility loci–i.e., there are major and minor loci, determining strong and weak antigens respectively. A difference between donor and host with respect to a single strong antigen (or allele at a major locus) normally incites a homograft reaction of near-maximal intensity, so that skin homografts are destroyed within about 11 days, or less. On the other hand a difference at only a minor locus may enable a graft to survive for upwards of a hundred days before it is eventually destroyed.

In the mouse, one major histocompatibility locus, the H-2, predominates over all the others in terms of the potency of its products. At this locus there are at least 20 alleles. Since, in addition to determining homograft incompatibility, this locus determines antigens that elicit the formation of humoral antibodies, it has been possible to study its products serologically. At least 33 serologically detectable specificities collectively characterize this locus. Some of these specificities are associated with the product of a single allele, others are shared in common by the products of 2 or more alleles. There is some argument as to whether the antigens of this locus are determined by true alleles, or by a series of closely linked genes or pseudoalleles. At any rate, the antigens are normally inherited on bloc as if they were the products of a single gene. Obviously an enormous degree of polymorphism is possible within the H-2 system itself simply because the antigens may be present in a variety of different combinations.

In rats and chickens evidence has also been forthcoming that a single locus, designated as the Ag-B and the B loci respectively, out-weighs the others with respect to the potency of the antigenic specificities it determines, and preliminary evidence indicates that a similar situation obtains in man where the Hu-1 locus (subsequently renamed the HLA locus) has recently been identified (Bach and Amos, 1967).

Where non-inbred populations are concerned, the survival times of homografts may vary enormously, being inversely related to the genetic disparity between donor and host, though over a wide range of species it is unusual for them to live longer than about 2 weeks.

## DISTRIBUTION AND CHARACTERISATION OF TRANSPLANTATION ANTIGENS

All the evidence presently available sustains the thesis that the full spectrum of antigens corresponding to an animal's histocompatibility genes are present on most, if not all, of its tissue cells. Each of a wide variety of tissues, normal or malignant, will sensitize a host in respect of others of the same genetic origin

(Barnes, 1964). Furthermore, animals made immunologically tolerant of homologous cells of one type of tissue are completely and specifically incapable of reacting against any other type of tissue or organ graft from the donor of the tolerance-conferring stimulus, or from another donor of similar genetic constitution (Billingham and Silvers, 1965).

Most of the available evidence concerning the quantitative distribution of transplantation antigens in different cell and tissue types pertains to the products of a few loci in the mouse and is based upon the capacity of tissue homogenates to absorb the appropriate isoantibodies. So far as it goes, the evidence indicates the existence of striking differences in the quantitative distribution of different isoantigens in different tissues (see Snell and Stimpfling, 1966). Whether transplantation antigens are present on the gametes is still undecided. With the aid of a fluorescent antibody technique capable of revealing the presence of H-2 antigens on the cell membranes of lymphoid cells, Barth and Russell (1964) were unable to detect these specificities on spermatozoa, nor to detect the rather weak Y-determined antigen. Nevertheless the latter, which occurs in a wide variety of tissues, does seem to be present on spermatozoa as evidenced by a report that adult C57BL/6 female mice can either be sensitized or rendered tolerant of subsequent skin grafts from isogenic male donors following injection with small or large members of sperm respectively (Katsh, Talmage, and Katsh, 1964).

Although the histocompatibility genes of the major loci in mice and rats determine antigenic specificities on red cells that are serologically detectable, there is no evidence that erythocytes can elicit sensitivity to normal tissue homografts. This may be because the relevant antigenic specificities are not present in sufficient quantity, or because they are not present in an immunogenic form. There is suggestive evidence of the presence of transplantation antigens in the platelets of rabbits and guinea pigs, but not in those of the rat.

Fractionation studies to isolate and characterize antigenically active material have centered mainly upon products of the H-2 locus in the mouse. These have established that the major part of the antigenic activity is located in an insoluble lipoprotein fraction derived from membranous structures of cells. As Nathensen and Davies (1966) point out, purification of these antigens for the purpose of determining the chemical nature of their immunologic determinants has been hampered by their association with the insoluble fraction of cells, by their lability to many extraction procedures, as well as the lack of a rapid quantitative assay procedure. It is not known whether the antigenic specificities determined by each of the different families of histocompatibility alleles are associated with macromolecules of similar biochemical constitution, nor do we know whether antigenic material is actually released or secreted by cells.

Various lines of evidence have indicated that effective transplantation antigens are present very early in development; in the chicken by the 4th day of embryonic life, and in mice certainly by the 15th and 12th days of gestation, and probably as early as the 4th day of gestation (see Billingham, 1964).

## MECHANISM OF HOMOGRAFT REJECTION

There is now a compelling array of evidence that the destructive immunologic response of a host against a solid tissue homograft, such as that of skin, is cell-mediated, closely analogous to sensitivity of the tuberculin type, to drug and bacterial allergies and certain experimental autoimmune diseases. The distinguishing features of this particular category of immunologic responses are, of course, their transferability to normal unimmunized animals by means of living cells of the lymphoid series, in contradistinction to putatively immune serum from specifically sensitized animals, and the fact that they all seem to be put into effect by blood-borne, immunologically activated cells of the lymphocytic series (see Wilson and Billingham, 1967).

Studies on graft-versus-host reactions have firmly established that immunologically competent small lymphocytes from the peripheral blood can interact directly with histoincompatible cells and initiate a primary response against them (Gowans, 1965; Billingham, 1968). This response involves a rapid transformation of some of the lymphocytes into so-called large pyroninophilic cells which divide to form lymphocytes of progressively decreasing sizes. These and other findings sustain the thesis that the host's response to a solid tissue homograft is initiated by recirculating small lymphocytes which, when confronted by antigen, settle out and develop into large pyroninophilic cells in the regional lymph nodes. Various lines of indirect evidence implicate these cells as the progenitors of small "activated" lymphocytes which leave the nodes, circulate in the blood and constitute the important immunologically specific component of the cellular effector mechanism. The characteristic mononuclear cell infiltration of the stroma of a homograft, which precedes its demise, is interpreted as the outcome of the mobilization from the blood stream of an effector cell population within the target tissue. There is an increasing amount of evidence that this cell population comprises a relatively small proportion of specifically activated or sensitized lymphocytes whose interaction with antigen has brought about the non-specific accumulation of unsensitized, immunologically uncommitted cells of the mononuclear series, including macrophages, which constitute the major portion of the immigrant cells. Exactly how these mononuclear cells procure graft destruction is still open to conjecture. Recent experiments _in vitro_ have shown that lymphocytes from sensitized donors can kill homologous target cells _in vitro_ in the absence of added complement or immune serum. This cytocidal effect is associated with a clustering of lymphocytes around the target cells, referred to as 'contactual agglutination' (see Wilson and Billingham, 1967). The idea is gaining ground that antibodies, cell-bound or otherwise, play little part in the genesis of the lesions in solid tissue homografts, and that the pathological changes are caused by the release from the mononuclear cells of some kind of non-specific pharmacologically active agent(s) (see Spector, 1967; Schild and Willoughby, 1967; Billingham and Streilein, 1968; and Benacerraf, 1968).

Where differences at major histocompatibility loci are involved the cellular response to a homograft is usually accompanied by a humoral one, reflected in the appearance of isoantibodies demonstrable _in vitro_ as hemagglutinins, haemolysins, leucoagglutins, cytotoxins, etc., corresponding to specificities determined by histocompatibility genes.

Although nearly all critical attempts to implicate these humoral factors in the rejection of solid tissue homografts have failed, it is well established that circulating antibody may play an important role in the destruction of monodisperse cellular grafts of various types, especially of lymphoid cells (see Snell and Stimpfling, 1966).

We still have a great deal to learn about the manner in which a homograft reaction starts. Once it was established that the regional lymph node draining a skin or solid tumor graft became "activated"—i. e., it acquired the capacity to transfer sensitivity to another animal—most workers assumed that sensitization took place by the percolation of antigenic material from the grafts into the regional nodes through peripheral lymphatics. However, Medawar (1965; see also Brent and Medawar, 1967) has raised the interesting alternative possibility that sensitization might take place peripherally. Blood borne lymphocytes may engage with graft antigens in the graft itself or at the level of its vascular endothelial cells, and then migrate via the graft stroma to the peripheral lymphatics and thence to the regional nodes where the effectors of the response are generated.

## SPECIAL SITES AND TISSUES

Before we consider embryos as homografts it is pertinent to ask whether any privileged or favored sites exist in the body in which homografts may acquire a blood supply but, for some reason or another, are exempt from a host's response, or whether there are any tissues or cells known that fail to express effective transplantation antigens.

Several privileged sites have indeed been discovered more or less empirically. The best studied examples are the area within the meninges of the brain, the anterior chamber of the eye, and within the connective tissue of the hamster's cheek pouch (see Billingham and Silvers, 1962; Russell and Monaco, 1964). Homografts of various tissues implanted into these sites normally acquire a rich blood supply yet may survive for anomalously long periods, if not indefinitely. The favored status of each of the three sites mentioned seems to turn upon the absence of draining lymphatic vessels. Thus there is no physiological pathway to transmit an antigenic stimulus to a seat of response or, alternatively, to transmit 'primed' small lymphocytes to a regional node, if peripheral sensitization occurs. It must be emphasized that in neither of these sites does a homograft enjoy any significant degree of protection from a state of pre-existing or subsequently evoked sensitivity. This is not surprising since the efferent limb of the immunologic reflex, afforded by the vasculature of the graft which transmits the effector cells, is present.

My colleague, Dr. Clyde Barker, and I have been studying a privileged site which can be produced artificially in guinea pigs (Barker and Billingham, 1967). Circular discs of skin, about 3 cm in diameter, are incised in the shaved flanks of adult animals in such a manner that only a single vascular bundle, with very little connective tissue, is left forming a uniting "umbilical cord" between the full-thickness skin flap and its host. After approximation of the margins of the wounds, the flaps are placed in protective plastic petri dishes glued to the hosts' skins. Using guinea pigs of the unrelated isogenic strains #2 and #13 it has been found that whereas skin homografts transplanted to shallow beds in normal skin are rejected within 8-10 days, similar homografts transplanted to beds prepared in the skin flaps heal-in normally and survive for as long as the host flaps themselves remain viable. Flap viability usually terminates abruptly after 25-30 days as a consequence of ischemia occasioned by accidental trauma to its vascular pedicle, though flaps occasionally survive for upwards of 50 days. Dye injection studies have shown that the privileged status of these flaps results from the complete interruption of their lymphatic drainage, which fails to become re-established when they are maintained in the plastic dishes. It need hardly be said that flaps prepared in specifically presensitized animals confer no protection upon subsequently implanted skin homografts.

However in contrast to the above situation with orthotopic skin homografts is that which obtains with renal homografts. These are able to sensitize their hosts via the vascular route even when special steps have been taken to prevent the establishment of lymphatic connections (see Wilson and Billingham, 1967). Strober and Gowans (1965) have presented cogent evidence that lymphocytes in the peripheral blood interact with alien cellular antigens in the graft as large numbers of them pass through the rich vascular bed. The 'primed' cells may then return to lymphoid tissues where they settle out and then set up the machinery of immunologic attack. The failure of peripheral sensitization to occur when small grafts are transplanted to the privileged sites described above may simply reflect the trivial extent of the exposure of host lymphocytes to alien vascular endothelium.

If homografts of the highly vascular 'skin' which forms the walls of hamsters' cheek pouches are transplanted to recipient areas prepared in normal trunk skin, they acquire a rich blood supply and the majority long outlive homografts of ordinary skin (Billingham and Silvers, 1962). Indeed some may survive indefinitely. This consititutes an example of an immunologically privileged tissue. Several lines of evidence indicate that its privileged status derives from peculiar properties of its rather mobile and slimy deeper layers of connective tissue which lacks lymphatic vessels and has a high content of mucopolysaccharides of 'fibrinoid' material (see Kirby et al, 1964). Apart from preventing the ingrowth of lymphatic capillaries from the wound bed into a pouch skin homograft, this connective tissue may function as a barrier, preventing the escape of antigenic material from the foreign cell population in the graft. Among the various lines of evidence sustaining this premise is the finding that the insertion of a layer of this pouch skin connective tissues between a thin homograft of ordinary skin and its bed affords complete protection to the graft, though it does not interfere with vascularization.

The classic example of a privileged <u>tissue</u> is afforded by cartilage. The long-term survival of the chondrocytes in cartilage homografts is well-documented both clinically and experimentally, as is the capacity of these cells to survive the transplantation of cartilage to specifically presensitized hosts (Craigmyle, 1960). The distinctive physico-chemical properties of the intercellular muco-polysaccharide matrix of cartilage homografts seem to underlie both their weak isoantigenicity as well as the exemption of the cells from immunological destruction. This matrix seems to function like a diffusion chamber, not only preventing the escape of transplantation antigens from the cells, but also preventing immunologically competent cells from the host establishing contact with them. Recent trans-plantation studies employing suspensions of chondro-cytes isolated enzymically from cartilage, as well as serological studies on the recipients of cartilage homografts, have indicated that chondrocytes do possess transplantation antigens. (Moskalowski et al., 1966, Stjernsward, 1965).

## 6. THE MAMMALIAN EMBRYO QUA HOMOGRAFT

In the light of the evidence reviewed in the fore-going sections it will be appreciated that to account for the successful development to term of the mam-malian fetus constituted a tremendous challenge to the ingenuity of students of transplantation biology. The challenge became even greater when it was es-tablished that embryos are also invulnerable to a state of immunity in their mothers specifically directed against transplantation antigens which they've inherited from their fathers (see Billingham, 1964). For example, if A strain fe-male mice are grafted once, or even several times, with skin homografts, or given multiple injections of cells, from strain C57 males, and then mated with males of the latter strain, they will give birth to litters of normal, healthy hybrid mice. Lanman and his associates (Lanman et al, 1962; Lanman, 1965) sensitized female rabbits by means of skin grafts from unrelated males and females. When the latter were subsequently mated and the resultant fertilized eggs transferred to the uterine horns of the sensitized females, which functioned as surrogate mothers, they implanted and developed normally to term.

Numerous hypotheses have been advanced to account for the survival of the fetus as a homograft (see Medawar, 1953; Billingham, 1964) of which we need consider only two:

i) The Uterus is an Immunologically Privilaged Site

Several lines of indirect evidence make it appear unlikely that any kind of privileged status of the uterine environment is responsible for the success of fetuses as homografts. In man, non-uterine tissues, such as the pelvic ileum or rectum, the fallopian tubes or the peritoneum may form implantation sites for fertilized eggs and subsequent attachment sites for the placcentas. Despite these heterotopic attachments, it is well-established that ectopic pregnancies may proceed more or less normally for considerable periods, and sometimes even to term. When fetal death has occurred under these conditions, no evidence has been forthcoming to incriminate homograft reactivity on the part of the mother.

In animals, naturally occurring ectopic pregnancies are rare. However, in various rodent species segmenting eggs have been caused to become attached to the mesenteries, or have been transferred beneath the renal or splenic capsules of histoincompatible hosts where they still developed into normal embryos without the slightest indication of inciting a homograft reaction.

As a direct test of the privileged status of the uterus, Schlesinger (1962) ingeniously implanted small tumor grafts into the uterine horns of rats and mice. If the tumors and their hosts were of similar genetic constitution, then the grafts grew successfully. However, tumor homografts survived only for a short time in normal hosts and underwent accelerated rejection if implanted into presensitized animals, irrespective of whether the latter were pregnant, pseudo-pregnant or non-pregnant in one uterine horn.

An inherent weakness of Schlesinger's experimental design is its failure to exclude the possibility that the tumor homografts may have outgrown the limits of the "physiological" uterus, penetrating the myometrium and the uterine lining. However, Poppa et al. (1964) subsequently showed that homografts of a normal, non-invasive tissue—parathyroid gland—transplanted to the uterus of pseudopregnant and non-pseudopregnant parathyroidectomized rats were almost uniformly rejected within 20 days. This evidence indicates that, so far as homologous cells of non-embryonic tissues are concerned, transplantation immunity is both incitable and expressible in the uterine milieu. All the evidence we've considered so far sustains the view that whatever it is that prevents a fetus from sensitizing its mother, or protects it from a state of sensitivity, _must_ be associated with components of the fetus.

### ii) There is a Physiological Protective Barrier Between Mother and Fetus

In those species with hemochorial placentae the resistance of the embryo to rejection as a homograft expresses itself in its most striking form, since here we have a relatively large expanse of cells of fetal origin—comprising the syncytiotrophoblast—chronically and directly exposed to the cellular mediators of transplantation hypersensitivity—i. e., lymphocytic cells in the maternal blood stream.

The only hypothesis that will satisfactorily account for the properties of the fetus as a homograft is that it is separated from its mother by some kind of complete anatomical barrier that not only prevents sensitization of the mother in respect of fetal transplantation antigens, but fully protects the fetus from an experimentally evoked state of sensitivity specifically directed against it. As one might anticipate, attention has long been focussed upon the fetal trophoblast as holding the possible key to the riddle, since this represents an unbroken frontier component. The idea that the placenta could function as a barrier if its trophoblast cells were non-antigenic was advanced nearly 40 years ago by Witebsky and his associates (Cottingne and Witebsky, 1928; Witebsky and Reich, 1932) on the basis of observations that human placental villi are deficient in blood group antigens (see Thiede et al, 1965). Other evidence that normal trophoblast may possess peculiar immunologic properties was forthcoming from subsequent studies on its malignant derivatives

--chorionepthelioma of gestational origin--in man. Despite their fetal origin and wide metastatic dissemination, these tumors rarely undergo spontaneous regression in affected women (see Billingham, 1964).

Direct experimental evidence in favor of the thesis that normal trophoblast possesses properties that would enable it to constitute an effective immunologically protective barrier or buffer zone between mother and fetus was first presented by Simmons and Russell (1962). They analysed the histocompatibility characteristics of mouse placental tissue at various stages of its development. They studied grafts from $F_1$ hybrid embryos transplanted to adult hosts of the maternal strain since, under these conditions, accidental inclusion of maternal cells in fetal tissue grafts cannot influence the host immunologically. It was shown that if seven-day mouse conceptuses were separated into their trophoblastic and embryonic moieties and implanted beneath the renal capsules of maternal-strain hosts presensitized to paternal strain antigens, the embryonic grafts were promptly destroyed, whereas those of trophoblastic tissue displayed marked proliferative activity on the part of the giant cells with the formation of typical blood spaces. These grafts survived just as well and as long as if they'd been transplanted to genetically compatible hosts.

Evidence that mouse trophoblastic cells are effectively deficient in transplantation antigens was forthcoming from studies on the fate of fertilized ova or blastocysts transplanted heterotopically beneath the renal capsule or the spleen (Simmons and Russell, 1962; Kirby, 1963). In a genetically compatible host such grafts develop into trophoblastic giant cell tumors with a life-span of about 2 weeks. When $F_1$ hybrid fertilized eggs were transplanted to normal, maternal strain hosts they failed to elicit a detectable level of sensitivity and their life-span gave no evidence of curtailment. Even more striking was the inability of such grafts to incite a local mononuclear cell response when implanted into specifically pre-sensitized animals.

The findings of an interesting serological study by Schlesinger (1964) are in accord with the above results. Whereas whole placentas of embryos from upwards of 10 1/2 days showed a constant and relatively high level of isoantigenicity (as measured in terms of their ability to absorb specific hemagglutinins), trophoblastic growths obtained from grafts of 2 1/2 - 3 1/2 day old fertilized eggs in the cryptorchid testes of adult homologous hosts had no demonstrable serologic reactivity.

In 1959 Bardawil and Toy made the interesting suggestion that a local deposition of fibrinoid substance, which usually separates fetal and maternal tissue in man and is known as the layer of Nitebuch, "may behave somewhat as an immunological no man's land, walling the fetus off from chemical interaction with its host." Recently, Kirby and his associates (Kirby et al.,1964; Bradbury et al.,1965) have presented various lines of circumstantial evidence lending support to this general hypothesis. On the basis of careful histochemical and electronmicroscopical studies of the fibrinoid of mouse placentas they claim that each trophoblast cell is surrounded by a layer of amorphous, electron-dense fibrinoid material which ranges in thickness from $0.1\mu$ to $2.0\mu$. This fibrinoid, which is closely similar to the intercellular matrix of hamster cheek pouch connective tissue, contains a mucoprotein rich in tryptophan with at least two non-sulphated acid mucopolysaccharides, probably hyaluronic and sialic acids. The amount of fibrinoid present was found to be related to the immunogenetic disparity between the mother and her conceptus. When there was no disparity, the placentae had <u>less</u> fibrinoid than those of $F_1$ hybrid embryos or embryos resulting from the transfer of blastocysts of one strain of mouse to the uterus of pseudopregnant mothers of a different strain. Since there is evidence that placental fibrinoid is secreted by trophoblast cells, the immunological quarantining of the placenta may be comparable with that of cartilage in the manner in which it is accomplished.

Currie and Bagshawe (1967) have also reported some interesting observations sustaining this thesis and suggesting that the trophoblast cells themselves are <u>not</u> isoantigenically inert. According to them, when trophoblast is grown <u>in vitro</u> in the presence of lymphocytes of maternal or homologous origin it undergoes gross cytolysis. Postgestational choriocarcinoma cells suffer a similar fate on exposure to host lymphocytes in culture. However, trophoblast cells are not lysed in the presence of lymphocytes of <u>isologous</u> (i. e., genetically similar) origin. This direct destructive action of lymphocytes from unsensitized donors upon homologous trophoblastic cells is attributed to the phenomenon of "allogeneic inhibition" or contact-induced cytotoxicity—an interesting phenomenon discovered and analysed by Swedish workers (see Möller and Möller, 1966). According to them intimate contact between unsensitized lymphoid cells and target cells having different surface structural properties, of the type determined by histocompatibility genes, may result in a contact-induced cytotoxicity in vitro which is not an immunological phenomenon. If one accepts this interpretation of Currie and Bagshawe's observations, it follows that trophoblast cells must indeed express transplantation antigens after their fibrinoid coating has been removed by trypsinization prior to culture.

Currie and Bagshawe have also adduced various lines of evidence that the peritrophoblastic layer of fibrinoid, or sialomucin as they identify it, confers a high electronegative charge on the surface of the cells by virtue of the free carboxyl groups on sialic acid. Since lymphocytes likewise carry a negative charge, they put forward the interesting suggestion that, in vivo, the trophoblast escapes interaction with, or attack by lymphocytes as a consequence of electrochemical repulsion of these cells of maternal origin.

It may be noted that Fikrig et al. (1967) subsequently questioned whether the susceptibility of trophoblast cells to cytolysis, observed by Currie and Bagshawe, is due to the presence of transplantation antigens. When peripheral blood lymphocytes are exposed in vitro to homologous cells bearing a major alien histocompatibility antigen, a significant proportion of the lymphoid cells are stimulated to undergo a transformation into blast cells (see Bach and Voynow, 1966; Wilson and Billingham, 1967). Fikrig and his associates failed to observe such a transformation in mixed lymphocyte-trophoblast cultures.

Although most authorities are now in agreement that the trophoblast, or something associated with it, fulfills an immunological barrier function, the thesis that this property is restricted to the fibrinoid material is still on probation. Its presence in the appropriate position needs to be established in a wide range of mammals. Simmons et al. (1967) have recently studied, with an electron microscope, ectopic implants of mouse trophoblast, originating from mouse blastocysts implanted beneath the renal capsules of isogenic male hosts on the one hand and of homologous males on the other hand. They were unable to find any difference between the genetically compatible and the genetically incompatible grafts, both of which invaded the host tissue, nor did they observe any electron-dense "fibrinoid" material associated with the trophoblast cells in this ectopic site. However, it may be noted that Kirby and Malhotra (cited in Kirby et al., 1964), in a similar study of trophoblast which had been actively invading host kidney for 2-10 days, reported that the fibrinoid layer was conspicuously present around the cells. In an electronmicroscope study of normal rabbit placenta, Tai and Halasz (1967) observed "prominent deposition of fibrinoid material in the intercellular area of the trophoblastic cell layer" but failed to demonstrate the presence of a fibrinoid layer on the trophoblastic microvilli. Clearly resolution of these disparate findings is of the utmost importance. If it can be shown, unequivocally, that trophoblast cells can grow in some heterotopic sites in an alien host <u>without</u> fibrinoid investment it will necessarily imply a shortcoming on the part of these cells to express transplantation antigens on their surface.

In an ultrastructural analysis of the fetal-maternal

cellular junctional zones of placentas of varying degrees of histologic intimacy, Wynne (1967) observed that the most highly invasive trophoblasts, as seen in guinea pigs and man, are associated with necrosis of both chorionic and endometrial tissue and with the deposition of an acellular barrier towards which both fetal and maternal tissues probably contribute. In epithelial-chorial placentas of mares and cows, where there is direct apposition between chorionic and endometrial epithelia and no extensive degeneration or deposition of fibrinoid material, he suggests that absence of isoantigenicity of trophoblast, rather than the presence of an acellular protective barrier, would account for acceptance of the placental homograft. According to him, a positive correlation exists between invasiveness of the trophoblast, ultrastructural complexity of the decidua, necrosis, and elaboration of an acellular barrier.

Finally, it may be mentioned that, according to Schlesinger and Koren (1966), relatively pure mouse trophoblast cells grown _in vitro_ contain PAS--positive material but do not secrete it extracellularly. However, it must be borne in mind that the conditions prevailing _in vitro_ may not have been conducive for synthesis of this substance. These workers have made the interesting observation that trophoblast cells are capable of phagocytosing isoantibody-coated thymus cells whereas they are unable to phagocytose cells suspended in normal serum. On the basis of this observation they make the interesting suggestion that phagocytosis may play a role in protecting the fetus against maternal cell-bound immunity.

## 7. THE ANTIGENIC STATUS OF PRE-TROPHOBLASTIC EGG STAGES

Simmons and Russell (1966) have studies the fate of fertilized C3H eggs, 2 1/2 days post-conception, transplanted beneath the renal capsules of C57 male hosts pre-sensitized to various degrees against the antigens of the C3H donor strain. They found that the proportion of eggs which developed into trophoblastic tissue was inversely related to the level of immunity in the host. Trophoblast failed to develop in hosts presensitized by two consecutive C3H skin grafts, followed by 8-12 spleen cell injections at weekly intervals. However, (C3H x C57) $F_1$ hybrid eggs transplanted to sensitized C57 hosts proved less susceptible to the immunity, suggesting a gene-dosage effect in a situation where the dosage of antigen is very small. It may be emphasized that when trophoblastic proliferation did occur in a sensitized host there was no evidence that its extent was impaired.

In striking contrast to the susceptibility of fertilized eggs in hyperimmune hosts was the complete resistance of grafts of trophoblast derived from the ectoplacental cones of 7-day C3H embryos. On the basis of their findings Simmons and Russell believe that transplantation antigens <u>are</u> present in pre-trophoblastic egg stages, and postulate that trophoblast represents a differentiated form of embryonic cell, incapable of manufacturing or expressing on its surface antigens which are displayed by its immediate cell precursors. In their opinion, the zona pellucida, which is selectively impermeable to many proteins and all cells, might, in a female who has somehow become sensitized against her mate, afford protection to the portion of the placenta.

fertilized egg prior to the formation of an effective trophoblastic barrier.

On the basis of a similar study Kirby et al. (1966) have confirmed Simmons and Russell's findings. In addition they demonstrated that, whereas C57 strain eggs or blastocysts failed to develop if transplanted to the kidneys of hyperimmune C3H hosts, normal development occurred if the eggs were transplanted 'orthotopically' to the uterine horns of pseudopregnant hyperimmune C3H females. This important finding is interpreted as indicating that the uterus can confer some protection upon the eggs against a level of immunity that will destroy them in the milieu of the kidney. They consider that the decidual cells, which don't develop in the kidney, may be responsible for this protection of otherwise vulnerable embryos until the latter have developed their trophoblast-associated protective fibrinoid layer.

Three comments are in order concerning the experimental work reviewed above. Firstly, in the light of evidence that the hyperimmunized host mice manifested high levels of hemagglutinins, it is possible that the impairment of development of the eggs transplanted to the kidney may have been caused by a humoral immunity rather than a cellular one. Secondly, the vulnerability of the blastocysts in the kidneys of hyperimmunized hosts may have stemmed from a trauma-augmented delayed allergy type of inflammatory response unlike that which occurs during the natural act of implantation. Thirdly, it should be emphasized that the level of hyperimmunization required to prevent the development of alien eggs transplanted to a mouse's kidney is of a much greater order of magnitude than is likely to develop either naturally as a possible consequence of multiple pregnancies, or artificially as, for example, a consequence of repeated blood transfusions in man.

## 8. INFLUENCE OF ANTIGENIC DISPARITY AND IMMUNOLOGICAL STATUS OF THE MOTHER ON THE PLACENTA

Finally, although as we have seen, conceptuses in the uterus seem to be totally invulnerable to sensitivity in the mother specifically directed against their foreign antigens, there is evidence that the growth of the placenta is effected by both the genetic disparity between mother and her embryos and also by her immunological status.

Billington (1964) has shown that in mice placental size tends to be greater when mother and fetus are antigenically disparate then when they are alike, hybrid fetuses having larger placentae than fetuses whose parents belonged to the same inbred strain. The possibility that this size disparity simply reflected hybrid vigor was effectively ruled out by the observation that fertilized eggs from homospecific matings transferred to a host female of a <u>different</u> strain produced larger placentae than when allowed to develop in their genetically similar mothers. In a subsequent study of mouse trophoblast of ectoplacental cone origin transplanted to the testis Billington (1965) found that trophoblastic invasion of the host tissue was greater when there was histoincompatibility than when there was compatibility.

The influence of the immunological status of the mother of hybrid embryos on their placental size was investigated by James (1965). He confirmed that hybrid fetuses tend to have larger placentae than purebred fetuses in C57 BL/6 mothers and showed that prior immunization of the mother to paternal strain antigens in an outbred mating resulted in a significant increase in the placental size of the $F_1$ hybrid offspring, whereas prior induction of a state of immunological tolerance of paternal antigens in the mother resulted in hybrid fetuses whose placentae were significantly smaller than these of normal mothers. As James points out, if placental size is dependent upon the extent of trophoblast invasion of the uterus, this invasion must be effected by the immunological status of the mother in such a way that it is more extensive in immune and less extensive in tolerant than in normal mothers.

Clearly it is important for an understanding of the immunology of pregnancy to determine whether similar results are obtainable in other species.

## 9. POSSIBLE BIOLOGICAL SIGNIFICANCE OF TRANSPLANTATION ANTIGEN POLYMORPHISM

On the basis of some of the observations outlined in the previous section Clarke and Kirby (1966) have suggested that fetuses which are genetically unlike their mothers, and therefore are larger at birth, may have a greater chance of survival. They have ingeniously postulated the existence of a selective system on this basis, capable of maintaining balanced polymorphism which might account for the great diversity of transplantation antigens within species of viviparous animals.

Pertinent evidence had previously been presented

by Hull (1964) who studied a stock of mice in which two genes of the agouti series, $a^t$ and +, were present. Examination of the progeny of matings involving all possible combinations of parents suggested that there was some kind of incompatibility between mothers and offspring of the <u>same</u> agouti locus genotype, leading to reduction of the viability of these offspring. Since there was no indication that total litter size was reduced where this incompatibility was operating, it seemed likely that the selective elimination was occurring at an early stage in utero, when there was an excess of embryos over those which the female could carry to term. Hull suggested that the observed incompatibility could either be ascribed to the effect of the two genes, $a^t$ and + themselves or to a closely-linked gene or genes, possibly histocompatibility genes.

Michie and Anderson (1966) have presented striking evidence of a very powerful selective effect associated with a histocompatibility gene in a substrain of Wistar rats. Despite a history of 72 generations of brother-sister matings, about 50% of skin grafts exchanged between members of this strain underwent fairly rapid destruction. Analysis revealed that this state of affairs resulted from a strong selective effect associated with a histocompatibility gene. Two alleles, $g_1$ and $g_2$, were segregating in the population and the survival value of heterozygous ($g_1/g_2$) individuals was superior to that of either of the homozygotes. Litter size data indicated that the selective elimination must act <u>before</u> implantation of the fertilized eggs, and Michie and Anderson favor the interesting hypothesis that selective fertilization occurs, whereby $g_1$ sperm unite preferentially with $g_2$ eggs, and $g_2$ sperm with $g_1$ eggs. As they point out, these results, if confirmed, would constitute the first direct evidence for the postulated immunological nature of the membrane surface phenomena of fertilization.

In an analysis of the Ag-B histocompatibility locus genotypes of the $F_2$ progeny of DA (Ag-$B^4$) and Lewis (Ag-$B^1$) rats Palm (1967) has also observed a powerful selective effect in favor of the heterozygotes though she has not yet determined when the presumed selective elimination occurs.

What appears to be a similar kind of heterosis occurs in chickens with respect to the B blood group and histocompatibility system, certain blood group genotypes being inferior and certain superior with respect to the overall mortality of the embryos. (Morton et al., 1965)

There are therefore grounds for belief that the exceedingly finegrained polymorphism provided by the multiplicity of alleleic series of histocompatibility genes may be biologically significant before implantation as well as after this event. This is not surprising in view of the fact that histocompatibility genes are present in non-vivparous vertebrates.

## ACKNOWLEDGEMENTS

I am indebted to my colleagues, Drs. Susan Heyner and J. Wayne Streilein for helpful criticism and advice.

The expenses of some of the work described were defrayed in part by U.S.P.H.S. Grant CA-07001.

## REFERENCES

1. Bach, F. H. and Amos, D. B. (1967) Hu-1 major histocompatibility locus in man. Science, 156: 1506.

2. Banfield, W. G., Woke, P. A., and MacHay, C. M. (1966) Mosquito transmission of lymphomas. Cancer, 19: 1333-1336.

3. Bardawil, W. A. and Toy, B. L. (1959) The natural history of choriocarcinoma: problems of immunity and spontaneous regression. Ann. N. Y. Acad. Sci., 80: 197-261.

4. Barker, C. F. and Billingham, R. E. (1967) The role of regional lymphatics in the skin homograft response. Transplantation, 5: 963-970.

5. Barnes, A. D. (1964) A quantitative comparison of immunizing ability of different tissues. Ann. N. Y. Acad. Sci., 120: 237-250.

6. Barth, R. F. and Russell, P. S. (1964) The antigenic specificity of spermatozoa. J. Immunol., 93: 13-19.

7. Benacerraf, B. (1968) Cell-associated immune reactions. Cancer Res., 28: 1392-1398.

8. Billingham, R. E. (1964) Transplantation immunity and the maternal-fetal relation. New Engl. J. Med., 270: 667-672, 720-725.

9. Billingham, R. E. (1968) The biology of graft-versus-host reactions. In "The Harvey Lectures, 1966-1967." Academic Press, New York.

10. Billingham, R.E. and Silvers, W.K. (1962) Studies on cheek pouch skin homografts in the Syrian hamster. pp. 90-108 In Ciba Foundation Symposium on Transplantation (G. E. W. Wolstenholme and M. P. Cameron, eds.) Churchill: London, 1962.

11. Billingham, R.E. and Silvers, W.K. (1965) Immunological aspects of tissue transplantation. pp. 172-187 In Immunological Diseases. (Max Samter, editor) Little, Brown, & Co., Boston.

12. Billingham, R. E. and Streilein, J. W. (1968) The roles of lymphocytes in homograft rejection Proc. VIth Int. Congr. Allergology, in press.

13. Billington, W. D. (1964) Influence of immunological dissimilarity of mother and foetus on size of placenta in mice. Nature, 202: 317.

14. Billington, W. D. (1965) The invasiveness of transplanted mouse trophoblast and the influence of immunological factors. J. Reprod. Fertil., 10: 343-352.

15. Bradbury, S., Billington, W. D., and Kirby, D. R. S. (1965) A histochemical and electronmicroscopical study of the fibrinoid of the mouse placenta. J. Roy. Microscop. Soc., 84: 199-211.

16. Brent, L. and Medawar, P. B. (1967) Cellular immunity and the homograft reaction. Brit. Med. Bull., 23: 55-60.

17. Clarke, B. and Kirby, D. R. S. (1966) Maintenance of histocompatibility polymorphisms. Nature, 211: 999-1000.

18. Craigmyle, M. B. L. (1960) A study of cartilage homografts in rabbits sensitized by a skin homograft from the cartilage donor. Transpl. Bull., 26: 150-152.

19. Currie, G. A. and Bagshae, K. D. (1967) The masking of antigens on trophoblast and cancer cells. Lancet, i: 708-710.

20. Fikrig, S. M., Valenti, C., and Kehaty, T. (1967) Masking of antigens on trophoblast. Lancet, 1: 1055.

21. Gowans, J. L. (1965) The role of lymphocytes in the destruction of homografts. Brit. Med. Bull., 21: 106-110.

22. Hull, P. (1964) Partial incompatibility not affecting total litter size in the mouse. Genetics, 50: 563-570.

23. James, D. A. (1965) Effects of antigenic dissimilarity between mother and foetus on placental size in mice. Nature, 205: 613-614.

24. Katsh, G. F., Talmage, D. W., and Katsh, S. (1964)

Acceptance or rejection of male skins by isologous female mice; effect of injection of sperm. Science, 143: 41-42.

25. Kirby, D. R. S. (1963) Development of mouse blastocyst transplanted to spleen. J. Reprod. Fertil., 5: 1-12.

26. Kirby, D. R. S., Billington, W. D., Bradbury, S., and Goldstein, D. J. (1964) Antigen barrier of the mouse placenta. Nature, 204: 548-549.

27. Kirby, D. R. S., Billington, W. D., and James D. A. (1966) Transplantation of eggs to the kidney and uterus of immunized mice. Transplantation, 4: 713-718.

28. Lanman, J. T., Dinerstein, J., and Fikrig, S. (1962) Homograft immunity in pregnancy; lack of harm to fetus from sensitization of mother. Ann N. Y. Acad. Sci., 99: 706-716.

29. Lanman, J. T. (1965) Transplantation immunity in mammalian pregnancy; mechanisms of fetal protection against immunologic rejection. J. Pediatrics, 66: 525-540.

30. Medawar, P.B. (1953) Some immunological and endocrinological problems raised by evolution of viviparity in vertebrates. Symp. Soc. Exp. Biol. VII, Evolution, 320-338, Cambridge University Press.

31. Medawar, P. B. (1965) Transplantation of tissues

and organs: Introduction. Brit. Med. Bull., 21: 97-99.

32. Michie, D. and Anderson, N. F. (1966) A selective effect associated with a histocompatibility gene in the rat. Ann. N.Y. Acad. Sci., 129: 88-93.

33. Möller, G. and Möller, E. (1966) Interaction between allogeneic cells in tissue transplantation. Ann. N.Y. Acad. Sci., 129: 735-749.

34. Morton, J.R., Gilmour, D.G., McDermid, E.M., and Ogden, A. L. (1965) Association of blood-group and protein polymorphisms with embryonic mortality in the chicken. Genetics, 51: 97-107.

35. Moskalewski, S., Kawiak, J., and Rymaszewaka, T. (1966). Local cellular response evoked by cartilage formed after auto—and allogeneic transplantation of isolated chondrocytes. Transplantation, 4: 572-581.

36. Nathenson, S.G. and Davies, D. A. L. (1966) Solubilization and partial purification of mouse histocompatibility antigens from a membranous lipoprotein fraction. Proc. Nat. Acad. Sci., 56: 476-483.

37. Oettingne, Kj. V. and Witebsky, E. (1928) Plazenta and Blutgruppe. München med. Wschr., 75: 385-386.

38. Palm, J. (1967) Personal communication.

39. Poppa, G., Simmons, R. L., David, D. S., and

Russell, P. S. (1964) The uterus as a recipient site for parathyroid homotransplantation. Transplantation, 2: 496-502.

40. Russell, P. S. and Monaco, A. P (1964) The Biology of Tissue Transplantation pp. 1-207. Little, Brown, & Company, Boston.

41. Schild, H. O. and Willoughby, D. A. (1967) Possible pharmacological mediators of delayed hypersonsitivity. Brit. Med. Bull., 23: 46-51.

42. Schlesinger, M. (1962) Uterus of rodents as site for manifestation of transplantation immunity against transplantable tumors. J. Nat. Cancer Inst., 28: 927-945.

43. Schlesinger, M. (1964) Serologic studies on embryonic and trophoblastic tissues of the mouse. J. Immunol., 93: 255-263.

44. Schlesinger, M. and Koren, Z. (1966) Mouse trophoblast cells in tissue culture. Fertility and Sterility, 18: 95-101.

45. Simmons, R. L., Cruse, V., and McKay, D. G. (1967) The immunologic problem of pregnancy II. Ultrastructure of isogeneic and allogeneic trophoblastic transplants. Amer. J. Obst. & Gynec., 97: 218-230.

46. Simmons, R. L. and Russell, P. S. (1962) Antigenicity of mouse trophoblast. Ann. N. Y. Acad. Sci., 99: 717-732.

47. Simmons, R. L. and Russell, P. S. (1966) The histocompatibility antigens of fertilized mouse eggs and trophoblast. Ann. N. Y. Acad. Sci., 129: 35-45.

48. Snell, G.D. and Stimpfling, J.H. (1966) Genetics of Tissue Transplantation pp. 457-492 In Biology of the Laboratory Mouse, 2nd ed. (Earl L. Green, editor). McGraw-Hill: New York.

49. Spector, W. G. (1967) Histology of allergic inflammation. Brit. Med. Bull., 23: 35-38.

50. Stjernswärd, J. (1965) Studies in the transplantation of allogeneic cartilage across known histocompatibility barriers. Proc. 10th Congr. Int. Soc. Blood Transf., Stockholm, 1964: 197-202.

51. Strober, S. and Gowans, J. L. (1965) The role of lymphocytes in the sensitization of rats to renal homografts. J. Exp. Med., 122: 347-360.

52. Tai, C. and Halasz, N. A. (1967) Histocompatibility antigen transfer in utero: tolerance in progeny and sensitization in mother. Science, 158: 125-126.

53. Thiede, H. A., Choate, J. W., Gardner, H. H., and Santay, H. (1965) Immunofluorescent examination of the human chorionic villus for blood group A and B substance. J. Exp. Med., 121: 1039-1050.

54. Wilson, D. B. and Billingham, R. E. (1967) Lymphocytes and Transplantation Immunity, Advances in Immunology, 7: 189-273.

55. Witebsky, E. and Reich, H. (1932) Zur Gruppenspezifischen Differenzierung der Placentaorgane. Klin. Wschr., 11: 1960-1961.

56. Wynne, R. L. (1967) Comparative electron microscopy of the placental junction zone. Obstet. and Gynecol., 29: 644-661.

## DISCUSSION

B. L. Lobel: There is at least a superficial similarity between the sequence of events leading to homograft rejection and certain events which occur in the rat uterus during progestation. Following mating, there is extensive infiltration of the uterus by polymorphonuclear leucocytes and subsequently by mononuclear cells. This infiltration takes place over a period of four days. Shortly after the blastocyst descends into the uterus the endometrial stroma becomes hyperemic and edematous and foci of decidual tissue develop in proximity to the blastocysts. No infiltration of the decidual nodes by leucocytes occurs until vascularization takes place, when polymorphs and mononuclear cells infiltrate the decidual tissue also. Following administration of labelled thymidine on days $L_4$, $L_5$, $L_6$, $L_7$ or $L_8$ of pregnancy, labelled mononuclear cells were regularly observed in the endometrium and, at the later stages of development, in the blood vessels of the decidual tissue surrounding the implanted blastocysts. No labelled mononuclear cells were observed in the uterus following labelled thymidine administration during the estrous cycle or the preimplantation period of progestation [B. L. Lobel, E. Levy and M. C. Shelesnyak, Acta Endocr. (Kbh.) 56, Supp. 123, 1967 ].

Thus, there is here a parallel to the events discussed by Prof. Billingham: first, polymorphonuclear and then lymphocytic infiltration. The decidual tissue, before it becomes vascularized, appears to bar access of the infiltrating cells to the implanting blastocyst, in a fashion analogous to that of the mesenchymal barrier in the hamster check-pouch.

Vascularization develops in the decidual nodes only after trophoblastic differentiation and penetration has begun. Since the embryo is apparently antigenic [R. L. Simmons and P. S. Russell, Ann. N. Y. Acad. Sci., 99, 717, 1962] the differentiated trophoblastic tissue may prevent access of infiltrating cells to the embryo when vascularization of the decidual tissue has taken place. I would like to ask Prof. Billingham to comment on the similarities and implications in these observations.

R. E. Billingham: Although it's tempting to ascribe immunological significance to a local accumulation of lymphocytic cells, particularly the labelled cells you've observed: the possibility that these cells may have other functions—e.g. trophocytic- should not be dismissed. I believe that pathologists sometimes observe lymphocytes in association with spontaneous tumors where weak tumor specific antigens may or may not be involved. Products of cell damage or injury might incite the presence of lymphocytes. I suppose even here one could argue that normally sequestered intracellular material, having potentially autoantigenic properties, might be involved.

Apart from the species specific antigens which Dr. Katsh described this morning and the transplantation isoantigens I've been talking about, there may be placenta-specific antigens, possibly specifically associated with trophoblast cells. So far, the evidence in favor of the existence of the latter is not very convincing. It is, of course, not inconceivable that escape of transplantation antigens from the embryo across its trophoblastic investment is responsible for inciting the formation and/or the gathering of the cells you have observed. If this is the case, then a more striking cellular infiltration should be demonstrable if female rats of one strain are sensitized against the tissue antigens of males of a different strain and then mated.

B. L. Lobel: But if you think of these findings in the light of the work of Simmons and Russell, the separate implantation of different moieties of the blastocyst under the kidney capsule and the observation of dense mononuclear infiltration around the embryonic tissue and not around the trophoblastic moiety, then you might think that transplantation antigens are given off by the embryo, and their access to the circulation prevented by the trophoblasts, or alternatively perhaps some do get through, excite a response, and that trophoblasts prevent the cells which are called in from reaching and destroying the embryo. This is the interpretation that we would put on it.

R. E. Billingham: This seems a very reasonable idea. Of course we must bear in mind that if transplantation antigens do escape through the trophoblast and incite sensivitity in the host, then females which have been repeatedly pregnant by the same male should acquire a detectable level of immunity against grafts from that male. I think it's well established that multiple pregnancies do not sensitize females against their mate's transplantation antigens—indeed they may have exactly the opposite effect [See Billingham, R. E., Silvers, W. K., and Wilson, D. B. Proc. Roy. Soc. B, 163, 61, 1965].

It's important to realize that when homografts of different types of tissue, or cells, are implanted in different sites in the body there may be local variations in the details of the cellular interactions between the host and graft and the manner in which the host response develops. For example, it seems clear that the exemption from rejection of small grafts transplanted to vascular privileged sites turns upon the absence of a lymphatic drainage, whereas renal homografts can sensitize their hosts and undergo rejection in the complete absence of lymphatic connections with their host.

G. J. Marcus: If you give labelled thymidine to an animal, after a reasonable time one expects to find a certain fraction of the lymphocyte population labelled. Have you compared the proportion of lymphocytes which are labelled in the pregnant uterus with that in a non-pregnant uterus after similar treatment with thymidine?

B. L. Lobel: We did not find any labelled lymphocytes in the uteri of cycling rats or rats in early progestation. In the later stages of pregnancy, when we did observe labelled lymphocytes, we observed them only 12 or 24 hours after administration of the label, so they would not likely have been formed in bone marrow, since they would not have had time to mature.

G. J. Marcus: I would be very much surprised if you did not get some proportion of the lymphocytes labelled after 12 or 24 hours, albeit even a small proportion [cf. J. L. Gowans, J. Physiol. 146, 54, 1959]. Also, I believe the turnover of lymphocytes in bone marrow is relatively rapid, so that a rather significant proportion would be labelled by a single injection of thymidine. Incidentally, it is worth noting that lymphocytes were observed in association with decidual tissue over 60 years ago [K. J. Wederhake, loc. cit. E. C. Amoroso, in Marshall's Physiology of Reproduction, ed. A. S. Parkes, 3rd edition, vol. 2, Longmans, Green and Co., London, 1952, p. 157]. But my point is that if you have no evidence that the percentage of lymphocytes in the uterus which are labelled is different from what would be expected on an overall basis due to simply catching a number of lymphocytes as they are about to synthesize DNA, you cannot state that the labelling you have observed is significant in terms of lymphocyte stimulation or activation in relation to their immunological function. But even if there are a greater number of labelled lymphocytes, this still would not be proof for an immunological response in the uterus since there are non-specific, that is non-antigenic agents which induce lymphocyte transformations, e.g. proteolytic enzymes and microwave irradiation [D. Mazzei, C. Novi and C. Bazzi, Lancet, 2, 802, 1966; W. Stodolnik-Baranska, Nature, 214, 102, 1967]. Of course, the infiltration of even non-specifically sensitized lymphocytes would be consistent with a reaction of the delayed hypersensitivity type [cf. R. T. McCluskey, B. Benacerraf and J. W. McCluskey, J. Immunol. 90, 466, 1963] which we have proposed [M. C. Shelesnyak and G. J. Marcus, these proceedings].

B. L. Lobel: Unfortunately we have not attempted any quantitative studies of the lymphocyte labelling.

R. E. Billingham: To help interpret the significance of your observations it would be helpful to have information concerning the proportion of lymphocytic cells in peripheral blood which have taken up the label. This would indicate whether there had been a selective gathering or formation of labelled cells at the putative target site. I need hardly point out the need to know more about the lymphatic drainage of the uterus, its regional node system, and especially its response to homospecific and to heterospecific pregnancies.

H. R. Lindner: In the sheep the uterus is drained by the lumbar lymph nodes and collection of lumbar lymph is not a very difficult thing in a pregnant ewe [H. R. Lindner, M. B. Sass and B. Morris, J. Endocrin. 30, 361, 1964]. It's probably very difficult in a pregnant rat.

U. S. von Euler: Is it possible to determine the antigenic properties of the proteins present in the ovum or in the embryo and see whether they are retained over a longer time or whether they are lost? This may be very naive thinking but this is what one thinks about, whether the antigenic properties of the proteins are constant during the whole time.

R. E. Billingham: This is a very pertinent question. Presently available techniques for detecting the antigens responsible for graft rejection are probably inadequate to answer this question, though a fluorescent antibody procedure recently developed by Drs. David Lubaroff and Byron Waksman might be applicable [Science, 157, 322, 1967].

H. R. Lindner: Are you referring to embryonic antigens, not necessarily antigens present in the trophoblast?

R. E. Billingham: I was talking about transplantation antigens, but this would also apply to embryo-specific antigens.

H. R. Lindner: You did not commit yourself as to whether such antigens might be present in the trophoblastic cells as well.

R. E. Billingham: I don't think that effective transplantation antigens are associated with trophoblast cells. Of course this doesn't exclude the possibility that histocompatibility genes determine isoantigenic specificites on these cells—specificities that might confer serological reactivity upon them, but which, for one reason or another, are ineffective in eliciting cellular immunity. The model I have in mind is, of course, the erythrocyte in rodents. These express certain specificities determined by major histocompatibility loci in a serologically effective manner but they are incapable of eliciting the cellular form of immunity responsible for homograft rejection.

M. Tausk: While I listened to this truly brilliant lecture, I got a feeling that an attempt to graft reproduction physiologically on this body of immunology was being refuted and that this graft was being rejected. In other words, I got the impression that what you said was all militating against the probability that the deciduoma reaction could be a reaction of sensitization of the uterus.

R. E. Billingham: Right.

M. Tausk: This was said in the introduction by Prof. Shelesnyak, which I could quote literally since I have not only a brilliant memory, but also I have the manuscript in front of me, but I believe I have quoted it in a fair way. This morning already it was said that this could be one of the mechanisms, not necessarily the universal mechanism of implantation. Well, at any rate, I was left with the feeling that everything Prof. Billingham has said was pointing towards the very strange and phenomenon that the blastocyst does not behave as a graft which causes antibody and which would therefore cause a reaction as one sees in the skin when a graft is rejected, sensitization.

Now, when I listened to this discussion between Dr. Lobel and yourself, I got the impression that what you were trying to show and what you were trying to agree on was that this lymphocytic infiltration might be part of an immune reaction perhaps directed against certain tissue antigens, but when the deciduoma would shield the trophoblast against further lymphocytic or other antibody aggression. Now, I thought what we were trying to do was to explain somehow, not how the lymphocytes got there, but how the decidual cells got there, how the deciduoma was generated. I take it for granted that we are talking about the rat. Unless I am greatly mistaken, which I may well be, I don't quite see how these data can be used to bolster the hypothesis, admittedly a hypothesis, that the delayed hypersensitivity reaction may be one of the mechanisms by which implantation is brought about.

G. J. Marcus: I would like to make some comments which may, in part, resolve some of the apparent paradoxes. First of all, lymphocytic infiltration occurs, particularly in the subepithelial endometrium before the decidual response begins, before the blastocyst sheds its zone pellucida. Therefore, from the chronological aspect, a role for lymphocytes in stimulating the decidual response is feasible. Now if the leucocytes are "activated" or "sensitized", they could well respond to antigen released by the blastocyst when the zona is shed, this resulting in local histamine-release and decidual induction [cf. J. L. Turk, Transplantation, 5, 952, 1967]. But, where do we go from here? Decidualization takes place and the decidual tissue may, for a time, confer upon the uterus a degree of immunological tolerance and at the same time protect the blastocyst from immunological attack. This barrier or tolerance doesn't exist before the decidual tissue develops. There have been several reports of attempts to transplant tumors into the uterus. Such attempts have usually been unsuccessful unless decidualization was induced [I. B. Wilson, Proc. Zool. Soc. London. 141, 137, 1963; R. V. Short and K. Yoshinaga, J. Reprod. Fertil. 14, 287, 1967], the tumor growing within the decidual tissue.

Now, if we assume that the decidual tussue provides a degree of tolerance, perhaps until the decidua become well vascularized, then by this time the trophoblast has undergone differentiation and development and invades the decidua. Schlesinger has shown recently, that trophoblastic cells _in vitro_ will attack or phagocytose other cells only if they are coated with antibody [M. Schlesinger and Z. Koren, Fertil. Steril. **18**, 95, 1967]. Since the trophoblast becomes invasive _in vivo_ only when the decidua become vascularized it may well be that this action indicates the presence of immunologically competent or "activated" cells, which were present previously but have access to the trophoblast only after vascularization of the decidua [see also D. A. James, Nature, **205**, 613, 1965].

R. E. Billingham: Prof. Tausk has given us a very fair appraisal of the situation. Dr. Lobel has noted a cellular phenomenon associated with the early events of nidation which has some of the hallmarks of an immunologic interaction. If it is an immunological phenomenon the nature of the antigen(s) involved is still open to conjecture. The evidence doesn't exclude a very low grade reactivity against transplantation antigens. However, the possible level of reactivity involved appears to me to be so trivial that it's hard to believe that very effective amounts of histamine, or other pharmacologically active agents, are likely to be produced.

E. S. Kisch: If a tissue, which otherwise cannot be grafted into a host without punishment, be first grafted on a deciduoma, would the tissue acquire any invulnerability so that if it were then grafted elsewhere it might be accepted or tolerated?

R. E. Billingham: In situations in which homografts of skin and certain other tissues are grafted to privileged sites where they become vascularized yet fail to become rejected, the grafts don't lose their potential vulnerability. This is evidenced by their fate if removed and grafted elsewhere on the animal, or upon another animal of similar genetic constitution. Likewise, skin or other grafts on immunologically tolerant animals do not lose their susceptibility to immunity of passively (more correctly, adoptively) acquired origin. You may recall that the skin homografts which flourished for considerable periods in the skin flaps, which Barker and I have been studying in guinea pig skin, did not lose their vulnerability. If the epidermis and some of the underlying connective tissue was excised from the undersides of these flaps and they were then sutured back into freshly prepared beds in the host's trunk skin, they were invariably rejected. This was almost certainly the outcome of restoration of a lymphatic drainage between the host flap tissue and the recipient's body.

However, pertinent to your question is Woodruff's evidence that certain types of tissue, particularly endocrine tissue, once established, do become progressively less vulnerable to immunological attack. After a certain critical period they may be capable of surviving in the face of a degree of resistance they would not have been able to withstand at an earlier stage. This hypothesis implies that grafts may be able to undergo some kind of adaptation, possible as a result of the surreptitious replacement of their vascular endothelial and possibly other cells by those of host origin [See M. F. A. Woodruff, in Biological Problems of Grafting, eds. F. Albert and P. B. Medawar, Blackwell Scientific Publications, Oxford, England, 1959, pp. 83-90].

E. S. Kisch: Does the host become sensitized to the presence of the skin graft in the guinea pig flap system so that when the flaps are replaced in the host's trunk skin the graft is rejected more quickly than if it had been grafted directly?

R. E. Billingham: No, it does not, under those conditions.

M. C. Shelesnyak: Perhaps I may help Dr. Tausk with his dilemma or question. It must be realized that when we speak of nidation, we refer to a complex sequence of events. As we visualize the mechanism, the initial response, the response in which we invoke the antigenicity of the blastocyst, essentially triggers the induction of decidualization, to aid the stroma to decidualize, and then the role of the antigenic interaction is finished. The deciduum forms and it initially acts as a protective barrier. The trophoblast, meanwhile, has time to develop in its role of protector. Thus, there is no real paradox as long as you extend the time sequence and realize that one phase or one step does one job and the other does another. This would also aid in accounting for Dr. Billingham's concern that the number of lymphocytes which appear in the uterus before the decidual response is not adequate.

The lymphocytes may be adequate to support the stimulus from the lumen to induce decidualization and give time to the trophoblasts to develop in their major role as the protectors.

S. Lamprecht: In relation to the barrier between the foetus and the maternal tissues, the theory of a fibrinoid layer around the trophoblast is very interesting. Kirby and his associates [D. R. S. Kirby, W. D. Billinton, S. Bradbury and D. J. Goldstein, Nature, 204, 548, 1964] have suggested that the chemical nature of the fibrinoid material is very similar to that of the slimy substance in the hamster's check pouch. However, Simmons [R. L. Simmons, V. Cruse, and D. G. McKay, Am. J. Obs. Gyn. 97, 213, 1967] recently presented very strong evidence against the existence of the fibrinoid layer. Would Dr. Billingham comment on this?

R. E. Billingham: I'm glad that Mr. Lamprecht has brought up the fact that Dr. Simmons and his associates have recently reported their investigations on the fate of genetically compatible and genetically incompatible fertilized eggs implanted beneath the renal capsules of mice. Unlike Dr. Kirby and his associates at Oxford, they failed to see any difference in the extent of infiltration of the host renal tissue by the trophoblast giant cells developing from the two types of implant. Furthermore, with the aid of the electron microscope, they were unable to find any fibrinoid or sialomucin material investing the trophoblast cells in either situation. The disparate results obtained by these two groups of investigators may be ascribable to differences of techniques for example, to fixation and processing of tissue. Exchange of information between these workers will probably resolve this problem. What is important is that, if it can be shown consistently that alien trophoblast cells can flourish in ectopic sites in normal or sensitized hosts, and that viable choriocarcinoma cells are present in the absence of a potentially protective layer of fibrinoid material in women with this tumor, the case for believing that trophoblast cells fail to express, or do not possess effective transplantation antigens will be greatly strengthened.

S. Tachi: We have been studying early implantation in the rat with the electron microscope and have made some observations which are relevant to the question of a trophoblastic barrier between the embryo and the uterus. By midnight between days $L_4$ and $L_5$ of pregnancy the trophoblast is thinly spread, measuring about one-third of a micron in thickness at some points [Fig. 1]. Arrays of fibrous material (plaques) characteristic of the developing blastocyst in the rat [A. C. Enders and S. J. Schlafke, in Preimplantation Stages of Pregnancy, Wolstenholme, G. E. W. and M. O'Connor, eds., CIBA Found. Symposium, 1965, p. 29] are still present. On the side facing the blastocyst cavity, the cell membrane of the trophoblast is clearly defined and as yet has no discernible coating.

By noon on day $L_5$, however, some amorphous

material appears on the inner side of the trophoblast [Fig. 2]. At this stage the trophoblast still contains fibrous plaques, and invasion of the uterus has not yet taken place.

Twenty-four hours later, the trophoblast has penetrated between the cells of the uterine epithelium and its basement membrane [Fig. 3]. Degenerating, engulfed epithelial cells are seen within trophoblastic cells [Fig. 4]. However, the feature I would like to call your attention to is the appearance of dense material forming a basement-membrane-like lining on the surface of the trophoblast facing the blastocyst cavity. The basement-membrane underlying the uterine epithelium is still intact so that the trophoblast appears to lie in a sandwich between two basement-membrane-like structures. These structures may be of significance as an immunological barrier during the early stages of embryonic growth. I would like to have Prof. Billingham's comments.

R. E. Billingham: Your observations and tentative interpretation of their possible immunological significance are very interesting. There are various observations which suggest that the mammalian epidermis, or its adnexae, may contain some tissue specific ingredient(s) which are normally quarrantined or sequestered from the host by virtue of its avascular nature and by the presence of a thin underlying basement membrane which may have important physiological and immunological properties. Our observation, that if homologous melanocytes are experimentally incorporated into the epidermis of white skin areas

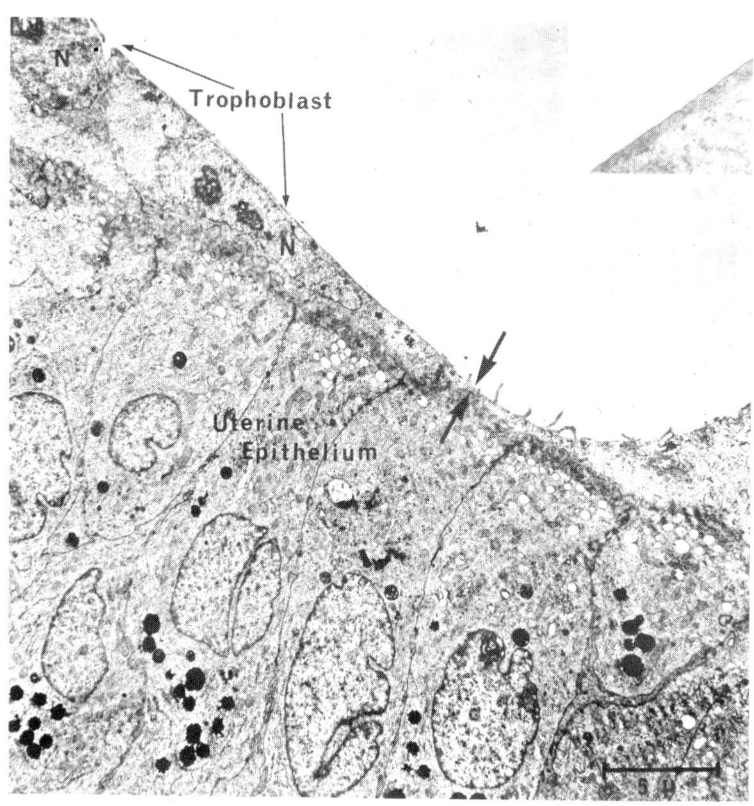


Fig. 1. An implanting blastocyst on day L4 midnight. The trophoblast surface facing the blastocyst-cavity remains clear (see inset). Thick arrows indicate the area of trophoblast spread thin. N; nucleus. Scale shows 5μ. Inset is x 5. 3 from the original figure.

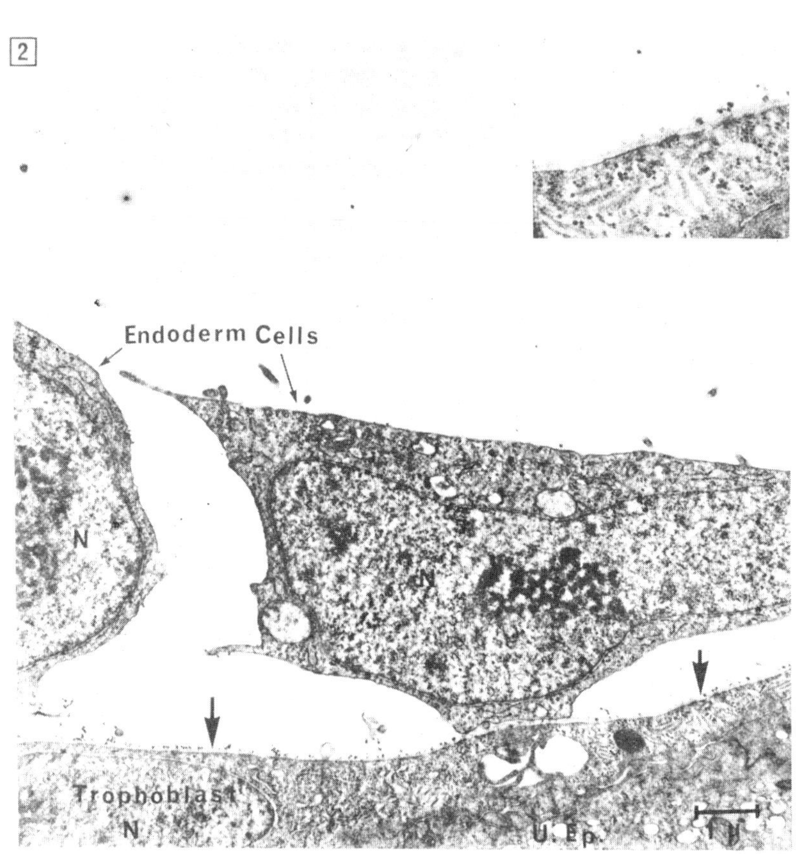


Fig. 2. Day L5 noon of pregnancy. Note the lining of the amorphous material on the trophoblast surface. N; nucleus. U. Ep.; uterine epithelium. The scale shows $1\mu$. Inset is x 2. 5 from the original figure.

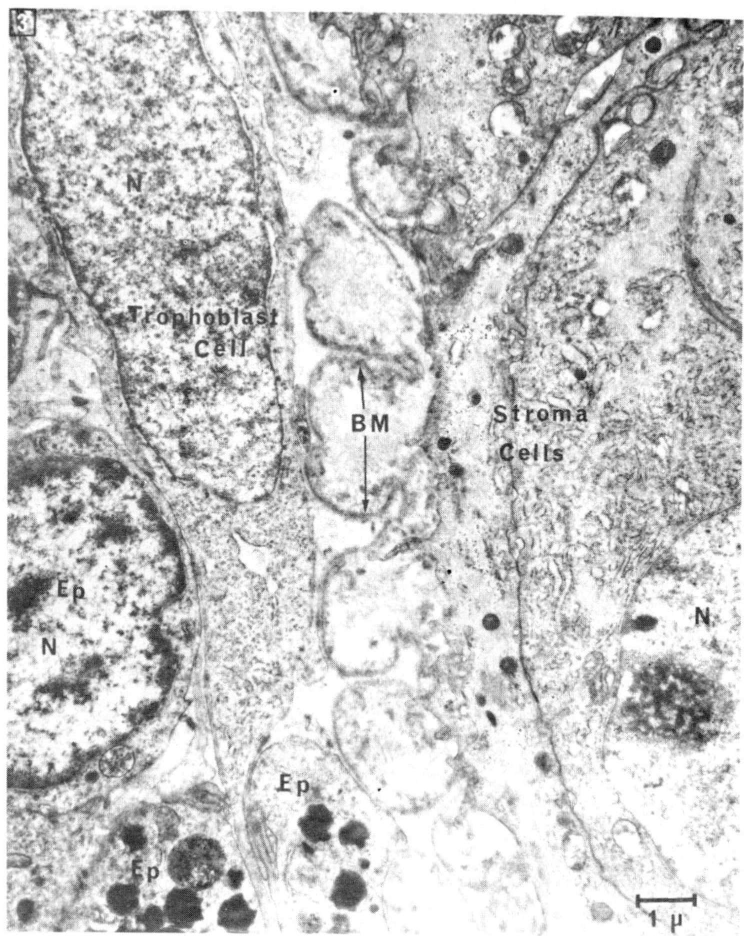


Fig. 3. Day L6 noon of pregnancy. The trophoblast penetrates between uterin epithelial cells ( Ep ) and basement membrane ( BM ). N; nucleus. The scale indicates $1\mu$.

4

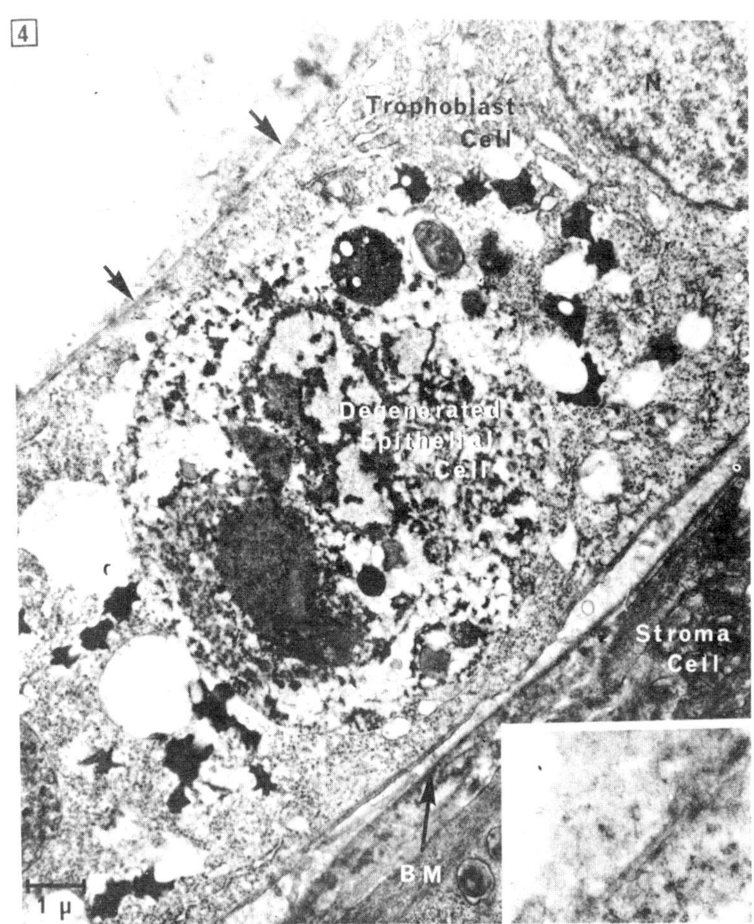


Fig. 4. The same stage as shown Fig. 3. Degenerating epithelial cell is seen within a trophoblast cell. Note the dense membranous deposit on the trophoblast cell surface. The scale shows 1$\mu$. The inset is enlarged from the original by x2. 5.

of spotted guinea pigs, they may survive for very considerable periods of time, is pertinent. Here we have an example of immunogenetically foreign cells being able to proliferate and migrate for prolonged periods in the host's epidermis without eliciting sensitization on the part of the host. However, they do undergo prompt rejection if the latter is sensitized experimentally-for example, by grafting it with skin from the donor of the grafted pigment cells [See Billingham, R. E. and W. K. Silvers, pp. 1-24 in "Biology of Skin and Hair Growth", edited by A. G. Lyne and B. F. Short. Angus and Robertson, Sydney, 1965].

In considering the possible significance of basement membranes of various kinds as immunological barriers, it is clearly important to find out whether lymphocytes are able to traverse them.

G. J. Marcus: Potts has recently published evidence that at least in the mouse, fusion between trophoblastic and maternal cells occurs over limited regions and that "tight junctions" or desomosomes link the trophoblastic and maternal cells in other regions [Am. J. Obstet. Gynec. 96, 1122, 1966]. Do Mrs. Tachi's observations provide evidence for such intimacy of contact in the rat?

S. Tachi: It is very difficult to state decisively whether fusion takes place between the cells. Pott's fixation method is different from mine. Potts fixed the tissues in osmium tetroxoid and embedded in celloidin to obtain thick sections from which he could pick out suitable specimens for electron microscopy. I fixed the tissues by perfusion with glutaraldehyde via the abdominal vein and then post-fixed in osmium tetroxide and embedded in Araldite. This is the procedure used by Reinius and by Enders and Schlafke. But even when the fixation is good, cell boundaries or membranes, if cut tangentially, would be very difficult to define.

C. Tachi: Do you suggest that differences in fixation procedures could account for the apparent disappearance of the membranes?

S. Tachi: It's a possibility, although I believe direct osmium-fixation would preserve the membranes adequately.

G. J. Marcus: But you believe that the fusion does not occur?

S. Tachi: I don't find evidence for fusion in my pictures nor have Enders and Schlafke mentioned fusion in their publications. I feel that in order to conclude that there is fusion, one must have evidence of transfer or exchange of material which could not ordinarily pass through membranes.

H. R. Lindner: Rightly or wrongly, the mind strives for simplicity. It is an intellectually unsatisfying situation, if one has to postulate two different rejection systems for monodisperse cells and for agglomerated cells or solid masses, as you described in your paper. Would you care to speculate on what the so-called non-specific lytic substance supposedly released by activated lymphocytes in contact with the graft might be? And to make the question relevant to Prof. Shelesnyak's paper, might histamine be involved, as has been suggested.

R. E. Billingham: Transplantation immunity is not unique in presenting both a humoral and a cellular candidate for consideration as immunologic effectors. A similar situation occurs in the case of delayed hypersensitivity to micro-organisms, such as the tubercle bacillus, and to simple chemicals, as well as in the case of the experimental autoimmune diseases.

So far as homografts are concerned, dissociated cells expose more of their surfaces, and consequently more antibody-combining sites, to facilitate the occurrence of complement-dependent cytotoxic reactions, than cells in intact tissues. Moreover, in the case of monodisperse cells both _in vivo_ and _in vitro_ there is evidence of variability in the susceptibility of cells of different histological types to humoral antibodies, lymphoid cells being peculiarly susceptible. However, even such robust cells as epidermal cells can be killed by cytotoxic antibodies in the presence of added complement.

_In vitro_ experiments have shown very clearly that lymphocytes from specifically sensitized animals can attack and destroy homologous target cells, as a consequence of some kind of intimate process involving contactual agglutination [See D. B. Wilson and R. E. Billingham, 1967, _Adv. in Immunology_ _7_ : 189-273]. This process probably contributes to the destruction of solid tissue homografts. However, in the light of increasing evidence that the majority of the cells constituting the mononuclear infiltrate associated with the destruction of solid tissue homografts are not specifically sensitized cells, one can no longer sustain the hypothesis that sensitized cells <u>per se</u> are the only direct mediators of the destructive process. In some way or another these cells may be able to coerce unsensitized cells, including macrophages, to release injurious immunologically non-specific but pharmacologically active agents which are believed to be principally responsible for graft destruction. Several candidates for this role are currently under study, [See R. E. Billingham and J. W. Streilein in Proceedings of the VIth International Congress of Allergology, 1968, in press].

S. Katsh: I suppose I should add a little bit. In culture, too, and we don't really claim to be culturing particular cells, one can take the testicular growth, new growth although it has passed through several serial transfers, and take humoral antibody, say from an heterologous or even an autologous source, and in culture show that it does have a cytotoxic effect. Incidentally, this is in the presence of complement, it's not effective without complement. I'm claiming, however, that this happens <u>in vitro</u>, that's why I didn't stick my neck out, because we don't really know whether the cell-fixed antibody, let's say that which may be present in the lymphocytes or plasma cell, might in proximity or perhaps even in contact cause the release of some x-factor which we still have an open mind about, which would, in turn, cause destruction of those cells.

H. R. Lindner: Do you feel that there is no evidence so far that histamine is involved in homograft rejection?

R. E. Billingham: The failure of all of the many attempts to prolong the lives of skin homografts by treatment of their hosts with a variety of antihistamines makes me disinclined to believe that this agent plays any significant role in graft destruction. Of course, as Dr. Schayer had previously stated, the failure of antihistamines to abbrogate a particular reaction might be due to their inability to get to the right place in appropriate concentrations.

H. R. Lindner: If you regraft an animal that has been sensitized by a previous graft, what is the time lapse before mononuclear infiltration can be demonstrated in the new graft?

R. E. Billingham: Second-set homografts are destroyed very rapidly, usually within about 6 days on highly sensitized hosts. Unlike first-set grafts, they never get a very rich blood supply and the feeble blood flow that does become established shuts down very rapidly. Thus, there isn't much opportunity for blood borne mononuclear cells to infiltrate such grafts. There is, however, an intense cellular infiltration of the graft bed, suggesting that the brunt of the immunological attack is centered here. Cellular infiltration is slight in the case of second renal homografts too.

S. Lamprecht: If I remember well, you said there are very few instances in which a tissue has no transplantation antigens. I would like to ask what is the situation of transplantation antigens in tumors. I ask this because, after all, the trophoblast is really an invasive, growing foreign body.

R. E. Billingham: Practically all tumors express all the transplantation antigens corresponding to the histocompatibility genes of the animal in which they arose. Some tumors possess, in addition, weak tumor-specific antigens. Moreover, there's no evidence of a qualitative deficiency in the antigen content of tumors. It's just worth mentioning that a very few murine tumors, with a very long history of propagation by transplantation behind them and which will grow in mice of practically any genetic constitution, have either lost certain important transplantation antigens or express them in a very feeble manner. From our point of view, it's fair to generalize that tumors are just as effective in provoking transplantation immunity and just as susceptible to it as non-malignant cells.

E. S. Kisch: I am not very happy with the comparison between the delayed hypersensitivity type of reaction that is postulated for nidation and the delayed sensitivity in homograft rejection, particularly from consideration of the timing. If one examines the timing carefully, the interval between copulation and attachment of the blastocyst is only five days. Isn't that a rather short interval for a delayed hypersensitivity reaction?

R. E. Billingham: The speed with which a host can develop an effective state of transplantation immunity to antigens of other types, is dependent upon three variables: the degree of "foreignness" of the antigen, or its immunogenicity; its dosage, and the route of its administration. As evidenced by the results of skin tests, guinea pigs can develop an effective level of transplantation immunity within 2-3 days of the intraperitoneal injection of homologous spleen cells. Sensitivity to orthotopic skin grafts takes longer to develop. Mice develop a detectable level of transplantation immunity following the parenteral inoculation of as few as 10,000 cells when major histocompatibility differences are involved.

Thus, in the light of these considerations, blastocysts would appear to be an extremely ineffective antigenic stimulus from the viewpoint of antigen dosage.

G. J. Marcus: But the blastocyst in our hypothesis is not the primary antigenic stimulus. A seminal component could provoke the sensitization.

M. Tausk: The supposition was that the animal is sensitized by the semen following coitus and not by the fertilized ovum. The blastocyst would only sometime later elicit the delayed reaction, after there had already been sensitization. This is in agreement with what Prof. Billingham said, because the blastocyst is not the sensitizing agent, but the semen is, and then you have large quantities available.

S. Lamprecht: Could a delayed hypersensitivity-like reaction occur in isogenic pregnancy?

R. E. Billingham: This is a most important question from the viewpoint of interpretation of Dr. Lobel's observations. In all pregnancies in which the mother and the father are genetically similar—i. e. members of the same inbred strain—the conceptuses possess no transplantation isoantigens against which the mother can become sensitized. Consequently, if Dr. Lobel's observations were made with inbred rats, we can exclude the possibility that the mononuclear cells infiltrate she observed had anything to do with transplantation immunity.

B. L. Lobel: Our observations were initially incidental to some of our studies of implantation. The rats, however, although originally of Wistar stock are definitely outbred.

P. F. Kraicer: And skin grafts between animals in our colony do not take. We have tried this several times.

H. R. Lindner: This is a point I had intended raising. If histocompatibility antigens were important and if an immune mechanisms were important in implantation, then you should at least have reduced fertility between mates which were tolerant for genetic reasons or because of an induced tolerance.

R. E. Billingham: If is a well-established fact that outbred mice tend to have larger litters than mice of inbred strains. I've never tried to mate mice of two different inbred strains which had previously been rendered tolerant of each other's tissue transplantation antigens, as a consequence of neonatal injection with homologous cells. However, I would be most surprised if they failed to produce offspring.

G. J. Marcus: Dr. Billingham pointed out earlier that even in highly inbred strains of mice, the H-2 antigen persists so that a certain degree of histoincompatibility remains. But, even so, need the postulated antigenic stimulus in nidation be of the histocompatibility type? Also we must not overlook the fact that normal mating requires the participation of a male and a female; there cannot be an absolute identity of genetic heritage in individuls of different sexes. In fact, Kirby has recently suggested that since male zygotes, by virtue of their Y-linked antigens, are always more dissimilar than female zygotes from their mother, an immunological influence favoring implantation of the male zygote might be a contributory determinant of the sex ratio

[D. R. S. Kirby, K. G. McWhirter, M. S. Teitelbaum and C. D. Darlington, Lancet, 2, 139, 1967].

One more question: Is there any evidence of the chemical similarity, between the slime of the hamster cheek pouch connective tissue and the fibrinoid material that Kirby has discussed?

R. E. Billingham: Kirby, in several of his papers, cites unpublished work that there is a similarity, but has not presented any of the evidence. I believe it's of a histochemical nature, but I think this is something he will produce.

S. Lamprecht: There is quite a difference between the systems because the cheek pouch of the hamster is sensitized by proxy.

R. E. Billingham: Right. Dr. Kirby and other workers have drawn an analogy between the immunologically privileged status of the hamsters cheek pouch, and that of the mammalian conceptus or embryo. However, even if the layer of slimy areolar connective tissue which seems to be responsible for the immunological peculiarity of the cheek pouch is similar, with respect to its biochemical constitution, to the fibrinoid material which, according to Kirby, invests and confers immunological protection upon trophoblast cells, the analogy applies only to unsensitized hosts. Pouch skin homografts are promptly rejected by sensitized animals, and pouch skin homografts hitherto accepted by normal animals are rejected if their hosts are sensitized by means of homografts of ordinary skin. The mammalian embryo in *utero*, however, is completely resistant to a state of sensitivity specifically directed against its antigens.

E. Nuriel: What is the nature of the reaction of a homograft against the host?

R. E. Billingham: If you take perinatal mice or rats of one inbred strain and innoculate them with suspensions of living cells derived from the lymphohaemopoietic tissues of adult donors from an unrelated strain, a peculiar wasting disease, often referred to as "runt" disease, may intervene. In rodents this disease may vary greatly in its time of onset and severity. Its onset is usually marked by the abrupt cessation of growth, often accompanied by diarrhoea and the appearance of cutaneous abnormalities. In the acute form these symptons usually occur within a week or so after innoculation, and the victims may die shortly thereafter. Milder, chronic forms of the disease can occur, with complete recovery after weeks or months. This disease can be caused in a wide variety of species, including rabbits, hamsters, chickens, and primates. An essentially similar syndrome may also develop in adult hosts subjected to procedures that abbrogate their ability to reject tissue or cellular homografts, and innoculated with immunologically competent cells from unrelated donors. There is overwhelming evidence that this syndrome, variously known as runt disease, homologous disease, transplantation disease, etc., according to the situation in which it occurs, is caused by the reaction of the innoculated mature immunologically competent cells against the foreign transplantation antigens confronting them in their new host—i.e., it is a graft-versus-host reaction. A necessary condition for the occurrence of graft-versus-host reactions is that the host must be incapable of reacting against and rejecting the innoculated putative "attacking" cells. The peculiar susceptibility of perinatal rodents turns upon the functional immaturity of their immunological response system.

Apart from systemic manifestations of graft-versus-host reactions, local, self-limiting graft-versus-host reactions develop following the innoculation of immunologically competent cells into the skin or beneath the renal capsules of appropriate, genetically alien hosts. Small lymphocytes from the blood or from the thoracic duct are highly effective in causing graft-versus-host reactions. On the basis of these various findings, several authorities have drawn attention to the potentially harmful immunological consequences of lymphocytes of maternal origin gaining access to the blood stream of the foetus. Indeed, there are now a few cases on record of babies who appear to have developed runt disease as a consequence of some kind of traumatic accident in utero which allowed them to become "innoculated" with an effective "dosage" of maternal immunologically competent cells.

A few babies transfused in utero with packed human blood cells as a therapeutic procedure in cases of Rh sensitization have developed the disease. Cytological studies have indicated the chimeric status of the lymphocytic populations of some of the affected infants. [For a full discussion of this subject, see Simonsen, M. (1962) Progress in Allergy 6 : 349-367; Billingham, R. E. in the Harvey Lectures, 1966/1967, Academic Press, New York, 1968].

I did not refer to graft-versus-host reactions, and runt disease, in my lecture since the events we have been considering in this conference obviously take place too early in ontogeny for graft-versus-host reactivity to be possible.

P. F. Kraicer: Am I correct in assuming that the proposed explanations of survival of foetus in uteru fall into two classes: either there is no antigenicity, or there is, and dispite this, there is a barrier.

R. E. Billingham: Right.

P. F. Kraicer: It strikes me, considering my own data, that I really don't understand. In the experiments that I described earlier, we observed, after certain treatments, much resorption of foetal material during about a week and a half of pregnancy. Embryo after embryo died and was resorbed; yet, a few survived in these uteri. Isn't that a little incredible?

R. E. Billingham: With what agent did you treat your animals?

P. F. Kraicer: Progesterone.

R. E. Billingham: It's possible that treatment of pregnant animals with certain drugs might compromise the postulated quarantining barriers of their embryos, so that with outbred populations and depending upon chance genetic segregation, some conceptuses might be "rejected" as homografts.

J. W. Everett: Wouldn't you get it even in an inbred strain?

R. E. Billingham: No, because in an inbred strain the foetuses cannot confront their mothers with any foreign transplantation antigens.

## NOTE

Probably the most direct evidence, to date, of an immunological factor operating in ovum implantation has been provided by the demonstration of inhibition of implantation in mice by post-coital administration of antithymocyte serum; the unimplanted blastocysts proved viable upon transfer and the failure of implantation was attributed to interference with the mechanism whereby the blastocyst initiates the decidual response since deciduomata could be provoked in one horn while blastocysts failed to implant in the other [D. R. S. Kirby, Nature, 216, 1229, 1967].

# CONCLUDING COMMENTS

# CONCLUDING COMMENTS

M. Tausk

It's comforting but also a little bit disquieting that there will be no discussion after this summary. This is a comfort because you won't be able to tear me to pieces here. On the other hand, it gives me a little uneasy feeling because if I should have misrepresented something, then people will go away from here bearing me a grudge and it won't be discussed. [However, this is, I believe, sufficient for an introduction].

I would like to begin my summary by stating that this has been a unique opportunity, an opportunity created by our chairman, not just now, nor when he conceived the idea of this workshop, but when he started his investigations, because he brought together a number of people whose work was focussed on one most important subject which is foremost in his mind. It has activated a number of investigations, here and elsewhere, and without trying to give a disproportionate view, I would venture to compare this in one respect with the effects of all the investigations undertaken with a view to space travel. Don't misunderstand me, I am not trying to equate the importance of what is being done here with the importance of all the work that is directed towards space travel. The _tertrium comparationis_ is this, that space travel has stimulated so much work on technology and electronics and telemetry, that it will have amply rewarded all the people who worked on it, even if man should never arrive at the moon. And now, si licet parva componere magnis, if you will permit me to compare things of unequal size, I will say: even if this group never achieves a full elucidation of what implantation is, so much work has been undertaken, so many people have been brought together, so many lines of investigation have been stimulated, that this certainly will always be a most rewarding accomplishment to look back on.

As you will remember, Professor Shelesnyak in his introductory paper outlined the main thoughts that have been guiding and directing his work. You will remember that the following features of nidation were most conspicuous and prominent in his expose. Number one, there is a very conspicuous factor of timing. To make this clear he wrote it out on the blackboard so that we would be continuously reminded of the timing that is essential in all the processes involved in nidation, and this presupposes the existence of some physiological clock, some central mechanism. He then arrived at the conclusion that nidation could be approached by studying a model, the deciduoma in the pseudopregnant rat. This, among other things, led him to the conclusion that some stimulus, some irritant, is needed to provoke this deciduoma. Now he said something in his paper which I would like to quote verbatim because I will come back to it in a few minutes. Having spoken about the irritant which causes a deciduoma, he says "the proposal of a non-specific stimulus for so specific a phenomenon as decidualization was rejected by us and a metabolic mediator was sought." Then he says, "Histamine early became a candidate". Here you can already see that things may take another turn than the originators of such an investigation may have thought. Presently when I briefly review what Dr.Schayer has said here, it will be shown that histamine, of all substances, is one of the least specific ones, and I think Dr.Schayer takes a certain pride in showing the universality of its effects. So it might be questioned whether the choice of histamine really was an answer to the problem as I just quoted it. But these things, of course, happen every day and only recently I got a reprint from a German pharmacologist with a title somewhat like "Right conclusions from wrong premises" or something like that. (Successful Errors and Other Odd Ways to New Discoveries, F. Lembeck, Medical History, 11, 157-164, 1967). Many times in the history of science it has happened that somebody starts from a certain premise, or belief in facts which turns out not to hold water when pursued. That really doesn't matter. One of the things you see is that an enormous amount of work has been done on histamine and we have an expert here who told us more about it.

The next thing that came to the fore was the famous estrogen surge; it was assumed that at the critical time there is an increased production of estrogen The increased production of estrogen was originally believed to cause the histamine-release, but our chairman has always been very critical towards his own ideas, and his paper bears out that he spared no trouble in attacking his own concepts when it looked as if they were no longer tenable. So it was shown that histamine and the estrogen surge were apparently not strictly related to each other in a cause and effect relationship, but that they were both required for the formation of a deciduoma as a model of implantation, and hence probably for implantation.

Now the estrogen surge has become a cornerstone in this concept and it is perhaps desirable to see briefly what the evidence for it is. First of all, when he starts talking about the estrogen surge the author says that perusal of the literature revealed that follicular activity reportedly occurred in the ovaries of the pregnant rat just prior to the time of maximal uterine sensitivity, that is on days L3 and L4. Then there is evidence such as the fact that the administration of an anti-estrogen, compound MER-25, or hypophysectomy just prior to that critical time would prevent decidualization, but afterwards would not. Furthermore, the concept was supported by changes in uterine vascularity, infiltration by eosinophilic granulocytes, increased DNA, etc.

Now the author quotes Clara Szego who proposed that histamine was an obligatory response of the uterus to estrogen and a mediator of estrogen action. Well, this sounds very plausible. We have heard, again from Dr. Schayer, that histamine is a substance which opens up the capillaries and so will produce hyperemia. Hyperemia is one of the effects of estrogen injection. On the other hand, it could not be foreseen or expected that histamine would in itself be a specific stimulator which would cause decidualization. That remained to be shown.

Now, as I have said, Dr. Shelesnyak himself has adduced objections to his own theories, such as for instance the fact that decidualization would occur if one gives an animal histamine parentally, without any local trauma, but it would not occur spontaneously when the animal was supposed to have a high endogenous stock of histamine. An anti-estrogen which would prevent decidualization would not necessarily antagonize histamine release. On the other hand, an antihistamine which does not prevent all the estrogen effects of the estrogen surge, might prevent decidualization, and so forth.

Well, the conclusion of all this was, as I said before, that apparently estrogen and histamine are both needed for decidualization. The sequence of events visualized would then be, that this estrogen surge would increase the mass of the uterus, and the number of binding sites, at least the quantity of compounds which could bind histamine, and thereby, by some still obscure mechanism, produce this highly interesting phenomenon, the deciduoma.

Certain features of implantation such as the behavior of a number of blood elements, lymphocytes and other leucocytic elements, etc. reminded the group of certain features of allergic reactions, and so the concept crept in that inflammation and particularly a local, delayed hypersensitive reaction may also be part of the picture.

So what does one do under such circumstances? One convenes a workshop conference, and one asks for one man who knows everything about histamine, another man who knows all about estrogen and how it is bound, and then another man who is supposed to know all about the time clock in the central nervous system and who should tell us how the central nervous system regulates hormone activities. Then what about immunology? Well, two men at least are needed for such a big field. And then, if we have hyperemia this can be brought about by an excess of substances which cause dilation of the small vessels but it may also be caused by a decrease in the quantity of substances which caused contraction, since in particular it has been shown here that there is a fall in the level of these contracting substances, the catecholamines. There is one great authority in Europe, perhaps in the world, who knows everything about catecholamines, so he was invited to enlighten us on that subject. And so the workshop started.

Dr. Schayer gave us a most comprehensive story about histamine. What he showed was the histamine opens up capillaries wherever more blood is needed. In this way it can really achieve a great deal. This story doesn't tell us specifically why under certain circumstances these capillaries will open, but Dr. Schayer has given us a great deal of highly interesting information about the production of histamine which is of course produced by splitting off a carboxyl group from its precursor. The enzyme which does this appears to be produced in greater quantities when there is a need for more blood in certain areas, and Dr. Schayer has also shown, or at least made it very probable, that there is an auto-regulatory mechanism which shuts these capillaries again because an increased blood flow washes out the histamine when it is no longer needed. He gave very interesting data about the binding of histamine and his theory really is comprised in these postulates: Histamine is continuously produced within smooth muscle and endothelial cells of small blood vessels; It acts primarily on intrinsic or intracellular receptors, and: The mechanism for histamine production can adapt to environmental requirements, i.e. histidine decarboxylase is an inducible enzyme.

Well, he shows us under what conditions this is

needed, but as I have said, alas and alack, this is fairly unspecific, and I don't see how Dr.Schayer's data can be used specifically to explain the role of histamine in the production of deciduomas and of implantation, except that where more blood is needed histamine will open the vessels. But more blood is needed for many things in life so I don't think it gets us very much nearer to the solution of the specific problem.

He also based a unified concept of the effects of glucocortico-steroids on their power to antagonize the effects of histamine. It would be unfair to elaborate on my objections to this unifying theory. This is beyond the point, anyway. It was certainly a highly stimulating and interesting lecture. One of the essential points perhaps is that Dr.Schayer believes that there is no evident reason why histamine produced intrinsically at gradually increased rates would not be the primary mediator of the inflammatory reaction. Now, the inflammatory reaction is a thing which has puzzled me for years. It is one of those universal reactions which nature uses to respond to all sorts of stimuli, and there is a certain analogy between inflammation, as we have again heard today, and the implantation of the blastocyst, but I don't think we can go any further than that.

Now we come to the closer of capillaries, to the catecholamines, and I am sure you were all impressed by Professor von Euler's paper, as much as I was. His demonstration that these substances like noradrenaline are encapsulated in tiny little containers, that these containers can actually be seen, in the sympathetic nerves, and that they are concentrated in little bulges, his studies on the way noradrenaline is bound and released, the quantitative aspects of all this, I found exceedingly fascinating.

I would like to quote a few sentences literally because of certain aspects of the language, and those of you who remember a discussion we had one afternoon, will understand what I mean when I say it. "By binding in a physiologically inactive form in submicroscopic structures, relatively large amounts of transmitter can be stored at strategic points and also, by binding in a large number of separate units, potentially form a very versatile system." I want to state that I do not wish to imply anything that the author did not wish to imply when he said this.

So, we heard that these highly potent compounds are stored there in these strategic positions and can have very important effects. We heard that their release is dependent on temperature, that there is probably a feedback which again leads to a certain equilibrium and we heard of the inactivation of the noradrenaline that comes out. Specifically with respect to the uterus, I can quote from Dr. von Euler's paper that "cervical ganglionectomy as shown by Barnea and Shelesnyak reduces the noradrenaline content of the uterus by 80%" and, "denervation does not prevent the estrous cycle nor the implantation of ova." So again, we have a number of highly interesting facts, difficult to integrate, difficult to use for a clear-cut explanation of the phenomenon we are faced with.

I hope you do not expect me to quantitatively repeat everything that has been said; apart from the fact that it would use too much time and you have all had a full day, I would feel ashamed to repeat so clumsily what has been said so elegantly by so many of the speakers.

The next paper I also found exceedingly stimulating

and fascinating. It was by Dr. Gorski on estrogen and the study of the estrogen receptors. This is the third pillar of wisdom on which this implantation mechanism has been built. Now, Dr. Gorski of course, like everybody, started out from the concept that there must be a receptor for estrogen, but as he said, nobody has seen this receptor, nobody has ever been able to identify and to characterize it. So he undertook this, and with most remarkable results. I am also quite sure that endocrinology, and particularly the study of steroid action, will never be the same again after this historic work. I am not exaggerating, I believe that this is a new development and much more, I am sure, will come out of it.

The main trick which he used an which, as he says has been done by others before him, was the use of an estrogen which was very highly labelled so that practically every molecule, was radioactive. The use of this very highly radioactive estrogen enabled him to follow the distribution of this compound in the various cell fractions and to see where it goes in the uterus, if and when small physiological quantities are used. A mistake that is often encountered in older studies is that people give animals relatively large quantities of estrogen or testosterone and then find that it goes to the liver, the lungs, and the kidney and everywhere except to the organs where it should go, because one gets an enormous overflow from very high doses, with those small doses which are highly active one does not get this overflow and then one sees where the really essential quantities of active substance go.

I was tremendously impressed by this work. As you will remember, Dr. Gorski told us that over fifty per cent of the labelled material goes into the nuclei of the cells. This has been suspected by many people who in the last few years have been operating more and more with these operators in the nuclear apparatus but now it has been shown. By using high speed centifugation he could fraction the various cell components. A very large quantity goes into the nuclei, but a remarkable fraction goes into the so-called supernatant or cytosol.

There is a large fraction which is obtained when these soluble fractions are centrifuged at 105,000 times gravity. Another highly interesting finding was also something that has been suspected all the time but has only now been shown. If you take an estrogen which is chemically unrelated to estradiol and which is not a steroid, the famous diethylstilbestrol, it binds with the same fractions; it does in fact use the same receptors. Dr. Gorski was also able to make a rough estimate of the number of sites that could be available in one cell, about 20,000. And there of course the estrogen would start to induce all those changes which we know as its effects.

So we have now, in a way, disposed of histamine, of the catecholamines, and of the estrogen needed for the estrogen surge. I repeat 'in a way' because this doesn't help us to understand what deciduum formation is, but it does help us a great deal in visualizing how estrogens start to work.

Then comes the time clock, the central synchronizing organization. This is one of the things which have always tremendously impressed me. In order to make reproduction possible it is necessary that the female ovulate exactly at the time when she is prepared to mate; this she signals to the male. In the case of the rat the mating will take place at a time which will make it possible for the spermatozoa to be deposited and to reach the Fallopian tubes a few hours before the ova, to sit there in that waiting hall and be ready to fertilize. The moment that happens, up comes the corpus luteum. It stops all further mating activities and says to the female: now you attend to your new business and take care of the fertilized ovum. Then this fertilized ovum is carefully handled in the Fallopian tube so that it goes to the uterus, neither too late nor too early. All these synchronized mechanisms fill me with awe and admiration, but that, of course, is an entirely unscientific attitude.

I am now coming to Dr. Everett whose name I have known for years and whose work I have always admired. Honestly, seeing his name on the list of invited people was one of the things that induced me to accept this invitation.

Well, you remember what he did and how he told us by what skillful method he found the areas in the brain which must be stimulated in order to make ovulation possible. Using an iron electrode he was actually depositing iron in those sensitive areas, so it wasn't really a purely electrical but also a chemical stimulation. He was able to show the location of the fibers, whose stimuli will ultimately reach the pituitary, but he has done much more than that. He discovered the highly interesting fact that certain narcotics or hypnotics will delay ovulation, that this period of delayed ovulation can very well be used to study the stimuli which will cause ovulation, and that this whole synchronizing clock can only achieve what it is supposed to accomplish (again an unscientific statement I suppose) by the very close interaction with the steroids that come from the ovary. Dr. Everett found that there are not only negative feedbacks, as we usually think but also positive feedbacks and that progesterone can not only inhibit ovulation but also induce it. He gave us a most exciting picture of this totality of central nervous happenings and their interaction with what happens in the ovary as a consequence.

I was greatly pleased to hear that he found a Dutchman in the United States, Zeilmaker, with whom he agreed on certain things. (Incidentally, Dr. Gorski also had a few Dutchmen, which may have significantly contributed to his success.) The point on which they both, Everett and Zeilmaker, agreed concerns prolactin which as you know has also been called a luteotrophic hormone in the rat. The function of prolactin in other animals than the rat is somewhat controversial; at any rate, the rat seems to need one hormone to make a corpus luteum and another hormone to make it function and produce progesterone. I quote: "He and I agree that the simplest interpretation of our results is that prolactin secretion is immediately elevated by the copulatory stimulus and that it cannot express itself until competent corpora lutea are present." Here, of course, we are getting very close to the core of the problem, to the mechanism of implantation where we wanted to get. So here is this interaction of hormonal and nervous action which is so characteristic for the entire central regulation of reproduction.

The next paper I can skip. That is my own, and it hasn't really contributed anything and not given you any more knowledge than you had because it was more or less a historical summary. All I want to quote from it is that Psychoyos has found that "a secretion of progesterone for at least 48 hours and the presence of estrogen at the end of this period is the basic hormonal sequence necessary for implantation." This is in marvelous agreement with the concept of Prof. Shelesnyak.

I'd like to pause here to answer a question which may have bothered you. How I ever got here? This will interest Dr. Billingham because it has something to do with grafting. I have permission to quote this. In March of this year, Dr. Shelesnyak wrote to my colleague Dr. Overbeek, assistant research director in Organon, where I was a director until six months ago, and asked him for a financial contribution to this workshop. (He asked for an amount which can be expressed only in six figures provided the unit is the cent.) Back came a reply from Dr. Overbeek that this would be an interesting thing but he was somewhat surprised to see that we were not offered an opportunity to send an observer to such a workshop. Then came Dr. Shelesnyak's answer saying: You do have a point and we shall be pleased to have a representative of yours. Would it be within the framework of your planning to consider having Tausk join us? We would be prepared to put up with him if he would give us a presentation on the historical roots of our current understanding of progestation. This I did not quote literally, but you can imagine it was something to this effect.

Now, we get to two most interesting papers on immunology, one by Dr. Katsh, and the other by Dr. Billingham. The last one is so fresh in our memory that I will not try to spoil the vivid impression we still have by a clumsy repetition. Dr.Katsh's paper is a little farther away so I will say a few things about that.

You know his paper was on immunological aspects of reproduction, but not with the purpose of showing that implantation is an allergic reaction. It was primarily concentrating on such questions as: do females become immune to the sperm of their husbands and if not, why not? I would like to quote one little sentence in this context where the speaker says: "The female presented with coital antigens is faced with the challenge of disposing of these materials." It is late in the day and therefore I take the liberty to quote such very serious things in a somewhat facetious way. It reminds me of the little story of the two English girls who came to the Continent for the first time and went to a hotel in Paris. In their bathroom they found a piece of furniture they had never seen before, called a bidet. One girl asked the other: "What's that, to wash your baby in?" "No," she replied, "to wash your baby out." (Forgive me for such indecent behavior on such an honorable occasion.)

As a matter of fact, the material presented by Dr. Katsh made us, made me at least aware of a number of problems which I had never thought of, irrespective of any practical applications which I am sure are in prospect and regardless of the relative contribution to the main problem of this conference. Apparently we can take it as established fact that antigens are formed to sperm and spermatic material and a number of highly interesting problems are involved in these questions. Dr.Katsh is just hinting at possible implications, both for the treatment of sterility and, what may be even more important, the treatment of fertility. I will refrain from more elaborate reproduction of this paper, but one of the interesting things is that there are apparently mechanisms at work which eliminate the antibodies, and which probably then could account for Sarah's pregnancy at the age of 90, as Dr.Katsh pointed out.

Then the last paper was that of Dr. Billingham It gave us a view on a field of which I knew practically nothing. I was introduced into a new world of rejection of homografts and of the privileged tissues like the anterior chamber of the eye and the still more privileged tissue of the cheek pouch of the hamster in which he probably keeps his tongue when Dr. Billingham studies him, and there is the slime sandwich which can be used to confer this privileged condition on pieces of skin which would otherwise be subject to rejection, but with this slime sandwich behave very properly and are not rejected.

So then to sum up this summary, I believe it is fair to say that while the various contributions may not have brought us very much nearer to the solution of the problems which are and were foremost in the minds of the organizers of this symposium, they certainly have not essentially undermined the soundness of their concepts, perhaps with some slight reservations as regards the immunological concepts where I have the impression that they may not have come out unscathed, but this may be my own impression and I will not elaborate on it. All these contributions have given us some fascinating views on a number of things which, I am sure, none of us was completely aware of, completely conversant with. I believe we have every reason to be most grateful for this very harmonious, hormonious Workshop.

# INDEX

# INDEX